Register Now for Online Access to Your Book!

SPRINGER PUBLISHING
CONNECT™

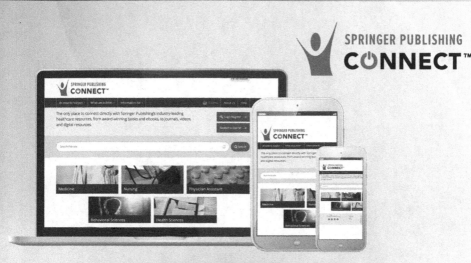

Your print purchase of *Sports Coverage: The Handbook for the Sports Medicine Clinician* **includes online access to the contents of your book**—increasing accessibility, portability, and searchability!

Access today at:
http://connect.springerpub.com/content/book/978-0-8261-4296-2
or scan the QR code at the right with your smartphone
and enter the access code below.

4NJE7C2T

*Scan here for
quick access.*

If you are experiencing problems accessing the digital component of this product, please contact our customer service department at cs@springerpub.com

The online access with your print purchase is available at the publisher's discretion and may be removed at any time without notice.

Publisher's Note: New and used products purchased from third-party sellers are not guaranteed for quality, authenticity, or access to any included digital components.

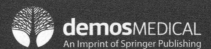

demosMEDICAL
An Imprint of Springer Publishing

View all our products at springerpub.com/demosmedical

SPORTS COVERAGE

The Handbook for the Sports Medicine Clinician

EDITORS

Gerardo Miranda-Comas, MD
Assistant Professor
Department of Rehabilitation and Human Performance
Icahn School of Medicine at Mount Sinai
New York, New York

Priya B. Patel, DO
Assistant Professor
Department of Orthopedic Surgery
Albert Einstein College of Medicine
The Bronx, New York

Joseph Herrera, DO
Professor and Chair
Department of Rehabilitation and Human Performance
Icahn School of Medicine at Mount Sinai
New York, New York

William Micheo, MD
Sports Medicine Fellowship Director
Professor and Chair
Department of Physical Medicine, Rehabilitation and Sports Medicine
University of Puerto Rico, San Juan, Puerto Rico

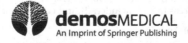

demosMEDICAL
An Imprint of Springer Publishing

Copyright © 2021 Springer Publishing Company, LLC
Demos Medical Publishing is an imprint of Springer Publishing Company.
All rights reserved.
First Springer Publishing edition 2021.

Springer Publishing Company, LLC
11 West 42nd Street, New York, NY 10036
www.springerpub.com
connect.springerpub.com/

Acquisitions Editor: Beth Barry
Compositor: Amnet

ISBN: 978-0-8261-4295-5
ebook ISBN: 978-0-8261-4296-2
DOI: 10.1891/9780826142962

20 21 22 23 / 5 4 3 2 1

Medicine is an ever-changing science. Research and clinical experience are continually expanding our knowledge, in particular our understanding of proper treatment and drug therapy. The authors, editors, and publisher have made every effort to ensure that all information in this book is in accordance with the state of knowledge at the time of production of the book. Nevertheless, the authors, editors, and publisher are not responsible for any errors or omissions or for any consequence from application of the information in this book and make no warranty, expressed or implied, with respect to the content of this publication. Every reader should examine carefully the package inserts accompanying each drug and should carefully check whether the dosage schedules therein or the contraindications stated by the manufacturer differ from the statements made in this book. Such examination is particularly important with drugs that are either rarely used or have been newly released on the market.

Library of Congress Cataloging-in-Publication Data
Names: Miranda-Comas, Gerardo, editor. | Patel, Priya, editor. | Herrera, Joseph E., editor. | Micheo, William, editor.
Title: Sports coverage : the handbook for the sports medicine clinician / [edited by] Gerardo Miranda-Comas, Priya Patel, Joseph Herrera, William Micheo.
Description: First Springer Publishing edition. | New York, NY : Springer Publishing Company, LLC, 2021. | Includes bibliographical references and index.
Identifiers: LCCN 2020016872 (print) | LCCN 2020016873 (ebook) | ISBN 9780826142955 (paperback) | ISBN 9780826142962 (ebook)
Subjects: MESH: Athletic Injuries | Sports
Classification: LCC RD97 (print) | LCC RD97 (ebook) | NLM QT 261 | DDC 617.1/027—dc23
LC record available at https://lccn.loc.gov/2020016872
LC ebook record available at https://lccn.loc.gov/2020016873

Contact us to receive discount rates on bulk purchases.
We can also customize our books to meet your needs.
For more information please contact: sales@springerpub.com

Printed in the United States of America.

CONTENTS

Section IV. Coverage Essentials for Limited-Contact Sports

Section V. Coverage Essentials for Noncontact Sports

CONTRIBUTORS

Joanne B. "Anne" Allen, MD, FAAPRM, FACSM   Founder, Allen Spine and Sports Medicine; Adjunct Professor, Department of Health and Physical Education, College of Health and Human Services, University of North Carolina Wilmington, Wilmington, NC

Walter Alomar-Jiménez, MD, JD   Clinical Lecturer, Department of Physical Medicine and Rehabilitation, University of Michigan, Ann Arbor, MI

Roxanna M. Amill-Cintrón, MD, FAAPMR   Physiatrist, Manatí Medical Center, Department of Physical Medicine and Rehabilitation, Manatí, Puerto Rico

Gautam Anand, MD   Vascular Surgery Resident, Department of Surgery, Lenox Hill Hospital, New York, NY

Ilya Aylyarov, MD   Resident Physician, Department of Emergency Medicine, New York University Medical Center/Bellevue Hospital, New York, NY

Michael R. Baria, MD, MBA   Assistant Professor, Department of Physical Medicine and Rehabilitation, The Ohio State University, Columbus, OH

Luis Baerga-Varela, MD   Assistant Professor, Department of Physical Medicine and Rehabilitation, School of Medicine, University of Puerto Rico, San Juan, Puerto Rico

Allison C. Bean, MD, PhD   Fellow, Sports Medicine, Department of Physical Medicine and Rehabilitation, University of Pittsburgh Medical Center, Pittsburgh, PA

Andrew Beaufort, MD   Physician, Department of Orthopaedic Surgery and Rehabilitation Medicine, State University of New York Downstate Medical Center, Brooklyn, NY

Tina Bijlani, DO   Resident Physician, Department of Rehabilitation and Human Performance, Icahn School of Medicine at Mount Sinai, New York, NY

Erik S. Brand, MD, MSc   Owner, Brand Performance Medicine, Bellevue, WA

Francisco E. Bentz Brugal, MD   Medical Director, Rehabilitek; Assistant Professor, Physical Medicine and Rehabilitation, Universidad Iberoamericana UNIBE, Santo Domingo, Dominican Republic

Eliana Cardozo, DO, CAQSM, FAAPMR   Assistant Professor, Department of Rehabilitation and Human Performance, Icahn School of Medicine at Mount Sinai, New York, NY

Brenda Castillo, MD   Attending Physician, Department of Physical Medicine and Rehabilitation, MossRehab, Elkins Park, PA

Lawrence G. Chang, DO, MPH Physiatry Resident, Department of Physical Medicine and Rehabilitation, Burke Rehabilitation Hospital, White Plains, NY

Richard G. Chang, MD, MPH, FAAPMR Assistant Professor, Department of Rehabilitation and Human Performance, Icahn School of Medicine at Mount Sinai, New York, NY

Andrew Chen, MD Family Medicine Resident Physician, Department of Family Medicine, Icahn School of Medicine at Mount Sinai, New York, NY

Michael Chiou, MD Resident Physician, Department of Rehabilitation and Human Performance, Icahn School of Medicine at Mount Sinai, New York, NY

Yusik Cho, MD Academic Chief Resident, Physical Medicine and Rehabilitation Residency Program, Burke Rehabilitation Hospital, White Plains, NY

Lisanne C. Cruz, MD, MSc, FAAPMR Physician, Synergy Sports Medicine and Rehabilitation, Toronto, Ontario, Canada

Francisco De la Rosa, MD Physical Medicine and Rehabilitation Residency Program Director, Hospital General Plaza de la Salud-Universidad Iberoamericana, Santo Domingo, Dominican Republic

Richard A. Fontánez-Nieves, MD Resident Physician, Department of Physical Medicine, Rehabilitation and Sports Medicine, School of Medicine, University of Puerto Rico, San Juan, Puerto Rico

Kevin Frison, MD Resident Physician, Department of Rehabilitation and Human Performance, Icahn School of Medicine at Mount Sinai, New York, NY

Juan Galloza-Otero, MD Assistant Professor, Department of Medicine, School of Medicine, Ponce Health and Sciences University, Ponce, Puerto Rico

Ariana Gluck, DO Physiatrist, Department of Rehabilitation and Human Performance, Icahn School of Medicine at Mount Sinai, New York, NY

Michael Harbus, DO Resident, Department of Rehabilitation and Human Performance, Icahn School of Medicine at Mount Sinai, New York, NY

Jasmin Harounian, MD Resident Physician, Department of Rehabilitation and Human Performance, Icahn School of Medicine at Mount Sinai, New York, NY

Jasmine H. Harris, MD Resident Physician, Department of Rehabilitation and Human Performance, Icahn School of Medicine at Mount Sinai, New York, NY

Liza M. Hernández-González, MD Assistant Professor, Department of Physical Medicine, Rehabilitation and Sports Medicine, School of Medicine, University of Puerto Rico, San Juan, Puerto Rico

Claudia Jimenez-Garcia, MD Post-Graduate-Year I, Department of Physical Medicine and Rehabilitation, School of Medicine, University of Puerto Rico, San Juan, Puerto Rico

Nathaniel S. Jones, MD, CAQ-SM   Assistant Professor, Department of Orthopaedic Surgery and Rehabilitation, Department of Family Medicine, Loyola University Chicago – Health Sciences Campus, Maywood, IL

Amie Kim, MD   Assistant Professor, Department of Emergency Medicine; Assistant Professor, Department of Rehabilitation Medicine, Icahn School of Medicine at Mount Sinai, New York, NY

Kevin Kuo, MD   Medicine Resident Physician, Emergency Department, Mount Sinai St. Luke's and West, New York, NY

Richa Lamba,   PGY-3 Resident Physician, Department of Physical Medicine and Rehabilitation, Temple University Hospital/MossRehab, Elkins Park, PA

Tiffany M. Lau, MD   Resident Physician, Department of Physical Medicine and Rehabilitation, Burke Rehabilitation Hospital, White Plains, NY

Vincent Lee, NMM/OMM   Pre-Doctoral Teaching Fellow, Western University of Health Sciences, Pomona, CA

Michelle Leong, DO   Physiatrist, Department of Rehabilitation and Human Performance, Icahn School of Medicine at Mount Sinai, New York, NY

Daniel R. Lueders, MD   Assistant Professor, Department of Physical Medicine and Rehabilitation, University of Pittsburgh Medical Center, Pittsburgh, PA

Adrian McGoldrick, FFSEM   Retired Chief Medical Officer, Irish Horseracing Regulatory Board, Kildare, Ireland

Gerardo Miranda-Comas, MD   Assistant Professor, Department of Rehabilitation and Human Performance, Icahn School of Medicine at Mount Sinai, New York, NY

Ana Ortiz-Santiago, MD   Chief Resident, Department of Physical Medicine, Rehabilitation and Sports Medicine, School of Medicine, University of Puerto Rico, San Juan, Puerto Rico

Robert Pagan-Rosado, MD   Resident Physician, Mayo Clinic, College of Medicine and Science, Rochester, MN

Lauren Paish, MD   Attending Physician, Department of Emergency Medicine, Wyckoff Heights Medical Center, Brooklyn, NY

Wilmar G. Pantoja, MD   Sports Medicine Fellow, Department of Rehabilitation and Performance, Icahn School of Medicine at Mount Sinai, New York, NY

Priya B. Patel, DO   Assistant Professor, Department of Orthopedic Surgery, Albert Einstein College of Medicine, The Bronx, NY

Juan C. Perez-Santiago, MD   Physiatrist, Wentworth-Douglass Hospital, Dover, NH

Courtney Pinto   Medical Student, New York Medical College, Valhalla, NY

Aditya Raghunandan, MD Sports Medicine Fellow, Department of Physiatry, Hospital of Special Surgery, New York, NY

Jonathan Ramin, DO Chief Resident, Department of Rehabilitation and Human Performance, Icahn School of Medicine at Mount Sinai, New York, NY

Ashwin L. Rao, MD Physician, Department of Family Medicine, University of Washington, Seattle, WA

Alexandra M. Rivera-Vega, MD Staff Physician, Physical Medicine and Rehabilitation, Michael E. DeBakey VA Medical Center, Houston, TX

Rebecca Rodriguez-Negron, MD, DABFM Associate Professor, Department of Family Medicine and Geriatrics; Associate Professor, Department of Physical Medicine, Rehabilitation and Sports Health, Center for Sports Health and Exercise Sciences, School of Medicine, University of Puerto Rico, Medical Science Campus, San Juan, Puerto Rico

Belmarie Rodríguez-Santiago, MD Physiatrist, Department of Physical Medicine, Rehabilitation and Sports Medicine, School of Medicine, University of Puerto Rico, San Juan, Puerto Rico

Raúl A. Rosario-Concepción, MD Senior Associate Consultant, Department of Physical Medicine and Rehabilitation, Mayo Clinic-Florida, Jacksonville, FL

Andres Arredondo Santana, MD Resident Physician, Department of Emergency Medicine, Icahn School of Medicine at Mount Sinai, New York, NY

Rachel Santiago, MD Resident, Department of Physical Medicine and Rehabilitation, Icahn School of Medicine at Mount Sinai, New York, NY

Fernando L. Sepúlveda-Irizarry, MD Assistant Professor, Department of Physical Medicine, Rehabilitation and Sports Medicine, School of Medicine, University of Puerto Rico, San Juan, Puerto Rico

Jeffrey Smith, MD Resident, Department of Physical Medicine and Rehabilitation, University of Pittsburgh Medical Center, Pittsburgh, PA

Daniel P. Spunberg, MD Chief Resident Physician, Department of Physical Medicine and Rehabilitation, Burke Rehabilitation Hospital, White Plains, NY

Anita Tewari, MD Physician, Department of Rehabilitation and Human Performance, Icahn School of Medicine at Mount Sinai, New York, NY

Iris X. Tian, DO Resident, Department of Rehabilitation and Human Performance, Icahn School of Medicine at Mount Sinai, New York, NY

Michael Turner, FFSEM Honorary Senior Lecturer, University College London, London, England

Julio Vazquez-Galliano, MD   Assistant Professor, Department of Rehabilitation Medicine, Montefiore Medical Center, Albert Einstein College of Medicine, The Bronx, NY

Jose R. Vives-Alvarado, MD   Post-Graduate-Year IV Senior Resident, Department of Physical Medicine and Rehabilitation, School of Medicine, University of Puerto Rico, San Juan, Puerto Rico

Fairen Walker-McCarter, MD   Attending Physician, Dynamic Pain and Wellness, Fairhope, AL

Bryant Walrod, MD   Assistant Professor, Department of Family Medicine, The Ohio State University, Columbus, OH

Nadia N. Zaman, DO   Fellow, Department of Sports Medicine, Icahn School of Medicine at Mount Sinai, New York, NY

Jason L. Zaremski, MD, CAQSM, FACSM, FAAPMR   Associate Professor, Divisions of Physical Medicine and Rehabilitation, Sports Medicine, and Research, Department of Orthopaedics and Rehabilitation; Co-Medical Director, Adolescent and High School Outreach Program, University of Florida College of Medicine, Gainesville, FL

As sports medicine practitioners, our primary responsibility is to provide optimal medical care for athletes on and off the field. The care continuum for the athlete includes injury/illness prevention, diagnosis, treatment, rehabilitation, and return to sport. In a practical sense, injury/illness prevention begins with preparticipation evaluations where the general health of the athlete is evaluated, specifically the assessment of any medical condition that might be not only detrimental to athletic performance, but also to the athlete's well-being. Following the care continuum is the on-the-field or clinic evaluation and diagnosis of an injury or illness which is often the first encounter with the patient/athlete. Prompt evaluation of an injured athlete on the field can expedite the diagnostic process, management, rehabilitation, and return to sport, frequently the most important outcome measure. Considering the importance of an early and accurate diagnosis, sideline or on-field medical coverage is essential.

The understanding of basic concepts related to sports coverage will help the practitioner provide high level care. Often the initial introduction to sports coverage occurs in didactic sessions where specific topics or cases are discussed. Although useful, this type of learning cannot replace first-hand experience; therefore, sideline coverage experience should be part of all educational training programs. Common avenues to start acquiring some sideline coverage experience is through volunteer work in local high schools, colleges, or club teams, or through involvement with specific sport–governing bodies, or at local mass participation events. These experiences can be very educational, but at times, or at least in our experience, covering sports or events new to the provider can be challenging and some educational points can be missed due to lack of familiarity with the sport and the particularities of the event or competition organization. The goal of this handbook is to provide a unified resource that covers the knowledge gaps that may be present when providing sports coverage.

The handbook is divided into several sections. The introductory section covers common topics that apply to all sports medicine providers providing sideline or event coverage independent of level of experience, for example: the role of the team medical provider; what to have in the medical bag; factors to consider when traveling with a team; medicolegal issues specific to the medical team member; how to assess and manage common medical emergencies; nutrition and hydration recommendations for pre-, during, and post-training or competition; preparticipation physicals; general concepts of adaptive sports; and lastly general concepts of doping in sports. The following sections will dive into sport-specific coverage divided by contact, limited-contact, or noncontact sport classification. We attempt to cover summer and winter Olympic sports and other popular sports that are practiced worldwide. The goal is to provide information on the history, participants, rules and regulations, equipment needed and/or required, medical coverage logistics, emergencies, medical bag essentials, epidemiology, and a brief discussion of common injuries for each individual sport. This will serve as an excellent resource for physicians in training or seasoned veterans from all specialties, athletic trainers, physical therapists, and any other healthcare providers who want to provide on-field, sideline, or event sports coverage.

We would like to thank all the authors for their time and effort in developing our ideas, with special thanks to our families for supporting us during this time.

Gerardo Miranda-Comas, MD
Priya B. Patel, DO
Joseph Herrera, DO
William Micheo, MD

GENERAL CONCEPTS IN SPORTS COVERAGE

1. THE SPORTS MEDICINE PROVIDER'S ROLE

Gerardo Miranda-Comas

The main role of the individual sports medicine practitioner is to provide the best care to the athlete as part of the sports medicine team. The team concept applies not only to the sport team, or organization, but also to the medical providers who take care of the athletes. The medical team is composed of several key players among whom very often the main player is not the head team physician, but the certified athletic trainer. He or she serves as the "gatekeeper" of the medical team, and the on-field provider for the most part. However, the team physician has the leadership role in the organization, management, and provision of care of athletes in individual, team, and mass participation sporting events. The team physician should possess the educational qualifications that include subspecialty training in sports medicine (in the United States) or specialty training in sports and exercise sciences (in most countries, except the United States), ideally with board certification and continued medical education. He or she must be proficient in the prevention and care of musculoskeletal injuries and medical conditions encountered in sports, especially on the field of play. The team physician recruits and integrates medical expertise with medical consultants, certified athletic trainers, and other allied health care professionals like nurses, physical therapists, occupational therapists, psychologists, nutritionists, exercise physiologists, chiropractors, and massage therapists. Aided by the athletic care network, the team physician also educates athletes, coaches, parents/guardians, and administrators. The team physician is ultimately responsible for an athlete's clearance to participate and the return-to-sport decision after an injury. Additionally, the team physician must ensure compliance with local, state, and/or federal rules, regulations, and laws, school and governing body guidelines, standards, policies, rules, and patient privacy laws. The head team physician oversees sideline preparedness which is the identification of and planning for medical services to promote the safety of the athlete, to limit injury, and to provide medical care at the site of practice or competition.

As a team, medical providers are responsible for the coordination of preparticipation evaluations, on-field injury management, medical care for off-field illnesses and injuries including rehabilitation, and safe return to sport. They also maintain open lines of communication with other team members to ensure continuity of care for the athlete, provide for appropriate education and counseling regarding nutrition, strength and conditioning, ergogenic aids, substance abuse, and other medical problems that could affect the athlete, and sustain proper documentation and record keeping.

Just like for the athletes, preparation starts during the preseason. Preseason planning promotes safety and minimizes problems associated with athletic participation at the site of practice or competition. During this time, prospective athletes should complete a preparticipation evaluation. The chain of command that establishes and defines the responsibilities of all parties involved is developed. The Emergency Action Plan (EAP) is implemented and rehearsed, policies for compliance of established standards for the care of the athletes and environmental assessment for event cancellation are revised, proper documentation practice and the recruitment of a network of providers are established. During actual game days or event days, the team physician coordinates all medical operations, prepares the medical bag and supplies, reviews the EAP with the whole team, assigns roles to each medical team member, and ensures proper communication with the medical team members and event/game personnel. Lastly, postseason evaluation of sideline coverage optimizes the medical care of injured or ill athletes and promotes continued improvement of medical services for future seasons.

▣ Further Reading

Callender SS. Being a team physician. *Curr Sports Med Rep*. 2018;17(2):39-40. doi:10.1249/JSR.0000000000000448.

Fu FH, Tjoumakaris FP, Buoncristiani A. Building a sports medicine team. *Clin Sports Med*. 2007;26(2):173-179. doi:10.1016/j.csm.2006.12.003.

Herring SA, Kibler WB, Putukian M. Sideline preparedness for the team physician: a consensus statement–2012 update. *Med Sci Sports Exerc*. 2012;44(12):2442-2445. doi:10.1249/MSS.0b013e318275044f.

Herring SA, Kibler WB, Putukian M. Team physician consensus statement: 2013 update. *Med Sci Sports Exerc*. 2013;45(8):1618-1622. doi:10.1249/mss.0b013e31829ba437.

2. MEDICAL BAG

Priya B. Patel

The medical bag is an essential tool kit for sideline sports coverage and the supplies included are directed toward the acute care of the athletes. It can be difficult to discern what should be included in your bag and therefore each sports chapter will include medical bag essentials. Prior to organizing the medical bag, inquire about the availability of an athletic trainer and/or Emergency Medical Services (EMS) and the supplies they are bringing. This will be important if you have limited space in your medical bag. The bag itself is an important decision. Bags should be big enough to store all necessary equipment; however, realistic in size and durability to allow portability. Most often, a duffel bag with various compartments is preferred because it is easy to transport and store.[1] If your bag is not water-resistant, then it is important to have the equipment in water-resistant containers/bags. Also, security locks may be needed if the bag contains medications, especially controlled substances. If you are frequently traveling, consider multiple bags with special attention to objects that may have to be checked in. It is important to pack the bag yourself and go over it with a checklist prior to sideline coverage so you are familiar with the location of the supplies.

The medical bag should be kept on the sidelines and you should have commonly used supplies available on you either using a fanny pack or in multiple pockets. The supplies included in this smaller bag should be at your discretion and sport specific. These may include gloves, bandages, gauze, trauma shears, a penlight, and cellphone.[1]

See the following comprehensive list of supplies.[1-3] Please refer to individual chapters for a more concise, sport-specific list.

General

- Blanket
- Blood pressure cuff
- Cell phone and/or walkie-talkies
- Eye shields
- Facemasks
- Flashlight or penlight
- Gloves
- Hand sanitizers
- Ice packs
- Injury sheets
- Oral fluids
- Paper and pen
- Pin for sensory testing
- Portable ultrasound (if available)
- Plastic bags
- Reflex hammer
- Scissors
- Stethoscope
- Sunscreen
- Tape
- Tape cutter
- Trauma shears

Emergencies

- Airway
- Automated External Defibrillator (AED)
- Cricothyrotomy kit
- Diphenhydramine
- Epinephrine 1:1,000
- Fracture immobilizers
- Ice baths
- IV fluids/D-50%-W
- Mouth-to-mouth mask
- Needles for pneumothorax (14- and 16-gauge needles)
- Rectal thermometer
- Short-acting beta agonist inhaler
- Stretcher

Wound Care

- Alcohol and Betadine swabs
- Bandages
- Bandage scissors
- Biohazard bag
- Disinfectant
- Needles (22, 25, 27 gauge)
- Normal saline
- Scalpels
- Sharps box
- Sterile gauze
- Sterile gloves
- Sterile lubricant
- Steri-strips
- Syringes
- Suture kit
- Tampons
- Topical antibiotics
- Topical corticosteroid cream
- Topical Lidocaine 1% or 2%
- Wound cleanser

Medications

- Acetaminophen
- Antihistamines
- Aspirin/nonsteroidal anti-inflammatory medications (NSAIDs)
- Glucose tablets
- Proton pump inhibitor
- Salt packets
- World Anti-Doping Agency (WADA) list of banned substances

Head and Neck

- Dental kit
- Eye kit
- Cervical orthosis
- Concussion evaluation form
- Contact lens solution and case
- Face mask removal tool
- Mirror
- Mouth guard
- Nasal-packing material
- Oto-ophthalmoscope
- Spine board and attachments
- Tongue depressors

Musculoskeletal

- Crutches
- Fracture immobilizers
- Knee brace
- Limb splints
- Slings

Special Considerations for Paraplegic Athletes[4]

- For autonomic dysreflexia
- Topical Nitroglycerin
  - Urinary Catheter
- For orthostatic hypotension
- Abdominal binder
  - Compression stockings

■ References

1. Daniels JM, Kary J, Lane JA. Optimizing the sideline medical bag preparing for school and community sports events. *Phys Sportsmed*. 2005;33(12):9-16. doi:10.3810/psm.2005.12.269.

2. Herring SA, Kibler W, Putukian M. Sideline preparedness for the team physician: a consensus statement—2012 update. *Med Sci Sports Exerc*. 2012;44(12):2442-2445. doi:10.1249/MSS.0b013e318275044f.

3. Yan CB, Rubin AL. Equipment and supplies for sports and event medicine. *Curr Sports Med Rep*. 2005;4(3):131-136. doi:10.1097/01.CSMR.0000306195.74864.cc.

4. Beutler A, Carey P. Medical considerations in adaptive sports. In: De Luigi A, ed. *Adaptive Sports Medicine*. Cham, Switzerland: Springer; 2018:59-70.

3. TRAVELING WITH A TEAM

Rebecca Rodriguez-Negron

▓ HISTORY

In the ancient Olympic Games, medical care was delivered mainly by trainers (paedotribes) and some physicians like Galen who were interested in sports.[1,2] In the United States, it was not until 1924 that the USA Olympic team assigned two physicians to cover the Olympic Games. Before that, medical care was given by nurses, trainers, and physicians who were at the Games as spectators.[1,3]

▓ MEDICAL TEAM AND SERVICE

The size and the composition of the medical team will depend on the philosophy and budget of the governing body, the number of athletes, type and number of sports, delegation or team support personnel, officials, administrators, coaches, and sometimes athletes' companions. Members of the medical team should include sports medicine physicians, orthopedists, nurses, physical therapists and athletic trainers, chiropractors, psychologists, and nutritionists. The International Olympic Committee (IOC) recommends one physician per 50 to 60 members of the delegation, but this number varies considering the need for 24-hour physician coverage (on-call) during the preparatory and competition periods. No specific recommendation exists for the other members of the multidisciplinary team.[4] This number will depend on philosophy, allowed licenses in the host country, budget, and delegation needs.

As clinicians, there are some basic things to consider in preparation to travel with a team or a multisport delegation. These factors include the budget, the specific sport(s) in which the athletes will participate, location of the sporting venues, transportation, security, organization at the venues, the available medical facilities at the venues, medical insurance for the athletes and delegation members, and the physician's liability insurance.

Each athlete should complete a preparticipation examination at least 6 weeks prior to the event or, if not feasible, at least provide basic medical information to the medical team.[5] Having medical information from the rest of the members of the delegation or team-support personnel is also desirable since medical attention will be provided not only to the athletes but also to the coaches, administrators, and other delegation officials.

The medical staff will offer basic medical services in a preset clinic, usually a separate hotel room or a designated apartment, and simultaneous on site coverage. During competition, a schedule should be established to ensure that all areas are covered especially high risk sports, and that the medical team gets proper rest and has the opportunity to support their teams as fan (Table 3.1).

Table 3.1 Suggested Schedule for Traveling Team Physicians

Time	Task
7 a.m. – Morning Meeting (15–20 minutes)	Discuss schedule for the day (clinic, field, and night call) Allow time for other members of the team to bring concerns and seek solutions
7 a.m.–11 p.m. (4-hour shifts are recommended)	Provide medical care in clinic and the field (prioritize high risk sports)
End of Day	Wrap up with Team leaders (Head Trainer, Head Psychologist, etc.) Assess concerns and areas for improvement

■ NATIONAL AND INTERNATIONAL TRAVEL LOGISTICS

Immunizations and Sanitary Issues: Every athlete should have his or her immunizations up to date in accord with the immunization schedule for age and medical conditions. Additional vaccines may be needed depending on the country that will be visited, like the yellow fever vaccine. These additional vaccines should be completed at least 1 month before traveling. It is also wise to know in advance if there are any sanitary issues or epidemics occurring in the countries or sites to be visited. Useful resources to accomplish this are: cdc.gov/vaccines/schedules, the Advisory Committee on Immunization Practices (ACIP), or smartphone applications like Shots Immunization App[6,7] as well as cdc.gov/travel or the World Health Organization (www.who.int). This will help you to prepare in advance, or in a worst-case scenario, to recommend cancelling a trip.

Security Issues: It is important to know if there is any concern for the security of the delegation in the country or cities to be visited. A useful Internet site for this is travel.state.gov. This will help you and the organizing body to prepare in advance, counsel the athletes, coaches, and other personnel, or in a worst-case scenario, to recommend cancelling a trip.

Licensing Issues: In the United States, since 2018, when traveling with a team between state lines, the liability insurance coverage of the team physician extends to another state for providing medical services to his or her own athletes, team members, and staff.[8] Prior notification to the insurer is required. But if you are traveling internationally, other regulations apply. You will need a temporary medical license to practice in a foreign country. Event organizers usually take care of this matter in conjunction with the credentialing body of the country that hosts the games. They will ask the team physician to submit his or her credentials including medical liability coverage.

■ MEDICATIONS AND SUPPLIES

Matters to consider when bringing medications and medical supplies to foreign countries include customs logistics in parent and traveling countries including issues with the transportation of controlled substances. Which medications and medical supplies to buy will depend on the expected weather and living conditions of the host country or region, possible illnesses, and musculoskeletal injuries.

When buying medications and medical supplies a decision of whether to buy them in the host country or bring them with your medical team should be made. If buying medications at the country of competition, be aware that names of medications can be different in several countries (e.g., paracetamol for acetaminophen, salbutamol for albuterol). Also, be aware that for some of these medications, like antibiotics, a prescription from local physicians is needed. It is recommended to buy the medications at home where you know their names, brands, and regulations of the manufacturing process. If buying supplies in the visiting country, be aware that after arrival, time constraint is a common issue. Therefore, an advanced research online or a local contact is recommended. A basic list of medications and supplies is included in Table 3.2, but specific needs of your team/delegation or issues in the country should be considered to modify this list accordingly.

Another issue with medications and medical supplies when traveling to foreign countries is customs regulations and logistics. Make a list with generic names, dose, and quantities for each medication and the medical supplies before traveling in or out. For large events, the organizing body will help with this and sometimes they will provide their own forms to be filled. Some countries will not allow transportation of controlled substances. Each country has its own regulations regarding this matter and it is recommended that you check this in advance. If an athlete or any

Table 3.2 Suggested Medications List

Analgesics – Non-NSAIDs[+]	Acetaminophen
	Urinary analgesics (e.g. Phenazopyridine)
	Antimigraine medication (e.g. Sumatriptan)
Analgesics – NSAIDs	Nonselective and COX 2 Selective NSAIDs
Anti-Infective Agents	Antiviral agent targeting HSV, HZV (e.g. Acyclovir)
	Penicillin: Amoxicillin, Amoxicillin-Clavulanate
	Macrolides: Azithromycin
	Cephalosporins: 1st generation (e.g. Cephalexin)
	Quinolones: (e.g. Ciprofloxacin)
	Clindamycin
	Doxycycline
	Metronidazole
	Trimethoprim-Sulfamethoxazole
	Antifungals: Oral Fluconazole, Topical antifungals
	Topical antibiotics (Mupirocin, Triple-antibiotic)
Antivertigo	Meclizine, Dramamine
Cardiovascular	Antihypertensives - ACE inhibitors (e.g. lisinopril), Calcium Channel Blockers (e.g. Amlodipine)
	Epinephrine Inj Ampules 1:1,000 (1 mg/mL)
	Nitroglycerin S/L 0.4 mg Tab
	Antiplatelet agents (e.g. aspirin)
Corticosteroids	Injectable corticosteroids (e.g. Triamcinolone 40 mg/mL)
	Prednisone (tablets)
	Dexamethasone (tablets)
	Topical HC
	Calamine lotion
	Dermoplast 2.75 oz.
	Antihemorrhoidal (e.g. Proctozone HC 0.5%)

(continued)

Table 3.2 Suggested Medications List (*continued*)

Gastrointestinal	Antiacids (e.g. Calcium carbonate, H2 blockers - Ranitidine, and Proton pump inhibitors-Omeprazole) Antispasmodics (e.g. Dicyclomine inj. and oral tabs) Antidiarrheals (e.g. Loperamide, Bismuth) Laxatives (e.g. Myralax, Docusate Sodium, Senna) Antiemetics (e.g. Ondansetron Inj and tabs)
Miscellaneous	Dextrose 50% SDV 50 mL Glucagon Injectable Kit Humulin R 100 u/mL Local anesthetics (e.g. Lidocaine 1%, 2%) Triamcinolone Dental Paste
Muscle Relaxants	Cyclobenzaprine, Tizanidine, Inj. Orphenadrine
Ophthalmic	Anti-infectives (Gentamycin Ophthalmic Solution 0.3%, Ciprofloxacin Ophthalmic Solution, Polytrim Ophthalmic Solution) Naphazoline & Pheniramine Ophthalmic Solution Topical anesthetics (e.g. Tetracaine Ophthalmic Solution 0.5%)
Otics	Anti-infectives (e.g. Acetic Acid Otic Solution 2%, Neomycin/Polymyxin B/HC Otic Solution Ofloxacin Otic Solution Analgesics (e.g. Antipyrine/Benzocaine Otic Solution)
Respiratory	Bronchodilators (beta-2 agonist: Albuterol soln Vials, MDI) Cepacol or Equivalent (18/Box) Antiallergics (e.g. Diphenhydramine Inj. and oral, Loratadine) Decongestants topical (e.g. Oxymetazoline Nasal Spray) Nasal corticosteroids (e.g. Fluticasone INH) Mucolytics/Antitussives (e.g. Guaifenesin DM) Inhaled corticosteroids (e.g. Q-VAR 40 mcg MDI)

+Consider various organs/system

ACE, angiotensin-converting enzyme; DM, dextromethorphan; HC, hydrocortisone; HSV, herpes simplex virus; HZV, herpes zoster vaccine; INH, inhaler; MDI, metered dose inhaler; NSAIDs, nonsteroidal anti-inflammatory drugs; SDV, single-dose vial; S/L, sublingual.

member of the delegation has a medical problem where a controlled substance is needed as part of the treatment, it will be better that the athlete's primary care physician give him or her a prescription. As the team physician, you should be aware of the use of these kinds of medications especially in your athletes, remembering that many controlled substances are already banned by the World Anti-Doping Agency (WADA).

■ COMMON MEDICAL PROBLEMS

International traveling and traveling between time zones increases the risk for some common medical problems.

Travelers' Diarrhea

Travelers' diarrhea (TD) is a common disease among travelers from resourceful countries or regions to less resourceful areas; 80% to 90% are related to bacterial infections. Transmission occurs via fecal-oral route, usually with contaminated water or food. *Escherichia coli* is the most common organism causing TD; its enterotoxigenic and enteroaggregative variants account for 50% to 60% of the infections. Enteroinvasive agents as *Campylobacter, Salmonella, and Shigella* make up 10% to 20% of the infections. *Campylobacter* is more common in South and Southeast Asia. Other related bacteria are *Yersinia, Vibrio, Aeromonas*. Viruses like norovirus and enteroviruses have also been linked to TD. If symptoms last more than 7 days, a parasite infection needs to be ruled out. Common parasites related to TD are *Giardia, Entamoeba, Cryptosporidium*. Prevention is the best treatment. It is recommended to maintain good hand hygiene, avoid raw foods, raw vegetables, nonbottle or nonboiled water, previously peeled fruits, unpacked sauces, and ice. Other methods of prevention are chemoprophylaxis and vaccines. Agents with proven benefit for chemoprophylaxis are the fluoroquinolones (FQ), bismuth subsalicylate (BSS), and rifaximin.[9] Of note, FQ are not recommended in athletes due to the risk of tendon rupture. Treatment is recommended according to this classification[10]:

Mild TD: Diarrhea that does not affect activities. Could be treated with loperamide or bismuth subsalicylate (BSS). Antibiotic use is not recommended.

Moderate TD: Diarrhea that is distressing or interferes with planned activities. Could be treated with loperamide or antibiotics, alone or in combination. FQ, azithromycin, or Rifaximin may be used empirically. Avoiding FQ in athletes and resistant area such as Southeast Asia is recommended. Caution is also advised for the use of Rifaximin in areas with high risk for invasive pathogens.[9]

Severe TD: Diarrhea that is incapacitating, completely prevents planned activities or has blood on it. Should be treated with antibiotics; azithromycin is preferred. Loperamide could be added.

Persistent TD: Diarrhea that lasts more than 2 weeks. Workup should be done to rule out parasitic infections or another organism. Residual irritable bowel syndrome (IBS) after a TD episode can also be seen.

High Altitude Illness

The risk of developing high altitude illness (HAI) increases as unacclimated individuals rapidly reach altitudes of 2,500 m (8,202 ft) above sea level or higher.

Acute Mountain Sickness (AMS) is thought to be caused by mild cerebral edema induced by hypoxia in a susceptible individual with tight space in the cranial vault, not allowing a small brain swelling without symptoms.[11] It is characterized by headache plus nausea, dizziness, fatigue or lassitude, and insomnia. Could present in mild, moderate, or severe form.

High Altitude Cerebral Edema (HACE) is considered a severe form of AMS with associated neurologic findings of ataxia, confusion, and altered mental status. If not treated rapidly, it could lead to coma and death. Its prevalence is low even at high altitudes (0.5%–1.0%) and is very rare at altitudes less than 4,000 m.

High Altitude Pulmonary Edema (HAPE) is a form of noncardiogenic pulmonary edema whose pathophysiology is thought to be related to maladaptive mechanisms leading to hypoxic pulmonary vasoconstriction, increased pulmonary pressures, damage of the alveoli by inflammatory mediators, and disruption in the fluid clearance mechanism of the alveolar capillary barrier. Fortunately, its prevalence is very low even at high altitudes.

Preventive Measures: These include ascent in stages, especially for sleeping altitude, and avoiding heavy exertion until acclimatized. Chemoprophylaxis is recommended for individuals with moderate to high risk of developing HAI. This includes those ascending rapidly to elevations of more than 2,800 m, individuals with a previous history of AMS and rapid ascent to elevation of 2,500 m or more, all individuals with history of HACE or HAPE, and for susceptible individuals at lower altitudes. Prophylactic medication should be started 1 day previous to ascent or the same day of ascent and continue for 2 to 4 days after arriving at the highest altitude or upon descent, whichever comes first. For AMS and HACE, the prophylaxis medication of choice is acetazolamide 125 mg orally every 12 hours. Acetazolamide, a carbonic anhydrase inhibitor, accelerates acclimatization by various mechanisms including enhancing diuresis and ventilation. These effects help in improving oxygenation and lessening the fluid retention associated with HAI. In patients with intolerance or previous allergic reactions to acetazolamide, oral dexamethasone (2 mg every 6 hours or 4 mg every 12 hours) is an alternate choice since it has been shown to be effective although it does not accelerate the acclimatization process. Prolonged use of dexamethasone can be associated to adrenal suppression and a tapering down schedule must be done. Oral ibuprofen has been studied with unclear results as a choice for AMS prevention, but it can be an alternative for those who cannot take acetazolamide or dexamethasone. Caution should be taken with ibuprofen and its possible renal and gastrointestinal adverse effects. For HAPE prophylaxis, nifedipine extended release (ER) 30 mg every 12 hours or 20 mg every 8 hours is the drug of choice. As a calcium channel blocker, nifedipine decreases pulmonary vascular resistance and pulmonary artery pressure and has also been seen to improve oxygenation. Other recommended medications are sildenafil 50 mg every 8 hours or tadalafil 10 mg every 12 hours. This phosphodieterases-5 inhibitors decrease the pulmonary vasoconstriction and hypertension associated to hypoxia in HAPE by increasing the availability of nitrous oxide, a potent pulmonary vasodilator.

Treatment: Mild AMS symptoms could resolve alone if measures of rest and no further ascent are taken. It is important to acknowledge that acetazolamide is considered a masking agent by the WADA and is prohibited at all times, in and out of competition. Systemic dexamethasone is a prohibited medication by WADA while in competition. If the use of these medications is absolutely needed in an athlete subject to WADA regulation, a Therapeutic Use Exemption form (TUE) must be submitted. Analgesics like acetaminophen and nonsteroidal anti-inflammatory medications (NSAIDs) and antiemetics could be used for those mild symptoms. In individuals failing to improve and those having severe AMS symptoms or suspected HACE or HAPE, the treatment of choice is to descend 300 to 1,000 m. Supplemental oxygen to a target of 90% in peripheral oxygen saturation is also recommended if descending is not immediately possible and in all cases of HAPE. The use of portable hyperbaric chambers can also be considered when immediate descent is not possible and there is no supplemental oxygen available.

▪ TRAVEL TIME ISSUES

Long traveling hours can be of medical concern even in healthy people including athletes. Venous thromboembolism (VTE) prevention and Jet lag (JL) are among those concerns.

Venous Thromboembolism

Predisposing risk factors for VTE in athletes are the same as for the general population. Among them are those of intermediate risk such as obesity, personal or family history of thrombophilia, pregnancy or postpartum period, age over 60, use of estrogen-containing oral contraceptives or hormone replacement therapy, and chronic venous insufficiency. High risk factors for VTE are recent major surgery, prior VTE, limb immobilization, and active malignancy.[12]

A road trip or flight for more than 3 hours could predispose some persons with intermediate or high risk to develop a VTE, especially if having more than one risk. So, for them it is recommended to wear under the knee compression stockings of 15 to 30 mmHg for VTE prevention. For those with high risk, if the trip is more than 8 hours, anticoagulation could be considered if there is no contraindications and the benefits outweigh the risks. Although the risk is low in low-risk individuals, it is advisable to encourage them to move their legs and have small walks every 1 to 2 hours during a journey of more than 3 hours. Risk of VTE can go up to 4 to 8 weeks after long travel.

Jet Lag

Jet lag (JL) is defined as a circadian rhythm disorder with difficulty in maintaining the sleep-wake cycle at appropriate times after fast transmeridian travel across time zones. Its pathophysiology is due to desynchronization between external cues and internal sensors at the suprachiasmatic nucleus (SCN) that regulates the body's circadian rhythm. When external stimuli such as light, temperature, and food availability are changed, patients can experience sleep disturbance, general malaise, gastrointestinal symptoms, daytime drowsiness, headache, mood disturbance, and impaired performance. Symptoms tends to be more severe when crossing more than five time zones, in eastward travels, and in more susceptible individuals.[13]

Treatment aims to restore the natural circadian rhythm. The SCN adapts slowly to the abrupt changes occurring in a patient experiencing JL. If no intervention is used, many persons will need 1 day for each hour of change in time zone to adapt to the new time zone. In some individuals, a combination of a stimulant to keep alertness, a chronobiotic and a short-acting hypnotic to induce sleep will be needed to advance adaptation. Among stimulants, bright light exposure at appropriate times, especially to sunlight, can be effective. Caffeine, a widely used stimulant, can also increase alertness and performance. Caffeine is allowed by WADA without restrictions since 2004. Melatonin and melatonin receptors agonist has also been recommended as chronobiotics near bedtime for moderate to severe symptoms. Some individuals can also take advantage of the sedative effects of these medications to promote sleep. Other less recommended alternatives are the use of short-acting hypnotics such as zolpidem to improve sleeping, although they have not proven effective on enhancing adaptation. Chronobiotics and hypnotics are allowed without restrictions by WADA, but caution must be taken because of their side effects and possible impairment in execution if given in high doses or at inappropriate times.

For short trips of 1 to 2 days duration, no manipulation in this adaptation is recommended since the SCN will not adapt that fast and could cause more harm than benefit. In this situation, taking short naps not close to bedtime and using caffeine as a stimulant to promote alertness could be of help to athletes.

Prevention includes avoiding sleep deprivation before travel and adjusting self-itinerary to the itinerary of the visiting country before traveling. It is also recommended to avoid alcohol, coffee, and dehydration during flight, as well as not doing heavy training upon arrival.

▇ SUMMARY

Traveling with a team can be a fun and fulfilling experience, but requires thorough planning to ensure the safety of the athletes and all the members of the traveling delegation or team. Several factors must be taken into consideration especially when traveling to a foreign country to prevent illness and life-threatening complications as well as to avoid problems with local law enforcement.

■ References

1. Tipton CM. Sports medicine: a century of progress. *J Nutr*. 1997;127(5 suppl):878S-885S. doi:10.1093/jn/127.5.878S.

2. Veith I. Galen of Pergamon. By George Sarton. [Logan Clendenning Lectures on the History and Philosophy of Medicine, Third Series.] (Lawrence: University of Kansas Press. 1954. Pp. 112. $2.50.) and Ancient Science and Modern Civilization. By George Sarton. (Lincoln: University of Nebraska Press. 1954. Pp. 111. $2.50.). *Am Hist Rev*. 1955;60(3):583-584. doi:10.1086/ahr/60.3.583.

3. Ryan A. Medical services for the modern Olympic Games. In: Ryan A, ed. *Sports Medicine*. New York, NY: Academic Press; 1974:24-26.

4. Crichton K. Putting together a medical team for the Olympic and Paralympic games. *Aust Fam Physician*. 2000;29:611-613.

5. Bernhardt DT, Roberts WO; American Academy of Pediatrics. *PPE: Pre-participation Physical Evaluation*. 4th ed. Elk Grove Village, IL: American Academy of Pediatrics; 2010.

6. Kary JM, Lavallee M. Travel medicine and the international athlete. *Clin Sports Med*. 2007;26(3):489-503. doi:10.1016/j.csm.2007.04.009.

7. American Academdemy of Family Physicians. Shots immunizations app by AAFP and STFM. https://www.aafp.org/patient-care/public-health/immunizations/shots-app.html.

8. Sports medicine licensure clarity act of 2017. S.808 — 115th Congress (2017-2018).

9. Riddle MS, Connor BA, Beeching NJ, et al. Guidelines for the prevention and treatment of travelers' diarrhea: a graded expert panel report. *J Travel Med*. 2017;24(suppl 1):S57-S74. doi:10.1093/jtm/tax026.

10. Libman M. Summary of the Committee to Advise on Tropical Medicine and Travel (CATMAT) statement on travelers' diarrhea. *Can Commun Dis Rep*. 2015;41:272-284. doi:10.14745/ccdr.v41i11a03.

11. Luks AM, Swenson ER, Bärtsch P. Acute high-altitude sickness. *Eur Respir Rev*. 2017;26:160096. doi:10.1183/16000617.0096-2016.

12. Watson HG, Baglin TP. Guidelines on travel-related venous thrombosis. *Br J Haematol*. 2011;152:31-34. doi:10.1111/j.1365-2141.2010.08408.x.

13. Jet lag and sleep phase disorders. *BMJ Best Practice website*. Updated February 07, 2018. https://bestpractice.bmj.com/topics/en-us/1017.

4. MEDICOLEGAL AND ETHICAL CONCERNS

Walter Alomar-Jiménez and Gerardo Miranda-Comas

▓ INTRODUCTION

The sports medicine physician should be familiar with the medicolegal aspects of sports medicine coverage. It is not uncommon to have questions regarding legal aspects while covering a sports event such as: healthcare responsibility, scope of practice, licensure, liability, and malpractice. There has been a significant increase in sports medicine litigation since 1990.[1] The most commonly discussed issue is the potential conflict of interest of the team physician.[2] On one side is the athlete's health and on the other, the team's, coaches', management's interests. However, the sports medicine physician's priority should always be the athlete's health.

The federal and state laws provide the framework for the medicolegal aspects of sports medicine coverage. The Article VI of the U.S. Constitution declares "that this Constitution shall be the supreme law of the land." This legal principle of supremacy implies that federal laws enacted by the U.S. Congress take precedence over state laws and apply to every state or territory under U.S. jurisdiction. Furthermore, a state law could not be contradictory to a federal law.

Several federal laws have direct implications in sports medicine coverage, such as the Health Insurance Portability and Accountability Act (HIPAA), the Family Educational Rights and Privacy Act (FERPA), and more recently, the Supporting Athletes, Families, and Educators to Protect the Lives of Athletic Youth (SAFE PLAY) Act (2015) and the Sports Medicine Licensure Clarity Act (2018).

The goal of this chapter is to familiarize the sports medicine physician with some of the medicolegal aspects to minimize the legal risks when providing coverage, and to incorporate these principles into the patient–athlete's care.

▓ RESPONSIBILITIES OF THE TEAM PHYSICIAN

The basic principles of medical ethics which guide every physician, such as autonomy, nonmaleficence, beneficence, and justice, also apply to the team physician. In addition, and to expand those principles, several sports medicine organizations, such as the International Olympic Committee (IOC), the International Federation of Sports Medicine (FIMS), and the American College of Sports Medicine (ACSM) have each delineated their own Sports Medicine Code of Ethics. The consensus of the different codes of ethics is that the principal priority or responsibility of the team physician must be the athlete's health.[3] It is imperative to never do harm and to always make objective medical decisions.

Some of the team physician's duties include: performing preparticipation physical examinations (PPE), determining athletes' eligibility, return-to-play decisions after injury, developing an emergency action plan (EAP) for practices and competitions, overseeing the staff providing healthcare services, and protecting against legal liability.[4]

■ CONFIDENTIALITY

Privacy and discretion are important values in all relationships. Patient–physician confidentiality is not the exception. Several federal laws establish the standards for protecting patient healthcare information such as the HIPAA and the FERPA laws. As an exception to the general rule, a team physician employed by a club may disclose an athlete's health information to the coaches and owners since this is not considered protected health information.[5]

FERPA is a federal law that protects the privacy of students' educational records. Treatment records are excluded from the definition of educational records under FERPA. Nonetheless, a school may disclose students' treatments records to another institution, without written consent, when legitimate educational interest is proven. In the absence of patient–athlete consent, a team physician should never disclose health information to the press or other entities.[6]

■ PHYSICIAN LIABILITY

Medical malpractice is a subset within tort law that deals with professional negligence.[7] In order to have a successful claim, the injured patient–athlete must prove four legal elements: professional duty owed to the patient–athlete; failure of the treating professional to use reasonable care executing that duty; failure resulted in damages; and causal link exists between the negligence and damages.[8] Negligence can be proven when the physician does not adhere to the standard of care. However, in the field of sports medicine, the standard of care might be difficult to establish because of the many different medical specialties involved in the care of the athletes such as orthopedic surgery, emergency medicine, family medicine, internal medicine, pediatrics, and physical medicine and rehabilitation.[9]

Adhering to the standard of care and practice guidelines is the best defense in a malpractice case. The court will also evaluate vital aspects in any medical decision such as: informed consent, discussion of benefits and risks of the proposed treatment and alternative treatment options. Jurisprudence has well established that signing a waiver liability would not prevent a malpractice lawsuit against a physician. Furthermore, some courts have invalidated those agreements because they violate public policy, See *Tunkl v. Regents of University of California* (60 CAL.2D 92).

Typically, malpractice cases have resulted from an adverse outcome in a surgery or procedure. Interestingly, the sports medicine physician could be found liable in return-to-play decisions as well. Concussion evaluation and management has been a hot topic in the recent years regarding sports medicine coverage. Some authors suggest that the legal system should hold team physicians responsible to alert football players about the risk of developing chronic traumatic encephalopathy (CTE).[10] We know that early return-to-play after sustaining a concussion or a cervical spine injury could have catastrophic effects.[11] The U.S. Congress addressed this concern, after many years of lobbying and many state laws, in the SAFE PLAY Act (2015). The federal law imposes a standard plan for concussion management: an athlete who sustained a concussion cannot return to play until written release from a healthcare professional (never on the same day). Moreover, the law requires that public schools educate parents, students, and coaches on concussion symptoms and risks.

■ THE TRAVELING TEAM PHYSICIAN

The traveling team physician faces many challenges and questions. Some of these are related to medical license and insurance coverage. Usually a physician possesses a medical license and malpractice insurance within his state/territory of practice. What happens when the team physician travels to another state? That was a longstanding debate that was recently addressed by the U.S. Congress in the Sports Medicine Licensure Clarity Act (2018). The Sports Medicine Licensure Clarity Act extends the liability insurance of a state-licensed medical professional to another state when the professional provides medical services to an athlete or athletic team. The interpretation and effect of this law is that the medical services provided are considered as they happened on the primary state in which the medical professional is licensed and insured. Prior to the event, the medical professional must disclose to his insurer the nature and extent of the medical services. It is important to mention that this liability insurance extension does not apply at a healthcare facility or while the medical professional is transporting an injured athlete to a healthcare facility.

▨ SUMMARY

The law regulates many aspects of our daily lives including the practice of medicine. The sports medicine field creates many medicolegal challenges for healthcare professionals. Although some federal laws have attempted to clarify some aspects, not all possible situations are covered. Sports physicians should understand the essential legal regulations and utilize the medical ethics principles to guide recommendations and decisions in the best interest of the patient–athlete's health. Our best defense always is to practice a high standard of care medicine.

▨ References

1. Mitten MJ. Emerging legal issues in sports medicine: a synthesis, summary, and analysis. *St John's Law Rev.* 2002;76(1):5-86. https://scholarship.law.stjohns.edu/cgi/viewcontent.cgi?article=1343&context=law review.

2. Koller DL. Team physicians, sports medicine, and the law: an update. *Clin Sports Med.* 2016;35(2):245-255. doi:10.1016/j.csm.2015.10.005.

3. Holm S, McNamee MJ, Pigozzi F. Ethical practice and sports physician protection: a proposal. *Br J Sports Med.* 2011;45(15):1170-1173. https://bjsm.bmj.com/content/bjsports/45/15/1170.full.pdf.

4. Pearsall AW 4th, Kovaleski JE, Madanagopal SG. Medicolegal issues affecting sports medicine practitioners. *Clin Orthop Relat Res.* 2005;(433):50-57. doi:10.1097/01.blo.0000159896.64076.72.

5. Testoni D, Hornik CP, Smith PB, et al. Sports medicine and ethics. *Am J Bioeth.* 2013;13(10):4-12. doi:10.1080/15265161.2013.828114.

6. Frenkel DA. Sports medicine and the law. *Med Law.* 2002;21(1):201-209.

7. Bal BS. An introduction to medical malpractice in the United States. *Clin Orthop Relat Res.* 2009;467(2):339-347. doi:10.1007/s11999-008-0636-2.

8. Pachman S, Lamba A. Legal aspects of concussion: the ever-evolving standard of care. *J Athl Train.* 2017;52(3):186-194. doi:10.4085/1062-6050-52.1.03.

9. Boggess BR, Bytomski JR. Medicolegal aspects of sports medicine. *Prim Care.* 2013;40(2):525-535. doi:10.1016/j.pop.2013.02.008.

10. Teo WZW, Brenner LH, Bal BS. Medicolegal sidebar: serving on the sidelines-the American Football Dilemma. *Clin Orthop Relat Res.* 2018;476(3):466-468. doi:10.1007/s11999.0000000000000188.

11. Cantu RC, Li YM, Abdulhamid M, Chin LS. Return to play after cervical spine injury in sports. *Curr Sports Med Rep.* 2013;12(1):14-17. doi:10.1249/JSR.0b013e31827dc1fb.

MEDICAL CONSIDERATIONS FOR SPORTS MEDICINE CLINICIANS

5. MEDICAL EMERGENCIES

Amie Kim, Ilya Aylyarov, Lauren Paish, and
Andres Arredondo Santana

The initial approach to the deteriorating patient utilizes the standard principles of the primary survey. Providers remain organized applying the Airway, Breathing, Circulation, Disability, Exposure (ABCDE) approach. The aim is to keep the patient alive, immediately intervene on life-threatening processes, and buy time until transport to definitive diagnosis and treatments. The key is to identify signs and symptoms of distress and treat life-threatening issues before continuing to the next stage of assessment. This includes physiologic systemic failure from exertion in sport, traumatic injury sustained in sport, and occult traumatic injury at the time of collapse. Perform a complete initial assessment and serially reassess as the athlete responds to treatment initiated or continues to deteriorate.

Emergency Action Plan (EAP) is a set of standardized protocols created by the medical and venue staff to prepare for an unexpected or catastrophic event that is established and rehearsed prior to the event. It consists of:

a) Mass Casualty Disaster (MCD) plan
b) Emergency personnel and roles (scene safety, equipment retrieval, first response)
c) Emergency communication (system within staff, between staff and Emergency Medical Services [EMS])
d) Emergency equipment (strategic Automated External Defibrillator [AED] placement, organized supplies)
e) Medical transport (ambulance, vehicle on standby)
f) Venue layout (EMS access, entry and exit routes, potential obstacles)[1]

▪ INITIAL APPROACH TO A COLLAPSED ATHLETE(S)

Step 1. Scene Safety. Confirm you and staff can access the collapsed athlete without endangering yourself or others.

> Apply personal protective equipment → Secure the environment → Remove the patient from immediate danger → Transfer patient and providers into safe location → Consider safe immobilization and transfer techniques if permitted

Step 2. Call for help

> Activate EAP/call 911 → Assign roles → Confirm equipment access → Communicate to event staff → Multiple victims - initiate MCD triage for quick classification. Simple Triage and Rapid Treatment (START) protocol is currently the most widely used system in the United States. First responders tag injured athletes by applying categories of injury severity[2]:

- BLACK: Deceased or expected. Injuries incompatible with life or without spontaneous respiration.

- RED: Immediate intervention. Severe injuries but high potential for survival. Prioritize to the collection point. Transition to ABCs.
- YELLOW: Collection point. Delayed transport. Serious injury but expected to deteriorate over hours.
- GREEN: Walking wounded. Minor injuries.

Step 3. Assess Airway, Breathing, Circulation, **Disability, Exposure** *(ABCDE). If no pulse or irregular pulse* **(Figures 5.1–5.3)**. Initiate CPR (advanced cardiac life support [ACLS] protocol). AED application and operation (basic life support [BLS] protocol). Follow the automated prompts. Special considerations include:

- *Exercise Associated Collapse (EAC)* is benign postural hypotension after completion of exercise. Abrupt cessation of strenuous exercise leads to blood pooling in the lower limbs. This decreases venous return that results in lightheadedness or syncope. It occurs in the absence of neurologic, electrolyte, or thermal abnormalities.

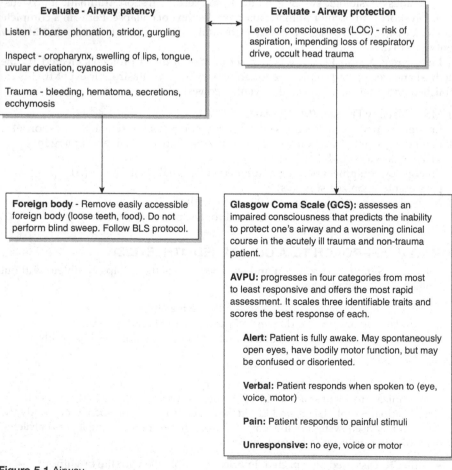

Figure 5.1 Airway.

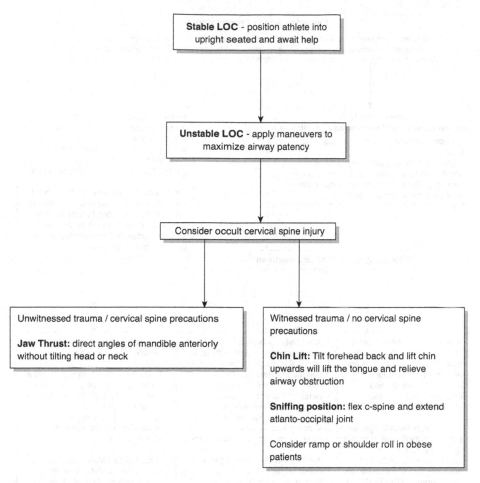

Figure 5.1 (continued)

- ○ Intervention:
    1. Position the athlete in Trendelenburg (supine with legs elevated).
    2. Titrate fluid intake to thirst.
    3. Older, at risk athletes should be evaluated for cardiac etiology.
- Patient in water: move patient to dry, safe location. Quickly dry as much water as possible. If shock is delivered while patient is immersed, electricity disperses through water and effectiveness is reduced. AED can be used safely for patient and provider if in a small puddle or in snow.
- Hairy chest: pads must have adequate contact with skin. Apply pressure to pads to enhance conduction.
- Pacemaker or implantable device: internal pacemaker or defibrillator is typically surgically placed in the chest upper region. AED pads should not be placed over or near the pacemaker.[3]

Continue chest compressions and intermittent defibrillation for three cycles prior to transferring patient from ground onto a stretcher or immobilization device.[3-6]

Evaluate - signs of respiratory failure

Inspect: symmetrical chest rise, retractions, accessory muscle use, diaphoresis, cyanosis
Auscultate: tachypnea, decreased or asymmetric breath sounds, wheezing, cough, rales

Absent breathing
Intervention - Positive pressure ventilation
- rescue breathing via pocket mask (BLS protocol).
*Caution. Applying positive pressure ventilation to a potential pneumothorax increases the risk of tension pneumothorax and cardiovascular collapse

Pneumothorax – is a life-threatening presence of air in the intrapleural space. Created by a communication from injury in the parietal pleural from chest wall trauma or from injury in the visceral pleural from a lung parenchyma injury.

Signs and Symptoms: include chest pain, dyspnea, tachypnea, tachycardia. There will be reduced breath sounds auscultated on one side of the chest, palpable crepitus from subcutaneous air in chest and/or neck.

Wheezing: evaluation and treatment

Asthma is an inflammatory response in the bronchioles that leads to constriction and air trapping. Patients will present with wheezing, dyspnea, and accessory muscle use.

Administer Beta-2 agonist (ex. albuterol) and steroids (prednisone). All selective and non-selective beta-2 agonists and glucocorticoids are banned on the WADA List of Prohibited Substances and Methods and require Therapeutic Use Exemption (TUE). In the case of emergency, retroactive TUE is possible

Anaphylaxis is an allergic reaction that presents with acute onset of wheezing plus fluid shifts into the skin (hives, pruritus), mucosa (facial swelling) or persistent gastrointestinal symptoms (bowel edema). Common etiologies include nuts, stinging insects, certain medications, or exercise-induced.

Administer Epi-Pen: if there is compromise of the airway, breathing, or circulation. All adrenaline is banned on the WADA List of Prohibited Substances and Methods and require TUE. In the case of emergency, retroactive TUE is possible.

Adult: Epinephrine (1:1000) 0.3mg IM Pediatric (less than 30 kg): Epinephrine (1:1000) 0.01mg/kg IM. EpiPen Jr and similar autoinjectors are 0.15mg per injection IM

Immediate decompression with needle thoracostomy.

Place the patient supine. Insert a 14 or 16-gauge angiocatheter at a 90 degree angle to the sterilized chest wall, in the second intercostal space at the midclavicular line, immediately above the third rib.

A rush of air through the needle can be heard. Attach an empty 10 mL syringe to confirm air. Reassess for clinical improvement.

Figure 5.2 Breathing.
Source: Roberts J. *Roberts and Hedges' Clinical Procedures in Emergency Medicine and Acute Care.* 7th ed. Philadelphia, PA: Elsevier; 2018.

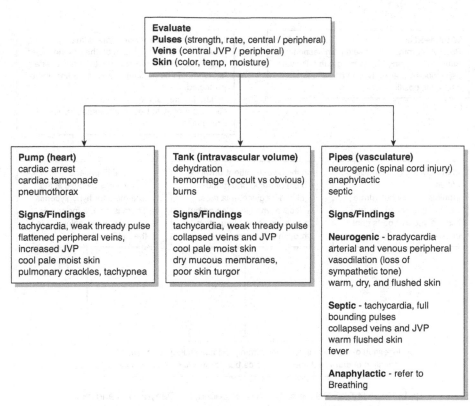

Evaluate
Pulses (strength, rate, central / peripheral)
Veins (central JVP / peripheral)
Skin (color, temp, moisture)

Pump (heart)
cardiac arrest
cardiac tamponade
pneumothorax

Signs/Findings
tachycardia, weak thready pulse
flattened peripheral veins,
increased JVP
cool pale moist skin
pulmonary crackles, tachypnea

Tank (intravascular volume)
dehydration
hemorrhage (occult vs obvious)
burns

Signs/Findings
tachycardia, weak thready pulse
collapsed veins and JVP
cool pale moist skin
dry mucous membranes,
poor skin turgor

Pipes (vasculature)
neurogenic (spinal cord injury)
anaphylactic
septic

Signs/Findings

Neurogenic - bradycardia
arterial and venous peripheral
vasodilation (loss of
sympathetic tone)
warm, dry, and flushed skin

Septic - tachycardia, full
bounding pulses
collapsed veins and JVP
warm flushed skin
fever

Anaphylactic - refer to
Breathing

Figure 5.3 Circulation: When there are problems in circulation and adequate vascular perfusion to vital organs cannot be maintained, the athlete may be in shock. The cause must be identified and treated primarily.

Step 4. Secure patient for evaluation. Assess disability (ABCDE; Figure 5.4). Level of consciousness or altered mental status (AMS) is often the only sign of occult trauma or profound metabolic processes. Collapse can be suggestive of hypoglycemia, dehydration causing hyponatremia or hypernatremia, or a postictal state from any of the above. If trauma is unwitnessed, a spinal cord injury and occult trauma are presumed, and the spinal cord is protected during evaluation.[7-9]

Cervical collar is placed to immobilize the cervical spine to prevent spinal cord injury in any unconscious athlete, any athlete with new neurologic complaints or findings (i.e. numbness, focal weakness), an athlete with significant midline spine pain with or without palpation, or an obvious spinal deformity. Two providers are required for application. The first provider places both hands on the sides of the athlete's head to maintain in-line stabilization, avoiding cervical traction. The second provider secures collar and confirms neutral position of head to neck.

Longboard helps immobilize the spine to prevent spinal cord injury from a possible occult spine fracture in any unconscious athlete, any athlete with new neurologic complaints or findings (i.e. numbness, focal weakness), an athlete with significant midline spine pain with or without palpation, an obvious spinal deformity, or after a high velocity mechanism of injury. The recommended techniques include the *Lift-and-slide*

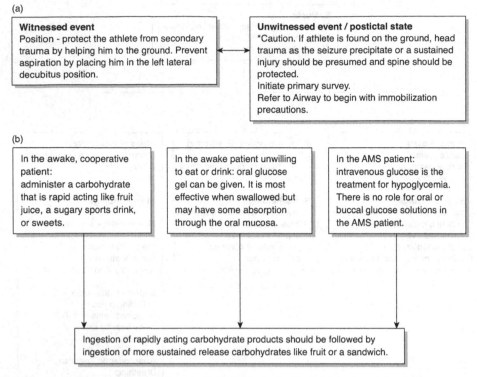

(a)

Witnessed event	Unwitnessed event / postictal state
Position - protect the athlete from secondary trauma by helping him to the ground. Prevent aspiration by placing him in the left lateral decubitus position.	*Caution. If athlete is found on the ground, head trauma as the seizure precipitate or a sustained injury should be presumed and spine should be protected. Initiate primary survey. Refer to Airway to begin with immobilization precautions.

(b)

In the awake, cooperative patient: administer a carbohydrate that is rapid acting like fruit juice, a sugary sports drink, or sweets.

In the awake patient unwilling to eat or drink: oral glucose gel can be given. It is most effective when swallowed but may have some absorption through the oral mucosa.

In the AMS patient: intravenous glucose is the treatment for hypoglycemia. There is no role for oral or buccal glucose solutions in the AMS patient.

Ingestion of rapidly acting carbohydrate products should be followed by ingestion of more sustained release carbohydrates like fruit or a sandwich.

Figure 5.4(a,b) Disability. (a). Seizures; (b). Hypoglycemia; (c). Dehydration and exercise-associated hyponatremia (EAH).
(a). **Seizures:** initial approach
(b). **Hypoglycemia:** rarely a sideline emergency, but hypoglycemia can be severe enough to cause brain injury or death. Early on, hypoglycemia can mimic dehydration. Signs and symptoms including sweating, pale and clammy skin, anxiety, headache, dizziness, and ultimately agitation, aggression, confusion, and focal neurologic deficits. If it progresses, it can lead to loss of consciousness, seizure activity, and cardiac arrest. Hypoglycemia must be ruled out in any athlete found unconscious by using a rapid fingerstick.[9]

technique (bridge lift) and the *Log roll technique*. The lift-and-slide technique is performed by 6–8 (the preferred technique involves 8) individuals: one at the head, two or three on each side and one controlling the spinal board. The other technique is the log roll and requires at least four providers: one controlling the head, two the body, and one the spinal board.

Pelvic binder - Major pelvic trauma can lead to severe hemorrhage. Early stabilization by compressing the bony pelvic ring is required. Aggressive pelvic rock can further cause venous plexus injury or clot disruption. Indications include: high mechanism of injury, pelvic pain endorsed, or tenderness identified, and any unconscious athlete.

Limb Bleeding may require the use of **tourniquets** if direct pressure fails to control hemorrhage. They are inexpensive, safe, and effective when applied early. Orthopedic surgeons frequently use pneumatic tourniquets in operative procedures for several hours without impact.[10]

It is applied by elevating the injured limb above the level of the heart → placed at long bone above area of injury to compress artery against long

(c)

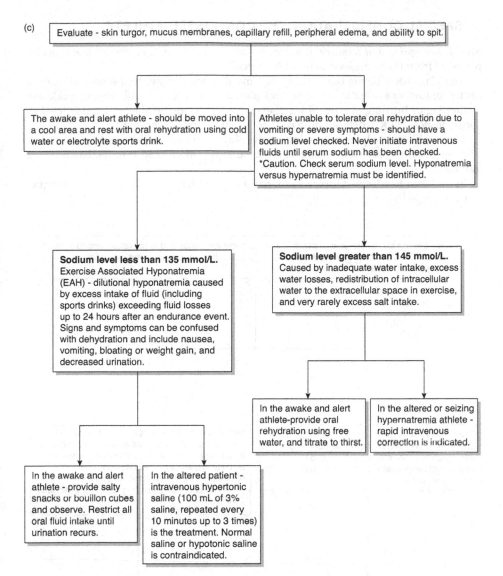

Figure 5.4(c) Dehydration: occurs in athletes who did not adequately prehydrate before the event or in unexpectedly high ambient temperatures combined with high humidity (high wet bulb globe temperature (WBGT)) which limits the ability to cool via evaporate sweating. It can be worsened in athletes with elevated blood glucose or a diarrheal illness. Symptoms of severe dehydration include thirst, fatigue, dizziness, headaches, lightheadedness, syncope, or seizure.

bone → tighten until hemorrhage ceases with loss of distal pulses → apply noncircumferential pressure dressing to site of ooze → record time of tourniquet application on athlete to relay to receiving facility.

A second tourniquet may be used adjacently to apply pressure over a wider distribution.

*Step 5. Exposure assessment (**ABCDE; Figure 5.5**).*[11,12]

■ SPECIAL CONSIDERATION: THE CONCUSSED ATHLETE

Step 1. Recognize and Remove. If a concussion is suspected, then the athlete must be removed from the game/competition/practice.[13,14]

Red Flags for a severe brain injury that merit quick transfer to the nearest trauma center for further evaluation include: neck pain or tenderness, double vision, weakness or tingling or burning in arms or legs, severe or increasing headache, seizure, level of consciousness (LOC), deteriorating conscious state, combative or agitated, vomiting.

Observable signs: lying motionless on the playing surface, slow to get up after a hit, disorientation or confusion, blank stare, facial injury after head trauma, balance and gait difficulty

Symptoms: headache, blurry vision, nausea, vomiting, sensitivity to light, fatigue, low energy, irritable

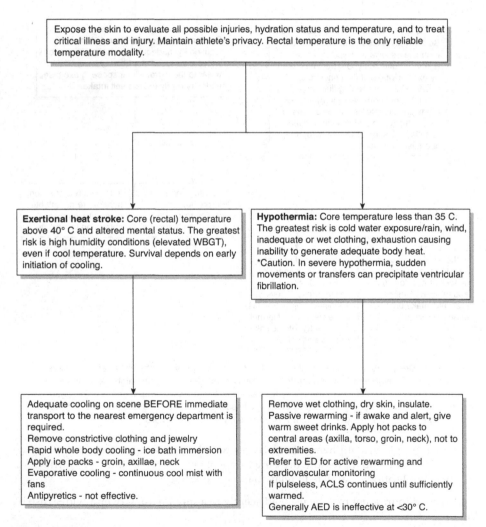

Figure 5.5 Exposure.

Memory assessment: use the Maddock questionnaire; "What venue are we at to-day?," "Which half is it now?," "Who scored last in the game?," "What team did you play last week?," "Did your team win last game?"

Step 2. Administer a Sports Concussion Assessment Tool. Using the SCAT 5 is recommended, but it is not the only assessment tool. The SCAT 5 is readily available online without cost. There is a pediatric version, Child SCAT 5 for boys/girls ages 5 to 12 years. The published document can be printed and used by any individual; it has step-by-step instructions as to how to administer.[10-12]

- Immediate or on-field assessment is the same as the Sports Concussion Recognition Tool discussed previously including a Glasgow Coma Scale and cervical spine assessment
- Office or off-field assessment

  o Step 1. Athlete Background Information

  o Step 2. Symptoms evaluation. Self-assessment evaluation of number of symptoms and severity of each

  o Step 3. Cognitive screening evaluating orientation, immediate memory, and concentration

  o Step 4. Neurological screen and balance examination

  o Step 5. Delayed recall

  o Step 6. Decision. Each domain is scored and documented with the date of the evaluation in order to assess progression and recovery. Scoring is not used as a stand-alone method to diagnose concussion, but as an aid in the decision-making process, especially return to sport.

■ SUMMARY

This chapter covered some of the more common emergencies that a sports medicine practitioner might experience during sideline, on-field coverage. These guidelines can be used to assess and provide initial treatment to an injured athletes, especially those who suffered life-threatening injuries.

■ References

1. Drezner, JA, Courson RW, Roberts WO, et al. Inter-Association Task Force recommendations on emergency preparedness and management of sudden cardiac arrest in high school and college athletic programs: a consensus statement. *J Athl Train.* 2007;42(1):143-158. https://www.ncbi.nlm.nih.gov/pmc/articles/PMC1896083.

2. Bazyar J, Farrokhi M, Khankeh H. Triage systems in mass casualty incidents and disasters: a review study with a worldwide approach. *Open Access Maced J Med Sci.* 2019;7(3):482-494. doi:10.3889/oamjms.2019.119.

3. American Heart Association. Part 3: adult basic life support. *Circulation.* 2000;102:I-22-I-59. https://www.ahajournals.org/doi/10.1161/circ.102.suppl_1.I-22.

4. Roberts J. *Roberts and Hedges' Clinical Procedures in Emergency Medicine and Acute Care.* 7th ed. Philadelphia, PA: Elsevier; 2018.

5. Link MS, Myerburg RJ, Estes III, M. Eligibility and disqualification recommendations for competitive athletes with cardiovascular abnormalities: task force 12: emergency action plans, resuscitation, cardiopulmonary resuscitation, and automated external defibrillators: a scientific statement from the Ameri-

can Heart Association and American College of Cardiology. *Circulation*. 2015;132:e334-e338. doi:10.1161/CIR.0000000000000248.

6. American Heart Association. Part 4: adult basic life support. *Circulation*. 2005;112:IV-19-IV-34. doi:10.1161/CIRCULATIONAHA.105.166553.

7. Gammon, M. Evaluation and treatment of trauma related collapse in athletes. *Curr Rev Musculoskelet Med*. 2014;7(4):342-347. doi:10.1007/s12178-014-9245-8.

8. Mills BM, Conrick KM, Anderson S, et al. Consensus recommendations on the prehospital care of the injured athlete with a suspected catastrophic cervical spine injury. *J Athl Train*. 2020;55(6):563-572. doi:10/4085/1062-6050-0434.19.

9. Villani M, de Courten B, Zoungas S. Emergency treatment of hypoglycaemia: a guideline and evidence review. *Diabet Med*. 2017;34(9):1205-1211. doi:10.1111/dme.13379.

10. Kauvar DS, Dubick MA, Walters TJ, Kragh JF Jr. Systematic review of prehospital tourniquet use in civilian limb trauma. *J Trauma Acute Care Surg*. 2018;84(5):819-825. doi:10.1097/TA.0000000000001826.

11. Belval LN, Casa DJ, Adams WM, et al. Consensus statement—prehospital care of exertional heat stroke. *Prehosp Emerg Care*. 2018;22(3):392-397.

12. Cappaert TA, Stone JA, Castellani JW, et al. National athletic trainers' association position statement: environmental cold injuries. *J Athl Train*. 2008;4(6):640-658.

13. Echemendia RJ, Meeuwisse W, McCrory P, et al. The Sport Concussion Assessment Tool 5th Edition (SCAT5): background and rationale. *Br J Sports Med*. 2017;51(11):848-850. doi:10.1136/bjsports-2017-097506.

14. Davis GA, Purcell L, Schneider KJ, et al. The Child Sport Concussion Assessment Tool 5th Edition (Child SCAT5): background and rationale. *Br J Sports Med*. 2017;51(11):859-861. doi:10.1136/bjsports-2017-097492.

6. NUTRITION AND HYDRATION

Michelle Leong and Gerardo Miranda-Comas

■ INTRODUCTION

The information provided in this chapter will provide clinicians with a general overview of nutrient and hydration needs in an athlete during training or competition. For individualized nutritional needs, athletes should seek guidance from a registered, board certified sports dietitian (RD, CSSD).

■ NUTRITION

Energy/Caloric Requirements: Appropriate caloric intake is vital for controlling body weight, maximizing performance, and maintaining overall health. Guidelines for recommended caloric intake are listed in Table 6.1.

Table 6.1 Guidelines for Recommended Caloric Intake

Gender	Calories (cal)/kilogram (kg) of BW
Male	8.6–10.5 cal/kg of BW
Female	7.7–9.1 cal/kg of BW
Individual Setting	Calories (cal)/kilogram (kg) of BW
Recovering from injury	6.8 cal/kg of BW
Low intensity activities or exercising 3–5 days/week	7.7–8.6 cal/kg of BW
Moderate training (5 days per week + conditioning 2–3 days/week)	8.1–9.1 cal/kg of BW
High/vigorous daily training	8.6–10.5 cal/kg of BW
Very high/Triathlon training/nonelite	10–11.4 cal/kg of BW
Very high/Competitive marathoners and triathletes	11.4–13.6 cal/kg of BW

BW, body weight.

Calories from carbohydrates should make up approximately 60%, protein 10% to 35%, and fats up to 10% or less of total caloric intake. Athletes should consume around 1.2 to 2.0 g of protein/kg of BW each day, with endurance and power athletes consuming amounts at the higher end of the range.

Training/Competition Diet: Athletic performance can be enhanced by nutrition. Typically, athletes follow a high-carbohydrate/low-fat diet. The goal of this diet is to meet training program energy requirements and to optimize restoration of muscle glycogen stores between workouts. Complex carbohydrates with a moderate to high glycemic index are favored.

Pre-exercise: Prior to training sessions or events less than 90 minutes, recommended carbohydrate intake is 6 to 12 g/kg of BW per 24 hours. This is appropriate for most sports, including power sports. For events lasting longer than 90 minutes, as in most endurance sports, recommended carbohydrate intake is 10 to 12 g/kg of BW per 24 hours starting 36 to 48 hours prior to the event. A meal consisting of high carbohydrate (1–4 g/kg of BW) and a moderate amount of lean protein is suggested 1 to 4 hours prior to training sessions/competition. The optimal amount of preactivity (within 60 minutes) food consumed is highly individualized. Physical activity on an empty stomach may result in cramping or indigestion. High fiber, high protein, and high fat items should be minimized to prevent gastrointestinal discomfort.

During exercise: Recommended carbohydrate intake is 30 to 60 g/hour for sessions 1 to 2.5 hours in duration, for endurance and intermittent high-intensity power sports, and up to 90 g/hour for sessions greater than 2.5 to 3 hours. Dividing the intake into smaller portions consumed more frequently can help avoid gastrointestinal discomfort. For athletes who do not have time to eat during an event, sports drinks may be used as an alternative. Drinking 150 to 300 mL (5–10 oz) of a 6% to 8% carbohydrate sports drink every 15 to 20 minutes is ideal. It is not necessary to consume fat during exercise.

Postexercise/Recovery: Endurance exercise sessions less than 1 hour do not require an increase in normal carbohydrate consumption postexercise. For sessions longer than 1.0 to 1.5 hours, it is recommended to eat or drink 1.0 to 1.5 g/kg of BW (100–200 g) of carbohydrates and 0.3 g/kg of BW (20–30 g) of protein within 30 minutes. For power and intermittent high-intensity sports, recommended intake is the same as just stated, even if sessions are less than 1 hour.

▦ HYDRATION

Optimum hydration via the consumption of water and electrolytes helps maintain body temperature, blood volume, and adequate muscle contraction. Sweat rates are highly variable and individualized. Sweat rates of 1 to 2 L/hour is typical for running sports, but may exceed 2 L/hour in warmer climates.

Hydration Assessment: The most viable assessment techniques include body weight change, urine specific gravity, 24-hour urine volume, urine color, and thirst. Total body water change should be less than 2%. Body weight change should be less than 1%.

General Fluid and Electrolyte Requirement

Pre-exercise: Prehydrating involves drinking 5 to 7 mL/kg of BW at least 4 hours before an event. If an athlete is unable to urinate or the urine is dark, an additional 3 to 5 mL/kg of BW should be consumed 2 hours prior to the event. This applies to all sports. Consuming beverages with 20 to 50 mEq/L of sodium, or eating small amounts of salty snacks may help stimulate thirst and retain consumed fluids. Overhydrating is not recommended as it can lead to hyponatremia.

During exercise: The amount and rate of fluid hydration varies depending on the individual sweating rate, climate, exercise duration, exercise intensity, and opportunity to drink. A suggested starting point is to drink when thirsty and to consume on average 0.4 to 0.8 L/hour. The aim for most sports is to minimize body weight loss to less than 2%. For endurance athletes, 0.15 to 0.35 L should be consumed every 15 to 20 minutes. For events less than 1 hour, pure water may be sufficient. For longer duration events, fluid replacement beverages should contain 20 to 30 mEq/L of sodium and 2 to 5 mEq/L of potassium in order to replace sweat electrolyte losses.

Postexercise/Recovery: To achieve effective rehydration following exercise, a rehydration beverage should contain moderately high levels of sodium (at least 50 mmol/L), and possibly some potassium. The volume of beverage consumed should be greater than the volume of sweat lost to provide for the ongoing obligatory urine losses. One and one-half L of fluid for every kg of BW (or 20–24 oz/lb) lost should be consumed to achieve rapid and complete recovery from dehydration. This applies to all sports. Intravenous fluid replacement after exercise is warranted if the individual has lost greater than 7% body weight or presents with nausea, vomiting, or diarrhea.

■ ENVIRONMENTAL VARIABLES

Heat and humidity: Exercise increases heat production and core body temperature. Fluid intake should be 6 mL/kg every 2 to 3 hours as sweat rates will be near maximal. Prehydration should begin 4 to 6 hours prior to competition and continue throughout the competition. Daily sodium intake should be increased to 5 to 10 g per day. Appropriate hydration can be monitored by maintaining weight within 2% of baseline. For every pound lost during exercise, 400 to 500 mL (~16 oz) of sodium-containing fluid should be consumed.

Cold: Exercising in the cold increases energy expenditure due to increased weight of protective clothing, increased energy consumption, and shivering. Athletes should supplement their typical diet with extra carbohydrates prior to and during exercising in cold temperatures. Athletes should follow the usual pre- and during-exercise hydration regimen.

Altitude: Energy requirements are increased in areas of high altitude, especially above 2,500 m (8,200 ft). Diet should be supplemented with extra carbohydrates pre- and during exercise. High fat foods can also be added to the athlete's typical diet to help overcome appetite suppression. The typical pre- and during-exercise hydration regimen should be followed.

Health Risks Considerations: There are several medical conditions that require a professional medical evaluation in order to avoid serious complications. **Exercise induced hyponatremia** causes headache, nausea, vomiting, restlessness, cramping, undue fatigue, disorientation and confusion, seizure, coma, and respiratory arrest. Risk factors include exercise duration greater than 4 hours or slow running, female gender, low body weight, excessive drinking over 1.5 L/hour, pre-exercise overhydration, and extreme hot or cold environments. **Rhabdomyolysis** causes severe muscle pain, muscle weakness, dark-colored urine. Risk factors include excessive, high intensity or increased duration of exercise, lack of warm up or gradual increase, extreme temperatures, electrolyte imbalances, low protein or glycogen diets, use of statins, alcohol use, acute illness. **Heat exhaustion** occurs when body temp is 100 to 104°F (38.3–40°C). Symptoms include difficulty continuing exercise, weakness, profuse sweating, pale skin, tachycardia, abdominal pain, nausea, vomiting, diarrhea. **Exertional heat stroke** happens when body temperature is greater than 104°F (40°C). Heat stroke symptoms are similar to heat exhaustion but also include collapse, confusion or disorientation, dizziness, difficulty walking, irritability, headache, hyperventilation, and dry mouth. Risk factors include dehydration, poor physical fitness level, little to no acclimatization to hot or humid conditions, obesity, older age, acute illness, excessive clothing or equipment during exercise.

■ SUMMARY

Appropriate nutrition and hydration are essential in an athlete to maintain overall health and to enhance performance. This chapter provides general recommendations regarding carbohydrate, protein, and hydration intake. Detailed nutrition and hydration plans should be discussed with a registered sports dietician.

■ Further Reading

Bonci LJ. Eating for performance: bringing science to the training table. *Clin Sports Med*. 2011;30:661-670. doi:10.1016/j.csm.2011.03.011.

Burke L, Hawley J, Wong S, Jeukendrup AE. Carbohydrates for training and competition. *J Sports Sci*. 2011;29(suppl 1): S17-S27. doi:10.1080/02640414.2011.585473.

Medeiros DM, Wildman REC. *Advanced Human Nutrition*. 4th ed. Burlington, MA: Jones & Bartlett Learning; 2019.

Phillips S, Van Loon L. Dietary protein for athletes: from requirements to optimum adaptation. *J Sports Sci*. 2011;29(suppl 1):S29-S38. doi:10.1080/02640414.2011.619204.

Sawka MN, Burke LM, Eichner ER, et al. American College of Sports Medicine position stand: exercise and fluid replacement. *Med Sci Sports Exerc*. 2007;39:377-390. doi:10.1249/mss.0b013e31802ca597.

Shirreffs S, Sawka M. Fluid and electrolyte needs for training, competition, and recovery. *J Sports Sci*. 2011;29(suppl 1):S39-S46. doi:10.1080/02640414.2011.614269.

Slater G, Phillips SM. Nutrition guidelines for strength sports: sprinting, weightlifting, throwing events, and bodybuilding. *J Sports Sci*. 2011;29(suppl 1):S67-S77. doi:10.1080/02640414.2011.574722.

Stellingwerff T, Maughan R, Burke L. Nutrition for power sports: middle-distance running, track cycling, rowing, canoeing/kayaking, and swimming. *J Sports Sci*. 2011;29(suppl 1):S79-S89. doi:10.1080/02640414.2011.589469.

Thomas DT, Erdman KA, Burke LM. American College of Sports Medicine joint position statement. Nutrition and athletic performance. *Med Sci Sports Exerc*. 2016;48(3):543-568. doi:10.1249/MSS.0000000000000852.

7. PREPARTICIPATION PHYSICAL EVALUATIONS

Brenda Castillo and Richa Lamba

INTRODUCTION

Approximately 30 million athletes younger than 18 years and another 3 million athletes with special needs receive medical clearance to participate in sports every year.[1] The primary goal of the preparticipation physical evaluation (PPE) is to maximize the health of athletes and their safe participation in sports. Although studies have not found that the PPE prevents morbidity and mortality associated with sports, it may detect conditions that predispose the athlete to injury or illness and provides strategies for injury prevention. A thorough history is critical to identify underlying medical conditions that may interfere with participation in sports and thus place the athlete at risk for injury. The physical exam, at minimum, should include assessment of the cardiovascular and musculoskeletal systems. Clearance to participate depends on the outcome of the evaluation and the general category of the sport. Our chapter intends to provide an overview on the principles and guidelines required to perform a comprehensive and systematized PPE in order to determine clearance for safe participation in sports.

GOAL AND OBJECTIVES

The overall goal of the PPE is to help maintain the health and safety of athletes. Its purpose is not to exclude athletes from participation, but to encourage safe participation. Its primary objectives are to: (1) detect any condition that could potentially endanger the health and/or safety of the athlete and his or her teammates and (2) meet legal and insurance requirements. The secondary objectives are to: (1) determine the athlete's general health; (2) counsel on health-related issues; and (3) assess fitness level for specific sports. For many young athletes who have limited prior contact with the healthcare system, the PPE may serve as an entry point to medical care.[2]

SUBJECTS

Medical associations, including the American College of Sports Medicine (ACSM), the American Heart Association (AHA), and the American College of Pediatrics (AAP), recommend that all potential athletes, competitive and recreational, should receive a preparticipation physical prior to initiating a new sport or season.[3] Every state requires some level of PPE for high school athletes and the National Collegiate Athletic Association (NCAA) recommends a PPE at entrance to a program for the college athlete. For the adult athlete (≥20 years of age) participating in recreational sports or fitness activities, the ACSM recently eliminated the recommendation for the need of a PPE. In turn, they developed an algorithm to guide the need for a medical evaluation before initiating physical activity.[4]

■ TIMING AND FREQUENCY

Recommendations regarding the optimal timeline and interval of the PPE are usually guided by consensus due to lack of lack evidence-based support. Six weeks prior to commencement of the sport season is the most frequently quoted timeline to perform a PPE. This allows for adequate time to address any concerns that may come up during the exam and permits for further evaluation, treatment, or rehabilitation of any problem identified that may limit eligibility for sport participation.[1,4]

For high school athletes, the current PPE intervals are based on state or organization requirements. The American Heart Association (AHA) recommends cardiac evaluation every 2 years based on the notion that cardiac changes are detectable at 2-year intervals as the heart matures. At the collegiate level, each department usually determines the PPE frequency policies using NCAA, National Association of Intercollegiate Athletics (NAIA), and National Junior College Athletic Association (NJCAA) recommendations and regulations.[4]

The AAP suggests a PPE evaluation every 2 to 3 years for grade school to high school and recommends a college athlete to have an annual evaluation with a focused history and problem-focused physical exam. Such recommendations are based on physiologic and psychological changes that occur as the athlete matures which require proper monitoring.[4]

■ EXAMINERS

State regulations may dictate who has authority to perform PPEs for public schools, with many states allowing healthcare providers other than physicians to perform evaluations at the high school level (e.g., nurse practitioners and physician assistants).[4] At the collegiate, professional, national, and international competition levels, the governing bodies will determine who may perform the PPE.[3] Providers performing the PPEs should have the knowledge and competence to screen athletes for problems that would affect participation or place an athlete at risk to adequately determine medical eligibility. Ultimately, the team physician should be responsible for the health and well-being of the athlete in collaboration with the healthcare team.[1,4]

■ SETTING

The PPE can be performed using a station or office-based model. The station-based model is best suited for screening of large numbers of individuals simultaneously by implementing multiple dedicated stations for addressing individual aspects of the exam. Parts of the exam (e.g.; vital signs and vision testing with eye charts) may be performed by nonmedical volunteers like team coaches and trainers, but the medical portions of the exam should be performed by a physician or nurse practitioner. Ultimately, the team physician should be the one to evaluate the results of all the components of the exam and make decisions regarding eligibility for participation. This approach is very efficient, can be inexpensive, and allows specialty care at each of the stations. Entire teams or schools can be evaluated in a single session, reducing the administrative burden of scheduling each athlete privately. However, there are significant disadvantages to the station-based approach including: continuity of care (e.g., access to previous medical records), coordination of care may be difficult for issues requiring follow-up, there is less privacy and time for anticipatory guidance, and the athlete may be less likely to discuss sensitive issues. Finally, athletes who previously have been disqualified from sports participation may attempt to take advantage of unfamiliar clinicians and use the station-based format as a second chance to get cleared.[3]

Another strategy commonly employed is the office-based PPE. The advantages of this strategy include improved continuity of care, access to medical records, time for anticipatory guidance, and ease of arranging follow-up diagnostic tests and treatment. A single provider is less likely to overlook known medical problems or family risk factors that would predispose the athlete to unnecessary risks. The primary disadvantages are the time burden and cost of an office visit in addition to the possible limited availability of appointments before the start of sports seasons.[4,5]

PPE COMPONENTS

History

A thorough history is critical to identify athletes with underlying medical conditions that may interfere with participation in sports. The history alone may uncover 88% of medical conditions and 67% of musculoskeletal problems. Ideally, a parent or guardian should be present to provide historical details for athletes younger than 18 years of age. All athletes undergoing a PPE should be questioned using the AHA's recommended inquiries about exertional symptoms, the presence of a heart murmur, signs of Marfan's syndrome, and a family history of premature serious cardiac conditions or sudden death. Other inquiries that need to be explored include a history or symptoms compatible with spinal and brachial plexus injuries, concussion, hematologic disorders, loss of paired organs, asthma or exercise-induced bronchospasm, neurologic disorders, heat illness, and musculoskeletal injuries.[1]

Other important components to review are: sports participation history, use of medications and supplements, menstrual history for female athletes, immunization status, dietary status, and health-risk behaviors.[2]

Physical Exam

The physical examination component should be performed by a skilled clinician and should emphasize an evaluation of vital signs, height, weight, BMI, dermatologic, pulmonary, cardiovascular, neurological, and orthopedic abnormalities that would help identify athletes at high risk of injury, disability, or death.[2] Routine genital examination is not recommended for female athletes, but may be indicated in symptomatic males or if a history of genitourinary problems is present. In addition, standardized orthopedic screening is not sufficient for athletes with known orthopedic injuries, for which a thorough joint-specific examination is recommended.

Diagnostic Test

Laboratory and imaging studies should be used as an extension of the history and physical examination when additional information is needed to evaluate a concern. Screening blood and urine tests are not recommended for asymptomatic athletes.

Significant controversy surrounds the use of screening echocardiography and/ or electrocardiography to detect occult congenital heart disease. A thorough history and physical examination based on the AHA screening recommendations remains the cornerstone of the cardiac preparticipation screening. It is important to recognize that further testing and referral should be considered for any athlete who has a personal or family history of sudden cardiac death or premature coronary disease, symptoms of syncope, unexplained dyspnea, chest pain, heart murmur, hypertension, or abnormalities suggestive of Marfan's syndrome or coarctation of the aorta. A routine ECG/EKG is recommended for master athletes as part of their PPE as atherosclerotic coronary disease is common in this population. Echocardiography and exercise stress testing are not suggested for routine screening.

No evidence-based guidelines exist as to the requirements for assessment of a previous head injury during the PPE. Baseline cognitive assessment such as the sport concussion assessment tool (SCAT) as well as baseline neuropsychological testing have been recommended for athletes who participate in high-risk sports (e.g., soccer, ice hokey, and football). However, neurocognitive testing (NCT) has poor specificity for concussion, and the utility of postinjury NCT in an athlete who does not have a baseline study is controversial.[5]

■ CLEARANCE FOR SPORTS PARTICIPATION

Fewer than 2% of PPEs result in disqualification of the athlete from sport and 3.1% to 13.9% of athletes subsequently require further evaluation before final clearance status is determined. Although disqualification from sport is rare, many medical conditions require adaptation or close monitoring for complications related to sports participation (e.g., bleeding disorders, asthma, concussion, epilepsy, and athletes with disabilities). Certain medical conditions may be incompatible with particular static or dynamic demands or with the risks associated with contact or collision sports.

Actions that may be taken include clearance to participate under one of four conditions: unconditional clearance (cleared for all sports and all levels of participation),

Table 7.1 Contraindications for Sports Participation

• Acute enlargement of spleen or liver
• Acute febrile illness
• Eating disorder
  • if athlete is not compliant with therapy and follow-up
  • evidence of diminished performance
• History of recent concussion and symptoms of postconcussion syndrome
  • no contact or collision sports until asymptomatic
• Hypertrophic cardiomyopathy
• Long QT syndrome
• Acute Kawasaki disease
• Active myocarditis or pericarditis
• Pulmonary vascular disease with cyanosis
• Hemodynamically significant right-to-left shunt
• Severe pulmonary stenosis (untreated)
• Severe aortic stenosis or regurgitation (untreated)
• Severe mitral stenosis or regurgitation (untreated)
• Vascular Ehlers-Danlos syndrome
• Catecholaminergic polymorphic ventricular tachycardia
• Uncontrolled severe hypertension
• Static resistance activities
	• Suspected coronary artery disease
	• Poorly controlled convulsive disorder
	  • no archery, riflery, swimming, weight lifting or powerlifting, strength training, or sports involving heights
	• Recurrent episodes of burning upper-limb pain or weakness, or episodes of transient quadriplegia
	  • no contact or collision sports
	• Untreated mental illness
	• Identified drug abuse
	• Down Syndrome with normal cervical spine radiographs
	  • no collision sports; no other restrictions
	• Cervical instability but no neurologic signs/symptoms
	  • disqualified from "neckstressing" sports like diving, gymnastics, butterfly stroke, high jumping, soccer, pentathlon, wrestling, judo, mixed martial arts, and other combat sports
	• Hemophilia
	  • restricted from contact or collision sports
	• Sickle cell disease
	  • no high-exertion, contact, or collision sports

Source: Data from Mirabelli M, Devine M, Singh J, Mendoza M. The preparticipation sports evaluation. *Am Fam Physician.* 2015:92(5);371-376. https://www.aafp.org/afp/2015/0901/p371.html.

cleared with recommendation for follow-up (including either evaluation or treatment), not cleared with clearance status to be determined after further evaluation, treatment, or rehabilitation, and not cleared in any sport or level of competition (see Table 7.1).[1,4]

ATHLETES WITH DISABILITIES

Athletes with a disability, either physical or cognitive, represent a population with a growing interest in physical activity and competition. The PPE preferably is performed by a healthcare professional who has been previously involved in the care of the patient and has access to the patient's full medical record. The medical history should contain additional questions to address the athlete's particular impairment. More emphasis is placed on the ocular, cardiovascular, musculoskeletal, neurological, and dermatologic systems during the physical exam. A qualified individual should inspect all prosthetic devices, orthoses, and assistive devices to determine adequate fit, proper use during sport-specific tasks, and assure they meet competition regulations. Deciding clearance for sports participation will take into consideration the athlete's medical condition, functional abilities, and the demands and safety of the sport.[4]

SUMMARY

The primary goal of the PPE is to timely identify a medical condition that could endanger the health and/or safety of an athlete. Based on expert opinion, the PPE is best performed at least 6 weeks prior to initiation of the competitive season. The medical history and physical exam of athletes with or without a disability follow the same guidelines and must be thorough. For the athlete with a disability, it is essential to evaluate any assistive device or special equipment being used. Clearance for sports participation will take into consideration the athlete's current health status and whether he or she will be able to safely tolerate the demands of the sport. Overall, more research is required to determine the efficacy of the PPE on preventing morbidity and mortality and to provide a standardized, evidenced-based methodology when performing the evaluation.

References

1. Mirabelli M, Devine M, Singh J, Mendoza M. The preparticipation sports evaluation. *Am Fam Physician.* 2015;92(5);371-376. https://www.aafp.org/afp/2015/0901/p371.html.

2. Hoffman S, Macri E. The preparticipation physical evaluation. In: Brukner P, Khan K, eds. *Clinical Sports Medicine.* 4th ed. Sydney, NSW, Australia: McGraw-Hill Education; 2011:1176-1181.

3. Sanders B, Blackburn T, Boucher B. Preparticipation screening—the sports physical therapy perspective. *Int J Sports Phys Ther.* 2013;8(2);180-192. https://www.ncbi.nlm.nih.gov/pmc/articles/PMC3625797.

4. Bernhardt D, Roberts W, eds. *Preparticipation Physical Evaluation.* 5th ed. Elk Grove Village, IL: American Academy of Pediatrics; 2019.

5. Peterson A, Bernhardt D. The preparticipation sports evaluation. *Pediatr Rev.* 2011;32(5):53-65. doi:10.1542/pir.32-5-e53.

8. ADAPTIVE SPORTS

Nadia N. Zaman

■ INTRODUCTION

The importance of physical activity and sports for health benefits has continually been shown for both able-bodied and disabled individuals; however, 56% of people with disabilities do not participate in sports.[1] With the advent and immense growth of the Paralympic Games, adaptive sports have become a platform for promoting health and wellness among those with disabilities. It has also led to studies on sports physiology, as well as injury and illness epidemiology, in athletes with disabilities to expand our understanding of how to keep them actively engaged.

■ HISTORY

The first official Paralympic Games were held in Rome, Italy in 1960 and was a multisport event involving athletes with a range of disabilities; there were approximately 400 athletes from 23 countries. Prior to this, a select number of athletes with specific physical disabilities competed in the Olympic Games amongst their able-bodied peers. Since its creation, however, it has grown into one of the largest international sporting events by the early 21st century, with over 4,000 athletes from 159 countries having competed in 22 different sports at the 2016 Rio Games, most of which was also broadcast on television worldwide.[1] The Paralympic Games have rapidly become a showcase of athleticism and skill in disabled athletes from around the globe. The rise of the Paralympic movement has led to the development of adaptive sports, defined by any modification that is made to a sport or recreational activity to accommodate an individual with a disability. The International Paralympic Committee (IPC) oversees and coordinates world and national championship competitions in nine of these sports (see Box 8.1).

In addition to this, local availability of adaptive sports across the United States has led to more than 60,000 individuals with disabilities having engaged in sports programs or activities in 2017.[2] At the community level, more than 30 different sports have been adapted to allow for the participation of athletes with disabilities through such organizations as Disabled Sports USA (see Box 8.2).[3]

Box 8.1 Sports Overseen by IPC
Paralympic athletics (track & field)
Paralympic swimming
Paralympic shooting
Paralympic powerlifting
Para-alpine skiing
Paralympic biathlon
Paralympic cross-country skiing
Ice sledge hockey
Wheelchair DanceSport

IPC, International Paralympic Committee.

Source: Adapted from Dehghansai N, Lemiz S, Wattie N, Baker J. A systematic review of influences on development of athletes with disabilities. *Adapt Phys Activ Q.* 2017;34:72-90. doi:10.1123/APAQ.2016-0030.

Box 8.2 Sports Adapted for Those With Disabilities		
Archery	Rafting	Surfing
Basketball	Rock Climbing	Swimming
Boccia	Running	Tai Chi
Canoeing	Sailing	Tennis
Cross-Country Skiing	Scuba	Triathlon
Curling	Skateboarding	Volleyball
Fishing	Sled Hockey	Waterskiing
Golf	Snowboarding	Wheelchair Racing
Hand Cycling	Snowshoeing	Yoga
Hiking	Strength Training	

Source: Adapted from Disabled Sports USA. *Annual 2017 Impact Report.* Rockville, MD: Disabled Sports USA; 2017.

■ EQUIPMENT

Wheelchairs[4]

Some aspects of wheelchair design are universal across sports, such as the fit of the wheelchair to the user to allow for efficiency; keeping the wheelchair lightweight while maintaining appropriate posture for play; and minimizing rolling resistance to allow for rapid acceleration and deceleration when necessary. In addition to the design of the wheelchair itself, the way an athlete is fitted for proper seating and propulsion also plays a large role in how well the athlete can perform. As the need for easy maneuverability and quick starts and stops increases for a sport, such as basketball, camber can be increased, and additional casters added for stability. These wheelchairs are still streamlined and kept lightweight to allow for movement. On the contrary, a rugby wheelchair is designed for high speeds, as well as a high level of impact, thus is larger and bulkier in comparison. Additionally, these wheelchairs often have added bumpers and hooks to obstruct opponents' paths to impede their progress.

Power wheelchairs are not often used in competitive team-based adaptive sports, though power wheelchair soccer has become a worldwide phenomenon. Life-sustaining medical devices like ventilators and tube-feedings can be attached to the wheelchair during play.

Handcycles have been adapted for use by athletes with disabilities to compete in racing sports. There are four major types of handcycles available, with the recumbent and kneeling types being the most commonly used in organized sports (see Table 8.1).

Table 8.1 Handcycle Designs

Arm-crank add-on	Attaches to an athlete's manual wheelchair
Upright arm-crank	Cycle designed with athlete sitting like he or she would in their regular manual wheelchair
Kneeling	Athlete sits in kneeling position with trunk upright or forward leaning above cranks
Recumbent	Athlete lies on back with cranks above chest

Prosthetics[5]

The availability of streamlined prosthetic limbs has allowed for the participation in sports for those with limb deficiencies. Sport-based prosthetics can be specifically designed and modified for the individualized needs of the athlete. Important aspects of design include the weight of the prosthetic limb itself, the allowance for volume change that may occur at the socket and the liner used (often elastomeric gel to reduce sheer stress). A number of different upper and lower limb prosthetic choices are available for a wide range of limb deficiencies to allow more opportunities to engage in a large number of sports. With the continued improvement in the way prosthetics are designed, however, there have been controversies regarding whether their energy-storing capacities and microprocessor advancements give the athlete a competitive advantage.

It is important to note that some athletes may choose to participate in sports without a prosthesis, and some sports do not require the use of a prosthesis in order to compete. Swimming, for one, can be performed without the need of a prosthetic limb, though swimming prosthetics are available for those who would like one. Additionally, the IPC actually requires that prosthetic limbs be removed before competition, and the International Amputee Soccer Association requires those with lower limb deficiencies to remove their prosthesis and use bilateral forearm crutches during play. When a prosthetic limb is removed for the sake of competition, athletes should make sure to protect the residual limb from exposure and injury.

▓ MEDICAL COVERAGE LOGISTICS

As with any other sporting event, a physician covering an adaptive sports event must make preparations before the game begins in order to ensure a safe environment for play including an Emergency Action Plan (EAP). Prior to the game, the provider should introduce himself or herself to both coaches, referees, and other staff including athletic trainers. The provider should also make sure he or she has good rapport with the emergency medical technicians (EMTs) on-site. He or she should make sure all essential equipment is available depending on what kind of impairments are expected; for example, if wheelchair athletes with cervicothoracic injuries are expected, there should be equipment readily available to check vital signs for anyone suspected of having a medical emergency. Please refer to the specific sports chapters for more details regarding medical coverage essentials.

▓ MEDICAL EMERGENCIES

Medical emergencies can occur in both able-bodied and disabled athletes and are often similar for both populations in a large number of sports. Those with functional impairments often have unique medical issues that may arise during play as a result of their impairment or adaptive equipment.

Autonomic dysreflexia (AD): This is a potentially life-threatening condition that occurs in individuals with spinal cord injury level T6 or higher; it is characterized by uncontrolled and uninhibited sympathetic excitation and arterial vasoconstriction causing a sudden and severe increase in blood pressure after exposure to a noxious stimulus.[6] While the most common causes of AD are usually bladder-, bowel- or skin-related issues, for athletes, AD can be triggered due to positioning, equipment, and contact-induced trauma during play. If AD is suspected, the athlete should be removed from the game and sat upright if he or she is supine with loosening of any restrictive gear or clothing. Blood pressure and heart rate should be monitored, and the patient should be transferred to the nearest acute care facility for management, which would include checking for bladder or bowel distention and providing oral or transdermal medications for sustained elevated blood pressures if necessary. *"Boosting"* is the term used when athletes with spinal cord injuries intentionally trigger an episode of AD in order to gain an advantage in physical competition. This is usually generated 1 to 2 hours before competition and done so by allowing the bladder to become distended or by sitting on hard objects to cause discomfort. Because AD can cause mortality, the IPC and World Anti-Doping Agency (WADA) banned the practice of boosting; now, an athlete with systolic blood pressure greater than 180 mmHg is withdrawn from competition if his or her blood pressure does not decrease upon rechecking.[6,7] This policy was made official in 1994 to stave off the unfair advantage, as well as for safety concerns.

Fractures: For those who are nonambulatory, immobility can lead to the development of decreased bone mineral density and osteoporosis over time. It has been reported that the "fracture threshold" for bone loss can be reached within 5 years of injury, which can mean even low-velocity and low-impact injuries can cause fractures in this population.[6] Furthermore, reviews have revealed that athletes with spinal cord injuries, spina bifida, and limb deficiencies had serum levels low in vitamin D, calcium and magnesium, regardless of gender.[2] Thus, athletes should be screened for vitamin D levels and adequately supplemented. Because many of these athletes will be insensate below the level of their injury, a high index of suspicion should remain if this athlete develops edema or erythema shortly after playing. Proper work-up should be performed with splinting for those who can be treated with conservative management, or surgery for those who need more immediate fixation for proper healing.

Thermoregulatory dysfunction: Individuals with spinal cord injuries have a higher risk of heat illnesses because of their impaired autonomic nervous systems. Due to impaired blood flow and inability to perspire in order to dissipate heat, this population of athletes can suffer heat exhaustion and heat stroke, where core temperature of the body can reach more than 104 degrees Fahrenheit. As a result, these individuals will need rapid cooling, oral or IV hydration and emergent transport to an acute care facility once properly cooled.[6]

EPIDEMIOLOGY[8]

As adaptive sports continue to rise, it becomes more and more paramount to understand the unique risks of injuries and illnesses in this specific population of athletes. Much of this research comes from studying the Paralympic movement itself. While this provides great insight into the most common risks overall, it is important to remember that still much information remains to be discovered, including the sport-specific risks that have not yet been well studied. Thus, the IPC's Injury Surveillance System (ISS) was established in 2002 in order to monitor incidence rates and exposure to risk.

COMMON INJURIES

Sports with the highest injury rates include football 5-a-side, goalball, powerlifting, wheelchair fencing, wheelchair rugby, Alpine skiing and ice sledge hockey; sports with the lowest injury rates included sailing, rowing, shooting, Nordic skiing and wheelchair curling.

Wheelchair athletes are prone to the same overuse and sports-based injuries that are common among their able-bodied counterparts. Upper limb injuries were more common than lower limb injuries, likely due to the demands of propelling the wheelchair. Shoulder injuries were the most prominently seen, followed by wrist/hand and then elbow. The knee was the most commonly injured region in the lower limb, followed by foot/ankle.

■ SUMMARY

Adaptive sports provide a safe and effective means of competitive play for those who have functional impairments that would not allow them to play otherwise. Understanding the unique characteristics of this population of athletes is important for providing adequate sideline coverage. Here, the main focus is to emphasize the participants' athletic achievements rather than their disabilities.

■ References

1. U.S. Department of Health and Human Services. *Healthy People 2010: Understanding and Improving Health*. Washington, DC: U.S. Department of Health and Human Services; 2000. https://files.eric.ed.gov/fulltext/ED443794.pdf.

2. Dehghansai N, Lemiz S, Wattie N, Baker J. A systematic review of influences on development of athletes with disabilities. Adapt Phys Activ Q. 2017;34:72-90. doi:10.1123/APAQ.2016-0030.

3. Disabled Sports USA. *Annual 2017 Impact Report*. Rockville, MD: Disabled Sports USA; 2017.

4. Cooper RA, Cooper R, Susmarski A. Wheelchair sports technology and biomechanics. In: De Luigi A, ed. *Adaptive Sports Medicine*. Cham, Switzerland: Springer International Publishing AG; 2018:21-34.

5. De Luigi AJ, Cooper RA. Adaptive sports technology and biomechanics: prosthetics. *PM R*. 2014;6:S40-S57. doi:10.1016/j.pmrj.2014.06.011.

6. Concannon LG, Bhatti OM, Fry AL, Harrast MA. Emergency assessment and care of the athlete. In: Mitra R. eds. *Principles of Rehabilitation Medicine*. New York, NY: McGraw-Hill; 2019:chapter 27. http://accessmedicine.mhmedical.com/content.aspx?bookid=2550&sectionid=206761017.

7. Gee CM, West CR, Krassioukov AV. Boosting in elite athletes with spinal cord injury: a critical review of physiology and testing procedures. *Sports Med*. 2015;45:1133-1142. doi:10.1007/s40279-015-0340-9.

8. Rudolph L, Willick S, Teramoto M, Cushman DM. Adaptive sports injury epidemiology. *Sports Med Arthrosc Rev*. 2019;27(2):e8-e11. doi:10.1097/JSA.0000000000000243.

9. DOPING IN SPORTS

Andrew Beaufort

■ INTRODUCTION

Sports doping is as old as competitive sport itself. This chapter aims to provide the sports medicine clinician with essential knowledge about doping substances, methods, and regulatory protocols across multiple levels of competition. Essential topics included are most recent epidemiology, medical coverage essentials based on level of competition, key doping substances and their level of prohibition including Cannabinoids, and selected doping methods, including gene doping.

■ HISTORY

Earliest accounts of sports doping date back to ancient Greece when athletes were known to consume mushrooms with performance-enhancing properties among other unusual practices.[1] The most important recent development to codify international efforts to maintain the integrity of sport through standards of antidoping occurred in 1999 with the creation of the World Anti-Doping Agency (WADA), an independent antidoping monitoring agency.[2]

■ ANTIDOPING AGENCIES AND ORGANIZATIONS

- International: WADA, UNESCO International Convention against Doping in Sport
- National: United States Anti-Doping Agency (USADA)
- Professional: Most leagues adhere to WADA standards
- College: National Collegiate Athletic Association (NCAA)
- High School: No agency or organization

■ WORLD ANTI-DOPING AGENCY

WADA is an independent, international organization founded by the International Olympic Committee and funded by national governments entrusted with the protection, oversight, and implementation of standardized antidoping programs.[3] The World Anti-Doping Code is the principle document for standardized antidoping programs and contains the Prohibited List among other codified tenets of a comprehensive antidrug policy including education, expected roles of national and individual stakeholders, and compliance measures.[3,4] The Prohibited List is updated annually in January and identifies substances and methods that are (a) prohibited at all times, (b) prohibited during competition, and (c) prohibited in specific sports. For more information regarding the substance's mechanism of action, common indications, risks associated with use, and detection visit the website: www.wada-ama.org/sites/default/files/wada_2020_english _prohibited_list_0.pdf.4 In addition to prohibited substances, WADA regulates methods such as blood manipulation, sample manipulation, and gene and cell doping. For the definition, purpose, common indications, risks associated with use, and detection visit the updated 2020 list (see link just mentioned).[4]

■ KEY BANNED SUBSTANCES

- *Anabolic Androgenic Steroids (AAS)*
  - ○ *Level of WADA Prohibition*: in-and-out of competition
- *Erythropoietin (EPO) and Agents Affecting Erythropoiesis*
  - ○ *Level of WADA Prohibition*: in-and-out of competition
- *Peptide Hormones and Their Releasing Factors*
  - ○ *Level of WADA Prohibition*: in-and-out of competition
- *Growth Hormone and Growth Factors Modulators*
  - ○ *Level of WADA Prohibition*: in-and-out of competition
- *Beta 2 Agonists*
  - ○ *Level of WADA Prohibition*: in-and-out of competition except with therapeutic use exemption (TUE). Exceptions include: inhaled salbutamol: maximum 1,600 micrograms over 24 hours in divided doses not to exceed 800 micrograms over 12 hours starting from any dose; inhaled formoterol: maximum delivered dose of 54 micrograms over 24 hours; inhaled salmeterol: maximum 200 micrograms over 24 hours.
- *Hormone and Metabolic Modulators*
  - ○ *Level of WADA Prohibition*: in-and-out of competition
- *Diuretics and Masking Agents*
  - ○ *Level of WADA Prohibition*: in-and-out of competition. Exceptions with TUE include: Drospirenone; pamabrom; and ophthalmic use of carbonic anhydrase inhibitors (e.g. Dorzolamide, brinzolamide); local administration of felypressin in dental anesthesia
- *Stimulants*
  - ○ *Level of WADA Prohibition*: in-competition
- *Narcotics*
  - ○ *Level of WADA Prohibition*: in-competition
- *Cannabinoids*
  - ○ *Level of WADA Prohibition*: in-competition; except Cannabidiol (CBD)
- *Glucocorticoids when administered by oral, intravenous, or rectal routes*
  - ○ *Level of WADA Prohibition*: in-competition
- *Beta-Blockers*
  - ○ *Level of WADA Prohibition*: in-competition in archery, automobile, billiards, darts, golf, shooting, skiing/snowboarding, underwater sports; and both in-and-out of competition in archery, shooting
- *Caffeine* (*not* in the 2020 list, but in the monitoring program 2019)

° *Level of WADA Prohibition*: Not Banned by WADA; NCAA has set a urinary threshold of 15 micrograms per milliliter, equivalent of 6 to 8 cups of brewed coffee, 2 to 3 hours before an event.

* *Sympathomimetic amines [phenylephrine, phenylpropanolamine, pipradrol,* and *synephrine], nicotine, caffeine, codeine, tramadol, inhaled glucocorticoids,* and *bupropion* among others as currently being monitored by WADA but not prohibited.

▨ KEY BANNED METHODS

* *Manipulation of blood and blood components*

  ° *Level of WADA Prohibition*: in-and-out of competition

* *Chemical and physical manipulation*

  ° *Level of WADA Prohibition*: in-and-out of competition

* *Gene and cell doping*

  ° *Level of WADA Prohibition*: in-and-out of competition

▨ OTHER REGULATING AGENCIES

Professional Coverage: This varies based on collective-bargaining agreements and/or league policies.

NCAA: The current administrator for all drug testing services is the National Center for Drug Free Sport, Inc. (Drug Free Sport).

High School: Currently, there is no governing organization for youth sports at the high school level tasked with implementation and monitoring of antidoping efforts. In 2017, the National Federation of State High School Associations Sports Medicine Advisory Committee (NFHS-SMAC) published a position statement on Appearance and Performance-Enhancing Drugs and Substances for reference.[5]

▨ EPIDEMIOLOGY

At the 2016 Olympic Games, 4,913 samples were analyzed (4,071 urine and 842 blood) among which 18 were reported as adverse analytical findings (AAFs). Among these, continuous erythropoietin receptor activator (CERA) was most frequently reported. At the Rio 2016 Paralympic Games, anti-doping testing was performed on 1,687 samples (1,396 urine and 291 blood). Of those samples, 12 were reported as AAFs;, methadone was the most common substance observed.[6]

Each academic year the student–athlete should sign a drug-testing consent form, in which the student–athlete consents to be tested for substances banned by the NCAA year-round for those in Divisions I and II.[7] Recent data from a cross-sectional survey of NCAA student-athletes (20,474) revealed that 3.1% (N = 399) of those surveyed had used performance-enhancing substances (PESs) within the past year, with nearly 25% reporting use of anabolic steroid use.[8] Rates of concomitant use of other dietary supplements and recreational drugs including amphetamines, tobacco, ephedrine, and (opioid) narcotics were higher in this cohort than among those who did not report PES use within the past year. There was no difference in the rate of reported usage among Divisions I, II, or III.[8] According to the latest NCAA survey, data from 23,000 student–athletes on substance use habits, overall alcohol binge drinking has continued to diminish since 2009 among males, 44% (down from 58% in 2009) and females, 39% (down from 51% in 2009).[9] Marijuana use has also increased among college student–athletes regardless of gender, with higher use occurring in states where the substance had been legalized. Among student–athletes, rates of cocaine use appear to be trending upward since 2009 while narcotic use, ADHD medication misuse, and amphetamine use have diminished.[9]

■ SUMMARY

Understating doping-control protocols, as well as legal and banned substances, is important in providing the best care to athletes by promoting their safety, performance, and fair competition.

■ References

1. Large DC. Everything bad about the Rio Olympics was much worse in ancient Greece. *Foreign Policy*. https://foreignpolicy.com/2016/08/03/everything-bad-about-rio-olympics-worse-ancient-greece-doping-cheating-zika. Published August 3, 2016.

2. Ljungqvist A. Brief history of anti-doping. *Med Sport Sci*. 2017;62:1-10. doi:10.1159/000460680.

3. World Anti-Doping Agency. World anti-doping code 2015 with 2019 amendments. https://www.wada-ama.org/sites/default/files/resources/files/wada_anti-doping_code_2019_english_final_revised_v1_linked.pdf. Published May 29, 2019.

4. World Anti-Doping Agency. Prohibited list January 2020. https://www.wada-ama.org/sites/default/files/wada_2020_english_prohibited_list_0.pdf. Published October 1, 2019.

5. National Federation of State High School Associations Sports Medicine Advisory Committee. Position statement on appearance and performance enhancing drugs and substances. https://www.nfhs.org/media/1018447/nfhs_position_statement_apeds_april_2017.pdf. Published July 31, 2017.

6. Pereira HMG, Sardela VF, Padilha MC, et al. Doping control analysis at the Rio 2016 Olympic and Paralympic Games. *Drug Test Anal*. 2017;9(11-12):1658-1672. doi:10.1002/dta.2329.

7. National Collegiate Athletic Association. NCAA drug testing program. http://www.ncaa.org/sport-science-institute/ncaa-drug-testing-program.

8. Buckman JF, Farris SG, Yusko DA. A national study of substance use behaviors among NCAA male athletes who use banned performance enhancing substances. *Drug Alcohol Depend*. 2013;131(1-2):50-55. doi:10.1016/j.drugalcdep.2013.04.023.

9. National Collegiate Athletic Association. NCAA National study on substance use habits of college student athletes. http://www.ncaa.org/sites/default/files/2017RES_Substance_Use_Executive_Summary_FINAL_20180611.pdf. Published 2018.

COVERAGE ESSENTIALS FOR CONTACT OR COLLISION SPORTS

SECTION III

COVERAGE ESSENTIALS FOR
CONTACT OR COLLISION SPORTS

10. BASKETBALL

Amie Kim, Andrew Chen, and Kevin Kuo

HISTORY

In the winter of 1891 in Springfield, Massachusetts, Canadian-American physician and physical education professor Dr. James Naismith invented the game of basketball as a means of keeping his students physically active while indoors during the harsh New England snow.[1] Initially played by shooting a soccer ball into an elevated peach basket, the game has since evolved into a sophisticated and technical game that is now one of the world's most popular sports.

GOVERNING ORGANIZATIONS

- International: International Basketball Federation (FIBA)
- National: USA Basketball
- Major professional leagues: National Basketball Association (NBA - US), Women's National Basketball Association (WNBA - US), Euroleague, Euroleague Women. Many countries have their own professional leagues.
- College: National Collegiate Athletic Association (NCAA), the National Association of Intercollegiate Athletics (NAIA), the United States Collegiate Athletic Association (USCAA), the National Junior College Athletic Association (NJCAA), and the National Christian College Athletic Association (NCCAA)
- High School: National Federation of State High School Associations (NFHS)

PARTICIPANTS

Basketball was the third most popular high school sport in male and female participation in the 2017 to 2018 season with nearly half a million athletes of both genders representing their schools in competition.[2] There are over 35,000 men and women who play competitive college basketball in the United States each year.[3] Approximately 450 and 150 athletes play professionally in the NBA and WNBA, respectively, each year.[4,5] Many people play recreational basketball across the nation and worldwide.

RULES AND REGULATIONS

Five players from two opposing teams are on the court at any given time. Players can advance the ball by dribbling, passing the ball to a teammate, or shooting the ball at the opponent's basket. Game time varies. U.S. high school games typically play four, 8-minute quarters. College men's games employ two, 20-minute halves. The NBA uses 12-minute quarters, whereas FIBA, Women's college games, and WNBA use 10-minute quarters.[6-10]

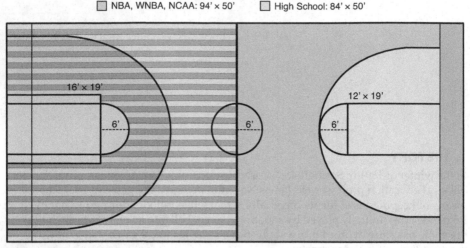

☐ NBA, WNBA, NCAA: 94' × 50'   ☐ High School: 84' × 50'

Figure 10.1 Court dimensions.

NBA, National Basketball Association; NCAA, National Collegiate Athletic Association; WNBA, Women's National Basketball Association.

>>> **Adaptive Sport Key Points: Wheelchair Basketball**

Wheelchair basketball retains the majority of the same rules as standard basketball with the exceptions of the use of modified wheelchairs by all players and variations in the definitions of dribbling and traveling. This version of the game is regulated by the International Wheelchair Basketball Federation (IWBF). Players are given a number depending on their functional ability and the five players on the court for a team should not surpass a total of 14.[11]

■ EQUIPMENT

The **basket** is 18″ in diameter and 10′ high. The regulation **backboard** is 72″ by 42″ (Figure 10.1). The men's **ball** is 29.5″ in circumference and the women's **ball** is 28.5″ in circumference. **Shoes** are commonly high-tops. The use of a **mouth guard** or **eye protection** is optional.

■ MEDICAL COVERAGE LOGISTICS

The role of the on-site physician leader is to organize and coordinate the medical staff, develop an emergency action plan (EAP), and interact with both coaches, referees, and other staff to help ensure the safety of the competitors and spectators. Prior to the basketball game, it is necessary to determine the available medical personnel and medical equipment. The physician should be familiar with the basketball gym or arena (its name and address) and where the emergency exits and Automated External Defibrillators (AEDs) are located. The most direct route for Emergency Medical Services (EMS) to access the court should be determined. Make note of the nearest hospital, preferably a trauma center with both orthopedic and neurosurgical physicians on call at all times. The medical equipment should be set up next to the home team bench near a door to the court for fast and easy access should a player require immediate medical attention. If an emergency occurs during the game, the physician cannot go out onto the court until the play has stopped and he or she is told to do so by the referee. Lastly, documentation is essential for review after the event to evaluate utilization and plan for future events.

MEDICAL EMERGENCIES AND MEDICAL BAG ESSENTIALS

The collapsed or unconscious athlete is considered a medical emergency and the established protocol must be activated including basic life support (BLS)/advanced cardiac life support (ACLS). Nontraumatic emergencies can include anaphylaxis, asthma, heat-related illness, specifically heat stroke, cardiac arrhythmias, and hypertrophic cardiomyopathy. Musculoskeletal injuries that may become medical emergencies include facial, upper, and lower limb fractures or dislocations with neurovascular compromise, traumatic brain injuries with or without spinal cord involvement, and blunt thoracoabdominal trauma with possible internal bleeding.

Medical Bag Essentials in Basketball	
Medical Emergencies:	**Wound Care:**
AED	Normal saline
14-and 16-gauge needles	Betadine swabs
Epi 1:1,000	Neosporin, mupirocin ointment
Diphenhydramine or another antihistamine	Moleskin
Albuterol inhaler	Elastic bandage
Head and Spine:	Tube stretch gauze
Concussion evaluation form	Sterile gauzes
Stretcher & Spine board	Vaseline
Cervical orthosis	Steri-strips
Save a tooth kit	Suture tray
	Lidocaine 1%
Fractures and Dislocations:	Skin stapler
Immobilizers and Slings	
Crutches	

EPIDEMIOLOGY

Although it has origins as a noncontact sport, basketball has become an increasingly physical game in which contact is expected and accepted. Injury rates among high school players in the 2017 to 2018 season were 1.77 per 1,000 athlete exposures in males and 2.21 per 1,000 athlete exposures in females.[12] Among NCAA male basketball players, a 15-year study saw injury rates of 9.9 per 1,000 athlete-game exposures and 4.3 per 1,000 athlete-practice exposures.[13] Sixty percent of all injuries were lower limb, with the ankle ligaments the most common injury and knee derangement the most common injury associated with a greater than 10-day absence from athletic participation. Relative to their younger counterparts, NBA players play at an older age, on a larger court, in longer games, more frequently per week, and for longer seasons. A 17-year survey saw an injury incidence in the NBA of 19.1 per 1,000 athlete exposures accounting for 59,179 games missed during this period. Nonbony injuries to the ankles, knees, and lumbar back were most frequently reported.[14]

COMMON INJURIES

Head and Spine Injuries

Head and spine injuries include concussion and lumbar spine injury. **Concussion** is the most common head injury in basketball.[15] Symptoms can include dizziness, blurry vision, headache, nausea, difficulty concentrating, or loss of consciousness. On-court evaluation includes a focused neurological and cervical spine assessment. More detailed locker room evaluation can incorporate standardized tools such as the Sport Concussion

Assessment Tool (SCAT). "Grading" is not the priority. Athletes suspected of concussion should not return to play on the day of injury. Graded return to activity with expedited follow-up is emphasized. Second Impact Syndrome is a rare and controversial entity, when a concussed athlete returns to play and suffers a second head injury associated with fatal brain edema.[16] *Low back pain* is a common complaint among athletes, and most causes are more benign *muscular strains, ligament sprains, and soft tissue contusions*. Bony *spondylolysis and spondylolisthesis* are common. Evaluate the athlete for red flag signs of spinal cord involvement. General management includes cold and heat compresses, non-steroidal anti-inflammatory drugs (NSAIDs), muscle relaxants, and physical therapy modalities. Opioids and glucocorticoids should be avoided. They are strictly banned by the World Anti-Doping Association and of questionable benefit. *Dental avulsion* of adult teeth requires immediate replant. Handle tooth by its crown to avoid injuring living structures on the root, gently rinse with saline, and replace into socket. Splint tooth to adjacent teeth using the metal insert from a nonrebreather respiratory mask and either apply derma-bond or if available 2-octyl cyanoacrylate (2-OCA) from the dental kit to secure. If replant is not possible, store the tooth in Hank's solution or milk.

Upper Limb Injuries

Upper limb injuries are relatively rare in basketball. Injury rates range from 1.9% to 2.7% of all injuries among high school athletes to 3.7% among NBA players.[12,14,17] These injuries are typically *glenohumeral sprains, acromioclavicular sprains,* and *shoulder contusions*. They often occur as a result of illegal activity (opponent foul) or via collision with another player. *Anterior shoulder dislocation*, although rare, is worth mention for sideline management. Anterior dislocations make up approximately 95% of all shoulder dislocations.[18] They can be caused by falling on an outstretched hand, but more frequently when there is trauma to the arm while it is extended, externally rotated, and abducted as a basketball player would do when attempting to block a shot. The player with this injury will present with a slightly abducted and externally rotated shoulder and will resist active or passive movement. A sensorimotor exam is needed to identify compromise to the axillary nerve or artery. Prompt closed reduction of the joint is recommended. Prereduction x-rays of the shoulder are not always necessary as in the second and third decade of life; less than 1% of patients with shoulder dislocations have concomitant fracture.[19] *Proximal interphalangeal (PIP) joint dislocations* occur with direct trauma or an axial-load "jam" to the finger. Dorsal dislocations are the most common and associated with hyperextension injuries. Concomitant volar plate disruption is a concern. Lateral dislocations cause injury to the lateral collateral ligaments. Volar dislocations are rare, and concomitant central slip (extensor tendon) injury is a concern. Dorsal dislocations are amenable to immediate closed reduction with axial traction to pull joint into alignment. Volar dislocation reduction requires both axial traction and gradual rotation with the wrist in slight flexion in order to avoid buttonhole entanglement of the middle phalanx lateral condyle with the collateral ligaments. After closed reduction, the finger must be immobilized to prevent delayed swan-neck (dorsal dislocation) or Boutonniere's deformity (volar dislocation).[20] A "jammed finger" typically occurs from forced lateral deviation of and subsequent injury to *radial or ulnar collateral ligaments* at the distal interphalangeal (DIP), PIP, or metacarpophalangeal (MCP) joints. Examination reveals tenderness at the joint and possible laxity on valgus and varus joint testing. Initial management is buddy tape immobilization. Advanced imaging and consultation to hand surgery is often considered for concomitant injury such as associated volar plate rupture, extensor tendon injuries, or radial ligament of index finger which is functionally significant for pincer grip. *Jersey finger* typically occurs when a finger is entangled on opponent's jersey or the basket netting, causing forced extension of the DIP joint and avulsion injury of the flexor digitorum profundus tendon. Examination reveals tenderness along the volar DIP and inability to actively flex the DIP joint. Radiographs may reveal associated volar avulsion fragment at distal phalanx. Management is typically operative. Immediately immobilize DIP joint into slight flexion with a dorsal blocking splint followed by hand surgery evaluation.[21] *Mallet finger* typically occurs from a direct axial load onto finger tip causing forced flexion of the DIP joint with rupture of the terminal extensor tendon. Examination reveals tenderness along the dorsal DIP joint, slight flexion at rest, and inability to actively extend the DIP joint. Radiographs may reveal associated dorsal avulsion fragment at the distal phalanx. Management is typically nonoperative. Immediately immobilize DIP joint into continuous and full extension for a minimum of 6 weeks.[21]

Lower Limb Injuries

Lower limb injuries are common. **Quadriceps contusion** is a common soft tissue injury in basketball caused by blunt trauma with another player. Initial symptoms include pain and swelling at the site of contact with delayed ecchymosis at 24 to 36 hours of injury. Immediate immobilization into 120° of knee flexion is recommended to gently increase quadriceps tension, limit intramuscular hematoma, and decrease myositis ossificans development. This is followed by continued ROM exercises and gradual advancement of activity. Return to play once quadriceps strength is equal to contralateral side.[22] **Anterior cruciate ligament (ACL)** injuries typically occur during noncontact planting and cutting, straight knee landing, or one-step stop landing with knee hyperextended.[23] Athletes will typically feel a "pop" followed by pain and rapid swelling around the knee. Examination reveals tenderness, large effusion, and a positive Lachman's and pivot shift test. MRI is the gold standard in preoperative planning and evaluating concomitant injuries, such as the "unhappy triad" (ACL, medial collateral ligament [MCL], and meniscus injury) of acute knee injury. Sideline management includes ice, hinged knee brace, and crutches for supported weight bearing. Surgical treatment is recommended in high-level athletes. **Meniscus injury** typically occurs on a flexed knee with cutting or pivoting, causing excess stress to the medial or lateral meniscus. Athletes can endorse lateralizing knee pain and mechanical symptoms such as knee "locking" or "catching." Examination reveals joint line tenderness, possible effusion, positive provocative tests such as Thessaly, McMurray, and Apley test. MRI is the most sensitive imaging modality; however, it carries the risk of false positives. Sideline management includes NSAIDs, ice, and rest. Depending on the severity of symptoms and classification of injury, competitive young athletes should be evaluated for surgical meniscal repair or resection. **Patellar tendinopathy** has a high incidence in basketball from overuse. Treatment for patellar tendinopathy begins with eccentric loading exercises. Additional management shows variable evidence and includes hyaluronan, platelet rich plasma (PRP), extracorporeal shock wave therapy, and arthroscopic surgery if conservative management fails. Patella strapping is a common treatment option although without strong evidence. **Ankle sprain** is the most common injury in athletes with lateral far more common than medial ligament sprains.[14] Players will typically report "ankle rolling" over another player or awkward landing. This creates a plantarflexion and inversion position where the mortise is at its most unstable. The most commonly injured ligament is the anterior talofibular ligament, followed by the calcaneofibular ligament and posterior talofibular ligament. **High ankle injuries** are more worrisome for associated syndesmotic injury and widening. Examination reveals ankle swelling, positive anterior drawer and talar tilt test. High ankle is discerned from low ankle sprains through Hopkin's squeeze test, Kleiger's test, and palpation of the syndesmosis. Radiographs may reveal concomitant avulsion fracture or joint space widening. MRI is the gold standard for grading ligament injury, although most low ankle sprains are nonoperative. Sideline management includes ice, elastic wrapping, early mobilization, and strengthening. The use of lace-up ankle braces and proprioception and balance-training programs are considered protective for repeat ankle injuries.[24,25] *Achilles tendinopathy* is tendon degeneration due to repetitive and excessive stress, such as explosive push-off and vertical jump. Athletes will typically endorse a recent increase in exercise load, with an insidious onset of stiffness and burning pain at the tendinous insertion point at the posterior calcaneus. Diagnosis is primarily clinical. Lateral ankle radiographs can reveal associated calcaneal spur or calcification patterns, and ultrasonography provides detailed evaluation. Management is typically nonoperative, and sideline management includes activity modification, NSAIDs, heel supports such as a heel lift or taping, and physical therapy.[26] *Achilles tendon rupture* occurs when the ankle undergoes sudden and forced, eccentric plantarflexion with acceleration such as when pushing off the foot. Athletes can report a painful "pop" at their posterior ankle. Examination reveals tenderness along the tendon with a possible palpable defect, gait difficulty, a positive Thompson test. Ultrasonography can distinguish grade of rupture, and MRI is the gold standard in preoperative planning. Sideline management includes NSAIDs, ice, rest, and ankle immobilization with short leg posterior splint. Complete rupture is typically surgically repaired. *Stress fracture* occurs from repetitive load to bone. Low risk stress fractures include the *posterior tibia, fibula, second and third metatarsal shafts*, and typically resolve with activity modification and unloading. High risk stress fractures seen in basketball include *fifth metatarsal base and shaft, medial malleolus, navicular,* and *anterior tibia*. These mandate particular attention due to prolonged healing times and higher likelihood of nonunion. Sideline management includes high index of suspicion, immediate immobilization, and nonweight-bearing restrictions. Tenuous vascular supply or high load location portends prolonged healing times, higher likelihood of nonunion, and possible surgical fixation.[27]

Blisters of the foot and ankle are common and difficult to treat. If not properly managed, they can become infected and lead to cellulitis. *Staphylococcus aureus* is a common bacterium in athletic facilities that cause skin infection. The key to managing blisters is to keep them clean and covered. Prevention is priority, by reducing friction and improving player comfort. This includes properly fitted shoes, cushioned socks with polypropylene, or applying a lubricant stick product to the area of high friction.[14]

SUMMARY

Basketball is an internationally popular sport that has evolved into an intensely physical game. Injuries from high contact as well as overuse occur at a high frequency requiring sideline physicians to prepare the knowledge and equipment for the injured basketball player.

References

1. Where basketball was invented: the history of basketball. https://springfield.edu/where-basketball-was-invented-the-birthplace-of-basketball.

2. National Federation of State High School Associations. High school sports participation increases for 29th consecutive year. https://www.nfhs.org/articles/high-school-sports-participation-increases-for-29th-consecutive-year. Published September 11, 2018.

3. Irick E. Student-athlete participation 1981-82–2015-16: NCAA® Sports Sponsorship and Participation Rates Report. http://www.ncaapublications.com/productdownloads/PR1516.pdf. Published October 3, 2016. Updated November 10, 2016.

4. NBA frequently asked questions. https://www.nba.com/news/faq.

5. Frequently asked questions: WNBA. https://www.wnba.com/faq.

6. Basketball. https://www.nfhs.org/activities-sports/basketball.

7. Men's basketball rules of the game. http://www.ncaa.org/playing-rules/mens-basketball-rules-game.

8. 2019-20 NBA rulebook. https://official.nba.com/rulebook.

9. 2018 official basketball rules: basketball rules and basketball equipment. http://www.fiba.basketball/documents/official-basketball-rules.pdf. Published January 5, 2019. Updated March 14, 2019.

10. Official rules of the Women's National Basketball Association 2018. https://ak-static.cms.nba.com/wp-content/uploads/sites/27/2018/06/2018-Rule-Book-FINAL.pdf. Published March 9, 2018. Updated March 14, 2019.

11. Wheelchair basketball. https://www.paralympic.org/wheelchair-basketball.

12. Comstock RD, Pierpoint LA, Arakkal A, Bihl J. National High School sports-related injury surveillance study: 2017-18 school year. http://www.ucdenver.edu/academics/colleges/PublicHealth/research/ResearchProjects/piper/projects/RIO/Documents/2017-18%20Convenience%20Sample.pdf. Published October 4, 2018.

13. Dick R, Hertel J, Agel J, et al. Descriptive epidemiology of collegiate men's basketball injuries: National Collegiate Athletic Association Injury Surveillance System, 1988-1989 through 2003-2004. *J Athl Train.* 2007;42(2):194-201. https://www.ncbi.nlm.nih.gov/pmc/articles/PMC1941286.

14. Drakos MC, Domb B, Starkey C, et al. Injury in the National Basketball Association: a 17-year overview. *Sports Health.* 2010;2(4):284-290. doi:10.1177/1941738109357303.

15. Daneshvar DH, Nowinski CJ, McKee AC, Cantu RC. The epidemiology of sport-related concussion. *Clin Sports Med.* 2011;30(1):1-17, vii. doi:10.1016/j.csm.2010.08.006.

16. Bey T, Ostick B. Second impact syndrome. *Western J Emerg Med.* 2009;10(1):6-10. https://www.ncbi.nlm.nih.gov/pmc/articles/PMC2672291.

17. Borowski L, Yard E, Fields S, Comstock RD. The epidemiology of US high school basketball injuries, 2005–2007. *Am J Sports Med.* 2008;36(12):2328-2335. doi:10.1177/0363546508322893.

18. Bass AB, Kortyna R. Shoulder dislocations. *Clin Rev.* 2017;27(1):32-35. https://www.mdedge.com/clinicianreviews/article/126527/orthopedics/shoulder-dislocations.

19. Orloski J, Eskin B, Allegra P, Allegra JR. Do all patients with shoulder dislocations need prereduction x-rays? *Am J Emerg Med.* 2011;29(6):609-612. doi:10.1016/j.ajem.2010.01.005.

20. Carruthers KH, Skie M, Jain M. Jam injuries of the finger: diagnosis and management of injuries to the interphalangeal joints across multiple sports and levels of experience. *Sports Health.* 2016;8(5):469-478. doi:10.1177/1941738116658643.

21. Bachoura A, Ferikes AJ, Lubahn JD. A review of mallet finger and jersey finger injuries in the athlete. *Curr Rev Musculoskelet Med.* 2017;10(1):1-9. doi:10.1007/s12178-017-9395-6.

22. Trojian TH, Cracco A, Hall M, et al. Basketball injuries: caring for a basketball team. *Curr Sports Med Rep.* 2013;12(5):321-328. doi:10.1097/01.csmr.0000434055.36042.cd.

23. Caplan N, Kader DF. Knee injury patterns among men and women in collegiate basketball and soccer: NCAA data and review of literature. In: Banaszkiewicz P, Kader D, eds. *Classic Papers in Orthopaedics.* London, UK: Springer; 2013:153-155. doi:10.1007/978-1-4471-5451-8_37.

24. McGuine TA, Brooks A, Hetzel S. The effect of lace-up ankle braces on injury rates in high school basketball players. *Am J Sports Med.* 2011;39(9):1840-1848. doi:10.1177/0363546511406242.

25. Taylor JB, Ford KR, Nguyen A-D, et al. Prevention of lower extremity injuries in basketball: a systematic review and meta-analysis. *Sports Health.* 2015;7(5):392-398. doi:10.1177/1941738115593441.

26. Alfredson H, Cook J. A treatment algorithm for managing Achilles tendinopathy: new treatment options. *Br J Sports Med.* 2007;41(4):211-216. doi:10.1136/bjsm.2007.035543.

27. Mayer SW, Joyner PW, Almekinders LC, Parekh SG. Stress fractures of the foot and ankle in athletes. *Sports Health.* 2014;6(6):481-491. doi:10.1177/1941738113486588.

11. BOXING

Aditya Raghunandan

HISTORY

Historically known as "pugilism," boxing was initially named as the "noble art" and is one of the oldest combat sports across all of human culture. The first evidence of boxing as a sport was discovered in Egypt that dates back to 3000 BCE. It was also a sport in earliest organized events of the ancient Olympic Games in 688 BCE. The first amateur competition took place in 1860, and the Amateur Boxing Association appeared in London in 1880.[1]

GOVERNING ORGANIZATIONS

- International: World Boxing Association (WBA), World Boxing Council (WBC), International Boxing Federation (IBF), World Boxing Organization (WBO)
- National: Association of Boxing Commissions (ABC), USA Boxing
- College: National Collegiate Athletic Association (NCBA) and the United States Intercollegiate Boxing Association (USIBA)

PARTICIPANTS

There has been a gradual rise in the number of athletes who participate in boxing in the United States since 2006. Approximately 6.53 million athletes (aged 6 years and older) participated in boxing in 2017.[2]

RULES AND REGULATIONS

The 10 Point Must System is the standard system of scoring a bout. All bouts are evaluated and scored by three judges. Most rounds end 10 to 9, with the more dominant boxer receiving 10 points, the other receiving 9. If a boxer is knocked down, he or she loses a point. If a boxer is knocked down twice, he or she loses two points. If both fighters are knocked down, the knockdowns cancel each other out. Intentional fouls may result in disqualification, unintentional fouls may result in point deduction. Fighters are judged based on effective aggression, ring generalship, defense, and the use of hard and clean punches. Absolute decisions occur if there is a technical knockout (TKO) or knockout (KO), both of which are determined by the referee on the canvas. If the fight does not end in a KO or TKO, results are determined by the judges' scorecards with four possible decisions: unanimous decision, split decision, majority decision, or draw. Each round is 3 minutes in duration, with a 1 minute rest period between rounds. Based on the specific match, there may be three to five rounds.[3]

EQUIPMENT

Gloves must be constructed under specifications approved USA Boxing guidelines with either a USA Boxing or Association Internationale de Boxe Amateur (AIBA) label in

>>> **Adaptive Sport Key Points: Boxing**

General rules and regulations are similar to able-body boxing, however there are fighter classifications based on level of disability. The classifications are as follows: 1 point player - no lower limb and little or no trunk movement; 2 point player - no lower limb but partial trunk control in forward direction; 3 point player - may have some limb movement and more control of their trunk, limited sideways movement; 4 point player - normal trunk movement but some reduced lower limb function; 4.5 point player - minimal lower limb dysfunction or single below knee amputation.[4]

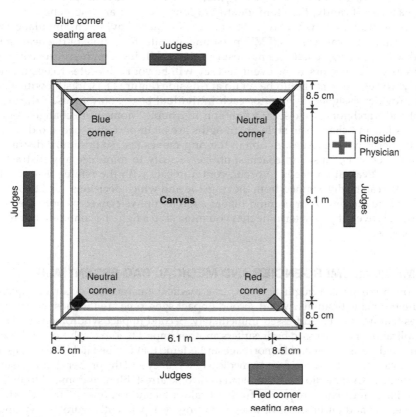

Figure 11.1 Boxing ring dimensions and positions

each glove. Gloves must be worn before entering the ring; tape or another flat binding material may be used to secure the cuff of the gloves. Boxers must wear 10, 12 or 16 oz. gloves based on weight class. *Mouth piece/mouth guard* is required. The round cannot begin without the mouth piece and the referee can pause the play if the mouth piece is dislodged. The mouth piece cannot be red in color. *Headgear* is not allowed in Elite Men competitions; however, it is mandatory for Senior Men's Competitions, Women's Competitions, Youth and Junior Competitions (Men and Women). *Gauzes and hand wraps* must meet USA Boxing specifications and equipment inspectors need to sign off directly on the hand wraps prior to a bout. The use of any substances on the hand-wraps is prohibited. Boxers must wear lightweight *boots or shoes* with socks no higher than knee length. Shorts must not be shorter than midthigh with a clear belt line that does not cover the navel. A *cup protector* must be worn by male boxers, women may wear an optional groin protector. A *breast protector* is optional item for women. A thin coat of pure *petroleum jelly* is allowed only on the face.[3]

▨ MEDICAL COVERAGE LOGISTICS

The medical director must establish an emergency action plan (EAP), define roles, and identify communication lines. On the day of the event, it is important to identify and introduce yourself to the emergency medical and support personnel. Venues can vary significantly; therefore identifying and clearing an emergency exit route is crucial prior to crowd arrival. Most events require having an ambulance with Emergency Medical Services (EMS) personnel on-site. Keep note of the nearest hospital with a trauma center and neurosurgical capabilities. Communicate early with referees and inspectors at the event, as they will be your advocates to ensure boxer safety. The equipment should be set up at ringside (Figure 11.1), ideally with a medical provider assigned to monitor each individual boxer. Stay focused during the fight and watch for cues to see if a fighter is in trouble. Momentum changes, signs of exhaustion and changes in style or strengths are all important aspects to determine if a fighter is having issues. Action in the ring moves fast, so minimize distractions from the crowds, fans, and coaches; utilize security to minimize any distractions. If medical evaluation needs to occur, communicate with the referee. Know which decisions can be determined from the ringside and which decisions need to be made from inside the ring. Bear in mind that as soon as a physician steps onto the apron, the bout is over. If you determine that you must stop a fight, be confident but remain reasonable.

▨ MEDICAL EMERGENCIES AND MEDICAL BAG ESSENTIALS

Although boxing is a pugilistic sport, true medical emergencies occur infrequently.[5] Acute traumatic brain injury and second impact syndrome are the most emergent injuries that need to be addressed immediately. Second impact syndrome is a possible complication if a concussed brain suffers another impact before resolution of the initial injury and leads to cerebral hemorrhage and edema that can be fatal. The collapsed or unconscious athlete is considered a medical emergency and the proper channels should be activated. Commodio cordis can lead to cardiac arrest. Blunt abdominal trauma can cause internal bleeding requiring further evaluation and treatment. Fighters who are knocked out and unconscious or those reporting neck pain with neurologic symptoms from trauma should have the cervical spine immobilized. Nontraumatic deaths are rare due to pre-event screening, but can be due to hypertrophic cardiomyopathy, cardiac arrhythmias, or asthma.

▨ EPIDEMIOLOGY

Boxing is a collision sport with a high incidence of traumatic and nontraumatic injuries. The rate of injuries among amateur and professional boxers ranges from 17 to 24 per 100 bouts. Open wounds or lacerations to the head and face account for 51% to 62% of injuries, 7% to 20% to the hands, wrists, or fingers with a minor number of injuries to the lower extremities.[5–9]

Medical Bag Essentials in Boxing	
Medical Emergencies:	**Fractures and Dislocations:**
AED	Immobilizers and Slings
Cricothyrotomy Kit	Crutches
14- and 16-gauge needles	**Wound Care:**
Nitroglycerin (sublingual)	Normal saline
Aspirin	Betadine swabs
Epi 1:1,000	Neosporin, mupirocin ointment
Diphenhydramine or another antihistamine	Moleskin
Albuterol inhaler	Elastic bandage
Head and Spine:	Tube stretch gauze
Concussion evaluation form	Sterile gauzes
Stretcher & Spine board	Vaseline
Cervical orthosis	Steri-strips
Save a tooth kit	Suture tray
	Lidocaine 1%
	Petroleum jelly

■ COMMON INJURIES

Head and Spine Injuries

Head and spine injuries, especially **concussion,** are commonly seen in boxing at all levels. Mechanism of injury is direct trauma to the head especially after a knockout. Symptoms include confusion, dizziness, headaches, nausea, and in severe cases, loss of consciousness. The fighter should be removed and evaluated in the locker room to rule out a more severe traumatic brain injury. Second impact syndrome is a possible complication if a concussed brain suffers another impact before resolution of the initial injury. Minimum time before returning to sport after a TKO, KO without loss of consciousness (LOC) and KO with LOC is 30 days, 60 days, and 90 days respectively.[6] **Cervical spine injury** can occur after a severe head injury from direct impact to the head and after a fall to the canvas or outside the ring.

Upper Limb Injuries

Upper limb injuries are mostly traumatic. **Hand fractures and contusions** represent the largest portion of injuries to upper limb. The metacarpophalangeal joints or knuckles are highly vulnerable to damage due to the clenched-fist posture along with the enormous forces generated by punching. The commonly referred to **"boxer's knuckles"** represent extensor hood disruption with derangement of the longitudinal central tendon and the transversely oriented sagittal fibers; surgical repair is required to maintain the integrity of the extensor unit and joint function. Traumatic destabilization of the carpometacarpal joint, referred to as **CMC boss**, can cause painfully large and tender bony prominences with or without cyst formation overlying the index and long finger CMC joints; this may eventually require surgical evaluation if not resolved with a conservative approach. The traditionally termed **"boxer's fracture"** involving **fracture of the 4th or 5th metacarpals** is actually not common in professional boxers. In contrast, the more typical **"professional boxer's fracture"** involves **fracture of the 2nd or 3rd metacarpals**; buddy taping and immobilization is the first line of treatment, but surgical correction may be needed in more complex fractures. **Wrist sprains** are also very common due to the indirect impact during repetitive punching. Fighters who learn proper punching technique during training coupled with precise taping, wrapping, and gloving increase shock-absorbing capacity while minimizing injury. **Shoulder injuries** occur as a tired fighter with fatigued rotator cuff muscles tries to throw hard punches to obtain a knockout; the structures around the shoulder can become injured due to sudden changes in direction upon impact of a punch. As a result, **rotator cuff injuries, labral tears, acromioclavicular joint dislocation** and **glenohumeral joint dislocations** can occur as a result. Neurovascular integrity should be confirmed, and the shoulder should be immobilized briefly until further evaluation is pursued.

Lower Limb Injuries

Injuries to the lower limbs are not common in boxing, but those that do occur are due to poor mechanics through the kinetic chain. Some of the common injuries include **thigh contusions, gastrocnemius injuries, tibial injuries,** and **ankle sprains.**[8] All of these can be handled conservatively at the ringside with use of ice and the fighter can usually be returned to the bout as long as he or she is able to demonstrate intact strength and balance.

Other Injuries

Facial and scalp lacerations are important to consider, especially if located in areas that obstructs vision of the fighter; these can render him or her more vulnerable to further injuries. **Oral, ocular,** and **ear/nose/throat traumas** are common; some may be potentially life threatening if the airway is involved. Mandibular fractures, isolated dental avulsions, epistaxis from nasal fractures and blunt trauma to the anterior neck causing laryngeal fractures could all pose a potential airway obstruction. **Blunt chest trauma** can cause **rib fractures** that are extremely painful and infrequently can lead to **splenic lacerations** or **tension pneumothorax. Commodio cordis,** caused by a direct blow to the chest is rare, but has the potential to cause cardiac arrest; this prompts the need for having Automated External Defibrillator (AED) present at all competitions. **Blunt abdominal trauma** causing direct blows to the solid organs have the potential to cause hematomas and insidious blood loss that may not be evident for hours to weeks after a fight. Liver injury is most likely to occur from an unprotected uppercut punch to the right costophrenic region or upper quadrant of the abdomen, whereas splenic injury is likely a consequence of unprotected body punches to the left upper quadrant. If an injury to the liver or spleen is suspected, abdominal CT should be pursued urgently due to potentially large volumes of blood loss into the abdomen. It should be noted that pregnant females are prohibited from fighting due to potential injury to the gravid uterus. **Genital injuries** can occur due to an accidental blow below the waistline. Testicles are usually not injured due to testicular mobility, cremasteric reflex, encapsulation of each testicle in a fibrous cover and use of protective equipment; however, if injured, testicular torsion should be high on the differential and needs to be ruled out with a doppler ultrasound.

■ SUMMARY

The sport of boxing has ancient roots and has gradually evolved to maximize fighter safety. A thorough understanding of the rules and regulations is necessary for the ringside physician to effectively protect boxers and make quick decisions about their continued participation based upon a limited examination.

■ References

1. Pleket HW. Ancient Combat Sports - M. B. Poliakoff: *Combat Sports in the Ancient World: Competition, Violence, and Culture.* Pp. xviii + 202; 97 illustrations. New Haven and London: Yale University Press, 1987. £16.95. *Classical Rev.* 1989;39:107-109. doi:10.1017/S0009840X00270613.

2. Lock S. Number of participants U.S. 2017. *Statista*. https://www.statista.com/statistics/191905/participants-in-boxing-in-the-us-since-2006. Published February 13, 2020.

3. Team USA. USA Boxing® National Rule Book. https://www.teamusa.org/usa-boxing/usa-boxing-national-rule-book. Published November 1, 2017. Updated Novermber 17, 2017.

4. Connors JL, Liadis JG, De Luigi AJ. Adaptive combative sports. In: De Luigi AJ, ed. *Adaptive Sports Medicine: A Clinical Guide 2018*. Cham, Switzerland: Springer International Publishing; 2018:333-342.

5. Loosemore M, Lightfoot J, Palmer-Green D, et al. Boxing injury epidemiology in the Great Britain team: a 5-year surveillance study of medically diagnosed injury incidence and outcome. *Br J Sports Med*. 2015;49:1100-1107. doi:10.1136/bjsports-2015-094755.

6. Neidecker J, Sethi NK, Taylor R, et al. Concussion management in combat sports: consensus statement from the Association of Ringside Physicians. *Br J of Sports Med*. 2019;53:328-333. doi:10.1136/bjsports-2017-098799.

7. Lemme NJ, Ready L, Faria M, et al. Epidemiology of boxing-related upper extremity injuries in the United States. *Phys Sportsmed*. 2018;46:503-508. doi:10.1080/00913847.2018.1516478.

8. Siewe J, Rudat J, Zarghooni K, et al. Injuries in competitive boxing. A prospective study. *Int J Sports Med*. 2015;36:249-253. doi:10.1055/s-0034-1387764.

9. Coletta DF Jr. Nonneurologic emergencies in boxing. *Clin Sports Med*. 2009;28:579-590. doi:10.1016/j.csm.2009.06.001.

12. FIELD HOCKEY

Anita Tewari

▉ HISTORY

While there is evidence of a hockey-like sport being played in ancient Egypt over 4,000 years ago, the modern-day version of the sport was developed in England in the mid-18th century and introduced to the United States in 1901.[1] Today, it is played globally in over 100 countries and remains quite popular, with growing interest in the United States.

▉ GOVERNING ORGANIZATIONS

- International: Fédération Internationale de Hockey/International Federation of Hockey (FIH)
- National: USA Field Hockey
- Professional Leagues: FIH Pro League
- College: National Collegiate Athletic Association (NCAA)
- High School: National Federation of State High School Associations (NFHS)

▉ PARTICIPANTS

In 2018, approximately 1.46 million individuals played field hockey in the United States,[2] including those playing in high school, college, and professional teams. Both men and women participate at all levels.

▉ RULES AND REGULATIONS

Each team may play with up to 11 players, one of which may be a goalkeeper at both the international and NCAA levels. Two umpires ensure the rules are followed. Traditionally the game is played on a rectangular grass or turf field. Field hockey may be played on a hard, indoor surface as well (there are no significant differences in the actual mechanisms of play between the two). The objective of the game is for the offence to move the ball up the field in order to score a goal. A goal can only be scored from within the defensive circle, which is marked on the field. Players may use only the flat side of their stick to play the ball. The ball can be raised only if it is safe to do so (i.e. the ball cannot be raised within 5 m of another player). Additionally, the ball cannot be played off the feet of any player, except the goalkeeper. Penalty corners may be awarded when a defender commits an offence within the circle. The game is played in 15-minute quarters with a 2-minute break between the first and second quarters, and then again between the third and fourth quarters. Halftime is 5 minutes in duration. These rules have been adopted at both the NCAA and IFH level, with the exception that halftime is 10 minutes at the NCAA level. At the high school level, games are played in two 30-minute halves with a 10-minute halftime break. At all levels, teams switch sides of the field after halftime.

Table 12.1 Typical Field Hockey Equipment for Goalkeepers and Players

Equipment Piece	International	NCAA	High School
Mouth Guards	Strongly recommended for players & goalkeepers	Required for players, recommended for goalkeepers	Required for players and goalkeepers
Shin Guards	Recommended (but required for tournaments)	Required	Required
Eye Protection	Optional with medical permission; must be nonprotruding	Optional with medical permission; must be nonprotruding	Required and must meet protection standard
Face Masks/Shields	Allowed only during a penalty corner; must be flat	Allowed only during a penalty corner; must be flat	Not allowed NCAA, National Collegiate Athletic Association.

■ EQUIPMENT

The **stick** has a handle on one end and a curved head on the other, which is flat on its left side. Sticks are traditionally made of a hard wood; however, they can also be combined with various materials including carbon, fiberglass, Kevlar, and graphite. The **ball** is spherical and made of a hard plastic. The ball must be of a color that contrasts with the playing field.[3]

Additionally, goalkeepers at the international level must wear protective equipment comprising of at least **headgear (with a facemask), leg guards and kickers**. Upper body protection is also allowed but not required. At the NCAA level, they must wear the same protection noted for the international level with mandatory **chest and throat protectors**. This protective gear must be worn by goalkeepers at the high school level in addition to mandatory donning of a **helmet with a fixed face mask, a mouth guard, and hand protection** (see Table 12.1).

> **》》 Adaptive Sport Key Points: Field Hockey**
>
> Field hockey for those with a physical disability is a newly evolving version of the sport. Although presently there is limited information on this version of the game, more will become available once it is further developed.[4]

■ MEDICAL COVERAGE LOGISTICS

Medical coverage should be provided on match days from at least 1 hour before the start until 1 hour after the final whistle and on training days from at least 30 minutes before training started until 30 minutes after it ends. The role of the on-site physician leader is to organize and coordinate the medical staff, develop an emergency action plan (EAP), and interact with the support personnel for the match, referees, and coaches to help ensure the safety of the competitors and spectators. Prior to a game or training session, it is important to identify available medical staff, support personnel, venue map, and the available medical equipment. Protocols and guidelines should include role definition of the medical staff, emergency transportation including personnel, routes and adequate facilities with the capacity to evaluate and manage possible injuries, and an outline of the chain-of-command and communication standards. Two equipped ambulances are recommended, in order to have one remaining if the other is needed to transport a player. Lastly, documentation is essential for review after the match to evaluate utilization and plan for future coverage.

■ MEDICAL EMERGENCIES AND MEDICAL BAG ESSENTIALS

Although field hockey is a limited-contact sport, it is important to be cognizant of potential medical emergencies that can result from an injury or the environment of play itself. An athlete who collapses or is unconscious would be considered a medical emergency and would require immediate attention. Nontraumatic emergencies can also result from heat stroke, cardiac problems (arrhythmias, cardiomyopathies), anaphylaxis, and asthma.

Medical Bag Essentials in Field Hockey	
Medical Emergencies: AED Nitroglycerin (sublingual) Aspirin Epi 1:1,000 Diphenhydramine or another antihistamine Albuterol inhaler Rectal thermometer Ice bath **Head and Spine:** Concussion evaluation form Stretcher & Spine board Cervical orthosis Dental emergency kit Eye emergency kit Nasal-packing materials	**Fractures and Dislocations:** Immobilizers and Slings Crutches **Wound/Laceration/Skin Care:** Normal saline Betadine swabs Neosporin, mupirocin ointment Moleskin Elastic bandage Tube stretch gauze Sterile gauzes Vaseline Steri-strips Suture tray Lidocaine 1%

■ EPIDEMIOLOGY

Field hockey is a fast-paced, limited-contact sport whose players wear minimal protective gear. Many injuries result from overuse; however, injuries from contact with a stick, ball, or other player can occur as well. The rate of injuries in high school field hockey players is 1.73 per 1,000 athletic exposures (AE), whereas in collegiate field hockey players the rate is 3.25 per 1,000 AEs.[5,6] Most injuries occur to the lower limbs, particularly the hip/upper leg, knee, and ankle; however, injuries to the head/face and neck are also common.[5] With the introduction of mandatory eye protection in high school field hockey, the incidence of eye injuries has decreased (approximately 90% reduction in the risk of eye injuries).[7,8]

■ COMMON INJURIES

Head and Spine Injuries

Concussions are among the most common injuries sustained to the head and neck region at all levels of play. The most common mechanism of injury resulting in a concussion is contact with another player; however head contact with either a raised ball or stick can also occur. Symptoms typically include confusion, dizziness, headaches, nausea and, in severe cases, loss of consciousness. It is advisable to remove the athlete from play and conduct a neurological exam including a concussion-specific evaluation with a standardized tool like the Sport Concussion Assessment Tool (SCAT) test. If there are no red-flag symptoms, the player may remain on the sideline; however, serial assessments should be conducted. Additionally, the player should follow up with a sports medicine specialist within 24 to 48 hours after the incident. Presently, USA Field Hockey allows the use of soft protective headgear for all field players; however, this is prohibited at the international level. Goalkeepers must wear hard protective helmets with fixed full-face protection.

Upper Limb Injuries

Upper limb injuries commonly occur on the distal aspect of the limb. **Wrist sprains** are a result of repetitive pronation, supination, wrist flexion, and extension when maneuvering the ball since players can use only one side of the stick. Depending upon severity, treatment will differ. Symptoms include pain, swelling, and limited range of motion. Mild sprains can be managed with ice and NSAIDs, with return to play occurring fairly quickly. Moderate sprains may require additional splinting or bracing to provide some degree of immobility and stability. Severe sprains may require surgical evaluation and additional imaging to rule out an occult fracture. **Phalangeal fracture** can occur. Since field hockey is played with the player's right hand positioned lower down on the stick, the fingers are susceptible to injury as the player can come into contact with the ball, which is often traveling at high speeds. Symptoms include pain, swelling, and limited ability (or inability) to flex/extend the digit. Closed fractures of the distal phalanx are typically treated by splinting for 2 to 3 weeks. If the fracture can be properly immobilized and protected, the athlete may be able to return to play, provided the pain is controlled. Open fractures require appropriate cleansing and orthopedic evaluation.

Lower Limb Injuries

Lower limb injuries are usually acute/traumatic in nature. **Thigh contusion** typically results from either direct contact with another player, his or her stick, or the game ball. **Contusions to the quadriceps** are fairly common. Symptoms include localized pain and swelling; more serious injuries can limit flexion of the knee. Treatment involves wrapping the thigh with an ACE bandage, applying ice to the area for 10 to 30 minutes, and stretching. For more severe contusions, crutches may be required to help alleviate pain with weight-bearing. Contusions should be monitored closely for 24 to 48 hours after the injury to ensure the hemorrhaging has stopped. A **muscle rupture** and/or **compartment syndrome** are important, serious conditions that must be thought of if the pain has not stabilized. Using a thigh-sleeve can be helpful with quadriceps stabilization when considering return to play. Typically, **ACL tears** occur as the result of sudden and repetitive deceleration or pivoting motions, whereas in contact sports, the main mechanism is usually direct trauma. Symptoms include feeling a "popping" sensation, pain, rapid swelling, loss of range of motion of the knee, and inability to bear weight on the affected leg. The player should be taken off the field. Ice and NSAIDs should be used to reduce swelling. Further management should include imaging (to explore any concurrent injuries) and surgical evaluation. Partial tears can sometimes be managed nonsurgically; however, surgical intervention is often required if the athlete intends to return to play, which usually occurs 9 to 12 months after the procedure. **Hamstring strains** can be seen due to trauma to the muscle belly, or sudden overloading of the muscle during an eccentric contraction. Symptoms include localized pain with possible swelling and bruising. Treatment includes adequate rest, ice, and stretching, followed by a strengthening program with return to play occurring when the patient is asymptomatic. **Ankle sprains** result from an inversion injury. Symptoms include pain, localized swelling, bruising, and limitations in ROM. Depending upon severity, treatment can include rest, ice, compression, elevation, and NSAID use. Crutches can be used to avoid weight-bearing. More severe injuries may require imaging, to rule out any associated occult fractures, and surgical evaluation. Return to play will depend upon severity of the injury.

Facial Lacerations and Contusions

Facial lacerations and contusions are relatively common (0.12–0.13 per 1,000 AEs), most often as the result of contact between the player's face and an elevated ball. Applying ice to the area of injury to reduce swelling and using NSAIDs to control pain are initial steps. Players can return to play if the swelling does not interfere with vision. Lacerations may require sutures to achieve hemostasis in addition to ice and NSAIDs. Whether or not an athlete can return to play after sustaining a facial laceration will depend upon the size, location, and severity of the injury. Facemasks, although allowed, are not commonly worn by field hockey players. **Corneal abrasions, eyelid lacerations,** and **orbital fractures** can occur, although less commonly. The typical mechanism of injury is contact between the eye and a raised ball. Localized pain and swelling can be seen with associated bruising and/or bleeding. While minor abrasions and lacerations can be taken care of on the sidelines, orbital fractures typically require ophthalmologic evaluation, and often athletes do not return to play until complete healing has occurred.

■ SUMMARY

Field hockey, although a sport with limited contact, is fast-paced and played with minimal protective equipment. Thus, it is important to be aware of the potential injuries that can occur when providing sideline medical coverage.

■ References

1. Maloney C. *Field Hockey: Understanding the Game.* CreateSpace Independent Publishing; 2013. Updated 2018.

2. Lock S. Participants in field hockey in the U.S. from 2006 to 2018. https://www.statista.com/statis tics/191655/participants-in-field-hockey-in-the-us-since-2006. Published February 12, 2020.

3. Maloney C. 2019 rule comparison table. http://www.teamusa.org/-/media/USA_Field_Hockey/2019 -Documents/Rules-Comparisons-Table-2019.pdf. Published May 22, 2019.

4. International Hockey Federation. Rules of para-hockey for athletes with an intellectual disability (ID). http://www.fih.ch/media/12236188/para-id-rules-2016.pdf. Updated June 30, 2016.

5. Lynall RC, Gardner EC, Paolucci J, et al. The first decade of web-based sports injury surveillance: descriptive epidemiology of injuries in US High School Girls' Field Hockey (2008-2009 through 2013-2014) and National Collegiate Athletic Association Women's Field Hockey (2004-2005 through 2013-2014). *J Athl Train.* 2018;53(10):938-949. doi:10.4085/1062-6050-173-17.

6. Barboza SD, Joseph C, Nauta J, et al. Injuries in field hockey players: a systematic review. *Sports Med.* 2018;48:849-866. doi:10.1007/s40279-017-0839-3.

7. Gardner EC. Head, face, and eye injuries in collegiate women's field hockey. *Am J Sports Med.* 2015;43(8):2027-2034. doi:10.1177/0363546515588175.

8. Kriz PK, Zurakowski D, Almquist JL, et al. Eye protection and risk of eye injuries in high school field hockey. *Pediatrics.* 2015;136(3):521-527. doi:10.1542/peds.2015-0216.

13. FOOTBALL

Priya B. Patel and Gerardo Miranda-Comas

HISTORY

Football emerged in the United States in the 1860s and 1870s as a direct consequence of the increasing importance of physical training and sport. Initially inspired by rugby in Great Britain, it soon rose to prominence and became America's "favorite pastime."[1]

GOVERNING ORGANIZATIONS

- International: International Federation of American Football (IFAF)
- National: USA Football and National Football League (NFL)
- College: National Collegiate Athletic Association (NCAA)
- High School: National Federation of State High School Associations (NFHS)

PARTICIPANTS

Approximately 1.8 million athletes participate in American football in the United States.[2] These include athletes ranging from high school to professional level. In addition, there are more than 3 million participants in youth football leagues.[3]

RULES AND REGULATIONS

General rules are very similar throughout the different levels of play and leagues. At the collegiate and professional level, the total game time is 60 minutes split into four quarters of 15 minutes each and a break after the 2nd quarter (break time can vary). There are two 11-person teams that are in play. The offense has four downs to advance the ball at least 10 yards and if they are successful, they earn a first down, at which time they continue to try to advance another 10 yards toward the end zone or attempt a field goal. If they are unsuccessful, the ball is turned over to the other team to have a chance as the offense. Generally, a team scores by either making a touchdown or a field goal.

EQUIPMENT

The National Operating Committee on Standards for Athletic Equipment (NOCSAE) has specific requirements for the helmet. It should be fit one to two finger-breadths above eyebrows and the chin strap can be secured as a four-point or two-point system. The face mask provides easy visibility and others offer additional protection from facial injuries. As extra eye protection, some may also wear nontinted plexiglass shields. Tinted shields may be allowed with physician approval. Custom-made mouth guards are mandatory in college and high school. Shoulder pads vary with position, flat pads worn by those that need greater glenohumeral motion and cantilever pads for those who need more protection due to greater contact. Lower limb pads are used to protect against direct contact to the thighs.[3]

Adaptive Sport Key Points: Wheelchair Football

Each team consists of six players and must include one female and one quadriplegic participant. The field measures 60 yards by 22 yards with 8 yards at each end zone. Games are split into two halves with each half consisting of 20 minutes. Halftime is 10 minutes. Play ends when the player holding the ball is tackled (a touch with one hand above the waist which includes the arm and hand).[4]

▪ MEDICAL COVERAGE LOGISTICS

The role of the on-site physician leader is to organize and coordinate the medical staff, develop an emergency action plan (EAP), and interact with the coaches and officials to help ensure the safety of the players and spectators. Prior to the game, it is important to identify available medical staff, support personnel, field map, and the available medical equipment. Sports medicine physicians and Emergency Medical Services (EMS) personnel, along with sports medicine fellows, residents, medical students, athletic trainers, or physical therapists can attend expected medical needs. Establishing an EAP is the most important task. Protocols and guidelines should include role definition of the medical staff, emergency transportation including personnel, routes and adequate facilities with the capacity to evaluate and manage possible injuries, and an outline of the chain-of-command and communication standards. Contingency plans should be made for extreme temperature, humidity, and other weather conditions that may lead to game cancellation or postponement, or in game modifications like extra water breaks, especially at the youth level. Lastly, prior to the start of the competition, the medical team should confirm that players are wearing proper equipment. During the game the medial team and equipment is set up on the home team's sideline. The referee will notify the head medical provider if an injured player needs to be evaluated on the field. Communication between individual members of the medical staff, coaches, referees, emergency medical staff, and local medical facilities is essential via two or more systems (e.g., hand-held radios and cell phones). Lastly, documentation is essential for review after the game/season to evaluate utilization and plan for future coverage.

▪ MEDICAL EMERGENCIES AND MEDICAL BAG ESSENTIALS

Medical Bag Essentials in Football

Medical Emergencies:

Automated external defibrillator (AED)
Tourniquet
Cricothyrotomy kit
14- and 16-gauge needles
Epi 1:1000
Diphenhydramine or another antihistamine
Albuterol inhaler
Rectal thermometer
Ice bath

Head and Spine:

Concussion evaluation form
Stretcher & Spine board
Cervical orthosis
Save a tooth kit
Protective equipment removal tools

Fractures and Dislocations:

Immobilizers and Slings
Crutches

Wound Care:

Normal saline
Betadine swabs
Neosporin, mupirocin ointment
Moleskin
Elastic bandage
Tube stretch gauze
Sterile gauzes
Vaseline
Steri-strips
Suture tray
Lidocaine 1%

The collapsed or unconscious athlete is considered a medical emergency that requires activation of the proper channels of communication and protocols including basic life support (BLS)/advanced cardiac life support (ACLS). Although rarely reported, non-traumatic emergencies can include cardiac conditions like arrhythmias and hypertrophic cardiomyopathy (HCM), anaphylaxis, asthma, and heat-related illness, specifically heat stroke. Musculoskeletal injuries that may become medical emergencies include, upper and lower limb fractures or dislocations with neurovascular compromise, traumatic brain injuries with or without spinal cord involvement, and blunt thoracoabdominal trauma with possible internal bleeding.

EPIDEMIOLOGY

Football is a high velocity collision sport with a high incidence of traumatic and non-traumatic injuries. The rate of injuries in high school football players ranges from 3.2 to 8.1 per 1000 athlete exposures, and the rate of injuries in college players ranges from 3.1 to 11.1 per 1000 athlete exposures.[2] The lower limbs are the most commonly injured body area, specifically the knee followed by the ankle. Injuries to the shoulders and head/neck are also common.[2,3]

COMMON INJURIES

Head and Spine Injuries

Head and spine injuries, especially **concussion,** are commonly seen in football at all levels. Mechanism of injury includes direct trauma to the head or due to an acceleration/deceleration force of the head due to trauma at another part of the body. Symptoms include confusion, dizziness, headaches, nausea and, in severe cases, loss of consciousness. Remove the player from play and conduct a neurological exam including a Sport Concussion Assessment Tool (SCAT) test.[5] If no red flags are observed, then the player may remain on the sideline without his equipment. Periodic assessment should follow until cleared to leave with a parent if under age. He will need to follow up with a sports medicine provider in 24 to 48 hours for further assessment. Second impact syndrome is a possible complication if a concussed brain suffers another impact before resolution of the initial injury. **Cervical spine injury** was more commonly seen prior to new rules and regulations against tackling head first. Players who are found to be unconscious on the field or those reporting neck pain with neurologic symptoms from trauma during play should have the cervical spine immobilized. The recommended technique to transfer the injured player with a suspected cervical spine injury is the lift-and-slide technique which requires eight individuals: one at the head, three on each side and one controlling the spinal board. The other technique is the log roll and requires at least four providers: one controlling the head, two the body, and one the spinal board.[6] Protective athletic equipment should be removed *prior* to transport to an emergency facility for an athlete–patient with suspected cervical spine instability. Equipment removal should be performed by at least three trained and experienced rescuers. If fewer than three people are present, the equipment should be removed at the earliest possible time after enough trained individuals arrive on the scene.[6] They should be transported to the ED for further evaluation.

Upper Limb Injuries

Upper limb injuries include traumatic and overuse injuries. Common shoulder injuries include labral tears, bony injuries, and neurologic injuries. **Labral tears** commonly include a tear in the superior portion of the labrum and extend anterior to posterior also known as "SLAP" tears. Mechanism of injury is due to repetitive injuries to the glenohumeral joint due to blocking or tackling. Symptoms include pain and weakness in the shoulder joint. Management includes removal from play; depending on the severity of injury, physical therapy and bracing may be used as well as surgery in some cases. **Bony injuries** include those to the glenoid labrum, known as a Bankart lesion, and to the humeral head, known as a Hills-Sachs lesion, often associated with glenohumeral joint (GHJ) dislocations and may require surgical management. **Brachial plexus neurapraxia,** also known as "stingers" or "burners," are due to a traction or compression of the brachial plexus. The mechanism of injury is usually the lateral flexion of the neck. Symptoms include unilateral burning pain, numbness or tingling down the arm, and weakness as well. These symptoms usually resolve quickly (minutes) and players can usually return to play after a thorough exam of the upper limb including range of motion and strength. Players with symptoms that do not resolve need further neurological testing to rule out cervical root avulsion. **Acromioclavicular (AC) joint** injuries are commonly seen in football and vary from sprain to tears of the ligaments around the AC joint. The mechanism of injury can be due to direct trauma to the lateral shoulder or falling on that point of the shoulder after a tackle. Symptoms include tenderness over the AC joint and you may feel a gap with displacement of the acromion from the clavicle. Players should be removed from play and obtain an x-ray of the shoulder. Depending on the severity of the injury, most will heal with conservative measures; however, some may require surgical intervention. **Mallet finger** is a flexion injury of the distal interphalangeal (DIP) joint. Mechanism of injury is due to trauma to the extensor tendon. Symptoms include difficulty to fully extend the DIP joint. Management includes obtaining x-rays to rule out a fracture and placing the DIP joint in mild hyperextension in splint for 6 weeks. **Jersey finger** is an avulsion injury of the flexor digitorum profundus. Mechanism of injury is due to extension of a flexed finger, usually when a player tries to grab a player for a tackle. Symptoms include inability to flex the DIP joint. Management includes surgical repair.

Lower Limb Injuries

The lower limbs are the most commonly injured body area in football. **Thigh contusion** is a common soft tissue injury in football. Mechanism of injury is usually blunt trauma. Symptoms include pain and swelling at the site. Ice and nonsteroidal anti-inflammatory medications (NSAIDs) are initially used. Players can return to play once strength is equal to the unaffected side. **Hip pointer** is a contusion of the iliac crest. Mechanism of injury is blunt trauma to the area. Symptoms include pain and inability to range the hip. Patient should be removed from play and immediately start icing area of pain. **Medial collateral ligament (MCL)** injury is the most common knee injury in football. Mechanism of action is a valgus load to the knee by direct trauma usually through tackling. Symptoms vary by grades of injury (Grades I–III), with Grade II as a partial ligament injury and Grade III as a full ligament tear. Valgus laxity testing at the knee will reveal if there is laxity with or without an end point. Management includes conservative treatment (rest, ice, NSAIDs). Some players may wear protective bracing. MCL injuries may occur concomitantly with **Anterior cruciate ligament (ACL)** and/or **medial meniscus tears** as part of the "unhappy triad." ACL tears can occur secondary to a direct valgus load, or without contact during a single leg landing from a jump, or during a cutting move while the foot is planted. An acute knee injury with immediate swelling after one of the mechanisms of injury mentioned, correlates with an ACL tear. The player cannot continue playing during the game and will need further imaging, MRI is the gold standard and possible surgical intervention. **Hamstring strain** is commonly seen due to noncontact sudden muscle contraction. Symptoms include tenderness over the area and players may have edema and ecchymosis as well. Management includes rest and return to play when patient is asymptomatic. *Lisfranc fracture* is commonly seen as a running injury. Mechanism of injury is due to twisting of the foot when a player is falling. Symptoms include pain and inability to ambulate on the affected foot. Player should be removed from play, sent to ED to obtain an x-ray. Management includes open reduction internal fixation (ORIF) surgery. *Turf toe* is an injury to the first metatarsophalangeal (MTP) joint. Mechanism of injury is due to trauma causing dorsiflexion of the planted toe. Symptoms include pain and swelling at the area and painful ambulation as a result. Management includes rigid shoe insert, donut padding, rest, and ice. Players can return to play when they are pain free.

■ SUMMARY

Football is a popular high-velocity contact sport that can be played at all levels. Understanding the game, positions, and most common injuries is essential for sideline coverage.

■ References

1. Collins T. Unexceptional exceptionalism: The origins of American football in a transnational context. *J Glob Hist*. 2013;8(2):209-230. doi:10.1017/S1740022813000193.

2. Shah S, Luftman JP, Vigil DV. Football: Sideline management of injuries. *Curr Sports Med Rep*. 2004;3(3):146-153. doi:10.1007/s11932-004-0062-5.

3. Rizzone K, Diamond A, Gregory A. Sideline coverage of youth football. *Curr Sports Med Rep*. 2013;12(3): 143-149. doi:10.1249/JSR.0b013e3182955d1c.

4. Wheelchair Sports Federation. Football. Updated December 11, 2009. http://wheelchairsportsfederation .org/adaptive-sports/football

5. McCrory P, Meeuwisse W, Dvorak J, et al. Consensus statement on concussion in sport—the 5th International Conference on Concussion in Sport held in Berlin, October 2016. *Br J Sports Med*. 2017;13(2):53-65. doi:10.1136/bjsports-2017-097699.

6. National Athletic Trainers' Association. Appropriate care of the spine injured athlete. Updated from 1998 document. Prof Rep. 2015. https://www.nata.org/blog/toddc/update-appropriate-care-spine-injured-athlete

14. HANDBALL

Roxanna M. Amill-Cintrón

▨ HISTORY

The origins of handball can be traced back to medieval times. Handball was first played in the late 19th century in Denmark. It was part of the Summer Olympics program in 1936. Men's handball was first played at the 1936 Summer Olympics in Berlin as outdoor handball, and in 1972 Summer Olympics in Munich as indoors. Women's team handball was added at the 1976 Summer Olympics in Montreal. Variations include Mini handball, Beach handball and recently wheelchair handball.

▨ GOVERNING ORGANIZATIONS

- International: International Handball Federation (IHF) - created in 1946
- National Members of the IHF include: African Handball Confederation (CAHB), Asian Handball Federation (AHF), European Handball Federation (EHF), North America and the Caribbean Handball Confederation (NACHC), Oceania Continent Handball Federation (OCHF), and South and Central America Handball Confederation (SCAHC).

▨ PARTICIPANTS

According to the IHF, currently there are about 27 million players and 128,000 teams worldwide.[1]

▨ RULES AND REGULATIONS

Playing court: 40 m by 20 m (131 ft by 66 ft), with a goal (2 m high and 3 m wide) in the center of each end. The goals are surrounded by a near-semicircular area, called the "zone" or the "crease," defined by a line 6 m from the goal. A dashed near-semicircular line 9 m from the goal marks the free-throw line. A middle line divides the court in 2 halves. A standard match has two 30-minute halves with a 10- to 15-minute halftime break. For youths, the length of the halves is reduced: 25 minutes at ages 12 to 15, and 20 minutes at ages 8 to 11. National federations of some countries may differ in their implementation from the official guidelines. Two teams of seven players (six field players and one goalkeeper) take the field and attempt to score points by putting the game ball into the opposing team's goal. The team that scores more goals wins. In case there is a tie, there are maximum two over-times, each consisting of a 5-minute period with a 1-minute break. Should these not decide the game, then a penalty shootout (best of 5 rounds) will determine the winning team. A handball player must follow certain rules while handling the ball. Outfield players can touch the ball with any part of their body that is above the knee. After receiving the ball, the players may pass, keep possession, or shoot the ball. If a player holds possession of the ball, the player can dribble or take up to three steps for up to 3 seconds at a time without dribbling. Only the goalkeeper can have possession of the ball inside the goal area (crease or zone).[2]

EQUIPMENT

The *ball* is spherical, made of leather or a synthetic material. Its official size varies depending on age and gender. The ball is intended to be operated by a single hand. No protective equipment is mandated, but players may use *mouth guards, pads,* and *soft protective bands*.

⟫⟩ Adaptive Sport Key Points: Wheelchair Handball

Created in 2005, wheelchair handball can be played in different ways. The most common is played by two teams of five players and one goalkeeper each. The other version substitutes the goalkeeper for a bouncing pyramid/wall or shooting wall. Matches will be played with two halves 20-minutes each, and a 10-minute half-time break. The court is the same although adaptations may be made. The goal size is adapted to that of Mini Handball. The wheelchairs shall be constructed in a safe and fair way to limit the risk for the player himself, his team colleagues, or the opponent team. Players must be strapped to the wheelchair at the upper and lower legs in order to avoid lifting or moving/using the legs.[3]

MEDICAL COVERAGE LOGISTICS

Medical coverage should be provided on match days from at least 1 hour before throw-off until 1 hour after the final whistle and on training days from at least 30 minutes before training started until 30 minutes after it ends.[5] The role of the on-site physician leader is to organize and coordinate the medical staff, develop an emergency action plan (EAP), and interact with the support personnel for the match, referees, and coaches to help ensure the safety of the competitors and spectators. Prior to a match or training session, it is important to identify available medical staff, support personnel, venue map, and the available medical equipment. The team is usually composed of a sports medicine physician, Emergency Medical Services (EMS), certified athletic trainer, and/or physical therapist. Protocols and guidelines should include role definition of the medical staff, emergency transportation including personnel, routes, and adequate facilities with the capacity to evaluate and manage possible injuries, and an outline of the chain-of-command and communication standards. Two equipped ambulances are recommended, in order to have one remaining if the other is needed to transport a player. Lastly, documentation is essential for review after the match to evaluate utilization and plan for future coverage.

MEDICAL EMERGENCIES AND MEDICAL BAG ESSENTIALS

The medical team leader and staff should be prepared to manage any medical emergency and trained in basic life support or advance life support. An unconscious or collapsed athlete is a medical emergency. Sudden cardiac death is the most common cause of sudden death in athletes. Musculoskeletal injuries that may become medical emergencies include upper and lower limb fractures or dislocations with neurovascular compromise, traumatic brain injuries with or without spinal cord involvement, and blunt thoracoabdominal trauma with possible internal bleeding.

Medical Bag Essentials in Handball	
Medical Emergencies:	**Fractures and Dislocations:**
Automated External Defibrillator (AED)	Immobilizers and Slings
Nitroglycerin (sublingual)	**Crutches Wound/Laceration/**
Aspirin	**Skin Care:**
Epi 1:1,000	Normal saline
Diphenhydramine or another antihistamine	Betadine swabs
Albuterol inhaler	Neosporin, mupirocin ointment
Rectal thermometer	Moleskin
Ice bucket	Elastic bandage
Head and Spine:	Tube stretch gauze
Concussion evaluation form	Sterile gauzes
Stretcher & Spine board	Vaseline
Cervical orthosis	Steri-strips
Dental emergency kit	Suture tray
Eye emergency kit	Lidocaine 1%
Nasal-packing materials	

■ EPIDEMIOLOGY

Handball, also known as "team handball," "field handball," "European handball," or "Olympic handball," is a physical sport with fast tempo, rapid changes in direction, and frequent contact and collisions between players,[6] in addition to overhead throwing. Three typical high-risk situations for injury in handball are throwing, player contact, and landing. The International Olympic Committee (IOC) injury and illness surveillance system rates handball among the Olympic sports with highest injury rates.[7] The most frequent location of injuries has been found to be in the lower limbs.[8] Acute injuries are common in the knee and ankle whereas overuse injuries are most common in the shoulder.[7] Most injuries occur in competition (matches) as compared to training sessions,[9,10] with a greater number of injuries occurring in the offensive phase of the game.[8,10] Sprains and contusions are the predominant injury types.[10,11]

■ COMMON INJURIES

Head and Spine Injuries

Head and spine injuries include **concussion** or **sports-related concussion (SRC)** seen in handball after a direct blow to the head, face, neck, or elsewhere on the body with an impulsive force transmitted to the head. It can present itself with almost no symptoms or may present as complete loss of consciousness in severe cases. Signs and symptoms may include headaches, dizziness, confusion, nausea, vomiting, amnesia, gait instability, irritability, slowed reaction, somnolence, and drowsiness. The affected player must be removed from the game immediately. Sideline evaluation is very important to assess for rapidly changing signs and symptoms. Periodic re-evaluation is important. If symptoms persist, the athlete should be taken out of sports until full recovery of symptoms. A gradual approach of return-to-sports has been recommended. The prevention and recognition of second impact syndrome is crucial to prevent more serious complications, which may be even fatal.[12]

Upper Limb Injuries

Upper-limb injuries in the shoulder and elbow are more often overuse injuries, while the wrist and hand are acute in nature. **Shoulder injuries**, predominantly from overuse, are a common source of shoulder pain in elite handball.[13] Glenohumeral internal rotation deficit (GIRD), excessive glenohumeral external rotation, and the presence of scapular dyskinesis are reported risk factors for shoulder injuries in handball. **Superior labral tear from anterior to posterior (SLAP) lesions, internal impingement**, and **rotator cuff tears** are conditions seen in this sport, due to the nature of overhead throwing. **SLAP tear** is an injury to the glenoid labrum that occurs due to repetitive traction forces on the labrum during abduction-external rotation and the biceps anchor pulling posteriorly (peel-back phenomenon). Symptoms include pain with overhead activities, feeling of catching, locking, popping or grinding in the shoulder, feeling of instability and loss of strength, or significant decrease in throwing velocity. MRI arthrogram is the diagnostic study of choice although new and more sophisticated MRIs have been developed that eliminate the need for contrast. Arthroscopy is the gold standard for diagnosis. There is evidence in the literature to support both surgical and nonsurgical forms of treatment. Most can be treated with rotator cuff and scapular stabilizer programs as well as stretching the posterior capsule with sleeper stretches to correct GIRD. Surgical arthroscopic repair may involve placement of suture anchors on torn labrum and may include biceps tenodesis. It may take 3 to 6 months to return to play. **"Handball elbow"** is a term used to describe a variety of chronic lesions occurring in and around the elbow.[14] Studies have identified two different patterns of elbow injuries in handball players: repeated hyperextension trauma to the extended arm while blocking a ball (typical for goalkeepers) and repeated overhead throwing (typical for field players). Both mechanisms cause similar overuse injuries. Goalkeepers present bilateral elbow injuries while field players complain of injuries mainly in the throwing arm.[14] Spectrum of injuries may include **ulnar or medial collateral ligament (UCL) sprains** or **tears, radiocapitellar overload syndrome** (lateral component of elbow injury due to incompetent UCL), **valgus extension overload syndrome** and **posteromedial olecranon impingement.** These syndromes are caused by repetitive valgus stress on the elbow during the acceleration phase of throwing in field players, and repetitive hyperextension trauma to the extended arm in goalkeepers.[14] This may predispose the athlete to acute (sudden "pop" while throwing) or chronic ligamentous injury. Symptoms include medial elbow pain, worse with throwing. Valgus stress to the elbow at 20 to 30 degrees of flexion may reveal increased laxity and pain compared to nonthrowing arm. X-rays may show bony hypertrophy and calcifications. Diagnosis is confirmed with MRI or diagnostic musculoskeletal (MSK) ultrasound. Most can be treated conservatively, but surgery is needed in cases of complete UCL tears or when partial tears remain symptomatic after a proper rehabilitation program. **Scaphoid fracture** occurs with a fall on the outstretched hand and the wrist in hyperextension with radial deviation and internal rotation. In handball a fracture may also occur from receiving a high-velocity ball in the hand forcing wrist extension or when blocking a shot. Pain in the anatomical snuffbox is the classic physical exam finding. X-rays, including anterior-posterior (AP), oblique, lateral and AP view with ulnar deviation, should be done initially. If negative and highly suspected injury, MRI, CT scan, or bone scan should be done. Treatment is based on injury classification (Herbert, Russe, or Mayo classifications).[15] Surgical versus conservative treatment will be based on location and degree of displacement of the fracture.[16] An acute injury to the thumb often results in **UCL sprain** or **tear** and involves risk of avulsion fracture. It occurs as a result of acute radial or valgus stress on the thumb. Diagnostic imaging may include plain films, MRI or MSK ultrasound. Conservative treatment through immobilization versus surgical repair will depend on extent of injury. **Proximal interphalangeal joint (PIP) sprains** and **dislocations** are common in contact sports that involve catching or hitting a ball, usually caused by hyperextension injury to the PIP. Dorsal dislocations are more common than volar dislocations. Plain radiographs may rule out associated fractures and assess stability. Stable injuries are treated conservatively, usually buddy taping. Unstable injuries are treated with surgery if reduction cannot be obtained by closed means.

Lower Limb Injuries

The lower limbs are the most commonly injured body area. **Anterior cruciate ligament (ACL) injuries** in handball occur mainly during no-contact plant and cutting movement or when landing from a jump and are the most common acute serious injury of the lower limb. Female athletes suffer ACL injuries more often than male counterparts,[17] with a higher incidence at elite level. The athlete may report hearing a "pop" followed by a feeling of instability. Immediate evaluation should include Lachman's anterior drawer or Pivot shift test, although it may be difficult in the acute phase due to pain and swelling. Hemarthrosis and swelling can develop very rapidly (within hours of injury). Radiographs should be done to assess for associated fracture such as tibial spine avulsion, tibial plateau, or Segond fractures. MRI, which is the gold standard, will demonstrate a classic contusion pattern in the anterior lateral femoral condyle and posterior lateral tibial plateau. Initial management (for both partial or complete ACL tears) should include rest, ice, compression, elevation (RICE), knee immobilizer with early gentle ROM exercises, and a proper rehabilitation program. Partial ACL tears can be managed conservatively. Complete ACL tears can be treated conservatively or surgically, depending on age and competitive level of the athlete. ACL injuries may occur concomitant with medial collateral ligament (MCL) and lateral meniscus injury (O'Donoghue unhappy triad). Long-term consequences include the development of knee osteoarthritis. **Lateral ankle sprains** occurred after landing on a single leg. The mechanism of injury involves inversion of a plantar-flexed foot when landing. Usually the anterior talofibular ligament is affected followed by calcaneofibular and posterior talofibular ligament. Signs and symptoms include lateral ankle pain, hearing a "pop" at time of injury, edema, ecchymosis, restricted ROM and, in some cases, weight-bearing difficulty. A positive anterior drawer test and talar tilt test may be evident. Radiographs are needed to assess for associated fractures. Musculoskeletal sonogram may show ligamentous injury and severity of sprain. Treatment is usually conservative. Recurrent sprains and poorly rehabilitated injuries may predispose the athlete to chronic ankle instability.

Orofacial Trauma

Orofacial trauma or direct trauma to the face with the ball or contact with another player may contribute to dental, nose, and/or periorbital injuries, facial lacerations as well as fractures of the jaw and facial bones. The athlete should be evaluated at sideline and the need for further management or treatment determined. If dental injuries are evident, then evaluation by a dentist should be done. Mouth guards have proven effective in preventing dental injuries such as tooth fractures and avulsion.[4]

■ SUMMARY

Handball is a throwing, dynamic, high-velocity contact sport, which is growing in popularity, and therefore is having an increasing trend of injuries. It is important for the medical provider to understand the sport's biomechanics and mechanism of injuries to properly assess and treat each athlete. Even though rules and regulations have been modified to increase player safety, it continues to be a high-risk contact sport.

▨ References

1. 8 things you didn't know about handball. Olympics. IOC. Published June 10, 2016. Archived from the original on 19 July 2018.

2. Rules and regulations IHF official site. https://www.ihf.info/regulations-team-types/355.

3. American Association of Adapted Sports Program. Wheelchair handball. http://www.adaptedsports.org/adaptedsports/members/pdf/WH_Handball_Rule_Book%20(Full%20Page).pdf. Published 2013.

4. Bergman L, Milardović Ortolan S, Žarković D, et al. Prevalence of dental trauma and use of mouthguards in professional handball players. *Dent Traumatol*. 2017;33(3):199-204. doi:10.1111/edt.12323.

5. Grimm K, Popovic N, D'Hooghe P. Medical coverage of major competitions in handball. In: Laver L, Landreau P, Seil R, Popovic N, eds. *Handball Sports Medicine*. Berlin, Germany: Springer; 2018:125-138.

6. Karcher C1, Buchheit M. On-court demands of elite handball, with special reference to playing positions. *Sports Med*. 2014;44(6):797-814. doi:10.1007/s40279-014-0164-z.

7. Aasheim C, Stavenes H, Andersson SH, et al. Prevalence and burden of overuse injuries in elite junior handball. *BMJ Open Sport Exerc Med*. 2018;4:e000391. doi:10.1136/bmjsem-2018-000391.

8. Bere T, Alonso J-M, Wangensteen A, et al. Injury and illness surveillance during the 24th Men's Handball World Championship 2015 in Qatar. *Br J Sports Med*. 2015;49(17):1151-1156. doi:10.1136/bjsports-2015-094972.

9. Giroto N, Hespanhol Junior LC, Gomes MR, Lopes AD. Incidence and risk factors of injuries in Brazilian elite handball players: a prospective cohort study. *Scand J Med Sci Sports*. 2017;27(2):195-202. doi:10.1111/sms.12636.

10. Laver L, Luig P, Achenbach L, et al. Handball injuries: epidemiology and injury characterization: part 2. In: Laver L, Landreau P, Seil R, Popovic N, eds. *Handball Sports Medicine*. Berlin, Germany: Springer; 2018:155-165. doi:10.1007/978-3-662-55892-8_12.

11. Åman M, Forssblad M, Larsén K. National injury prevention measures in team sports should focus on knee, head, and severe upper limb injuries. *Knee Surg Sports Traumatol Arthrosc*. 2019;27(3):1000-1008. doi:10.1007/s00167-018-5225-7.

12. McCrory P, Meeuwisse W, Dvořák J, et al. Consensus statement on concussion in sport—the 5th International Conference on Concussion in Sport held in Berlin, October 2016. *Br J Sports Med*. 2017;51(11):838-847. doi:10.1136/bjsports-2017-097699.

13. Andersson SH, Bahr R, Clarsen B, Myklebust G. Preventing overuse shoulder injuries among throwing athletes: a cluster-randomised controlled trial in 660 elite handball players. *Br J Sports Med*. 2017;51:1073-1080. doi:10.1136/bjsports-2016-096226.

14. Popovic N. Elbow injury in handball: overuse injuries. In: Laver L, Landreau P, Seil R, Popovic N, eds. *Handball Sports Medicine*. Berlin, Germany: Springer; 2018:217-225. doi:10.1007/978-3-662-55892-8_16.

15. Ten Berg PW, Drijkoningen T, Strackee SD, Buijze GA. Classifications of acute scaphoid fractures: a systematic literature review. *J Wrist Surg*. 2016;5(2):152-159. doi:10.1055/s-0036-1571280.

16. Li H, Guo W, Guo S, et al. Surgical versus nonsurgical treatment for scaphoid waist fracture with slight or no displacement: a meta-analysis and systematic review. *Medicine*. 2018;97(48):e13266. doi:10.1097/MD.0000000000013266.

17. Anderson MJ, Browning WM 3rd, Urband CE, et al. A systematic summary of systematic reviews on the topic of the anterior cruciate ligament. *Orthop J Sports Med*. 2016;4(3):2325967116634074. doi:10.1177/2325967116634074.

15. ICE HOCKEY

Lisanne C. Cruz

HISTORY

The contemporary sport of ice hockey was developed in Canada from European and Indigenous influences. In 1896, the first ice hockey league in the United States was formed. Men's ice hockey has been played at the Winter Olympics since 1924 and women's ice hockey was added to the Winter Olympics in 1998.

GOVERNING ORGANIZATIONS

- International: International Ice Hockey Federation (IIHF)
- National: USA Hockey
- Major professional leagues: National Hockey League (NHL), The American Hockey League (TheAHL), National Women's Hockey League (NWHL)
- College: National Collegiate Athletic Association (NCAA)
- High School/Junior League: United States Hockey League

PARTICIPANTS

In the 2019 to 2020 season, there were a total of 561,700 registered ice hockey players in the United States according to USA Hockey[1]; 85% were men and 15% were women. The majority of players were youth and kids (18 and under), making up 68% of players enrolled in hockey.[1]

RULES AND REGULATIONS

The game is played in an ice rink (Figure 15.1). A professional game consists of three periods of 20 minutes with the clock running only when the puck is in play. The teams change ends after each period of play, including overtime. Recreational leagues and children's leagues often play three shorter periods. Each team has about 20 players with six players on the ice at the same time including three forwards (two wingmen and one center), two defensemen, and a goalie. The objective of the game is to use a hockey stick to shoot a puck into the net of the opposing team. Players can reach speeds of 30 miles/hour and pucks can reach speeds of up to 100 miles/hour. The game is fast paced without breaks in play unless there is an icing call, the puck leaves the ice, there is a penalty, or the goalie stops it. The faceoff is used to begin every game, period, and play. It occurs when a referee drops the puck between the sticks of two opposing players.

EQUIPMENT

A **helmet with a strap** is required for all ice hockey players. They are made of a flexible thermoplastic outer shell with foam padding inside. A **face cage** or **visor** is used optionally depending on level of play. **Mouth guards** vary from standard plastic guards to custom-mouldable "boil and bite" compounds. **Neck guards** typically consist of a series

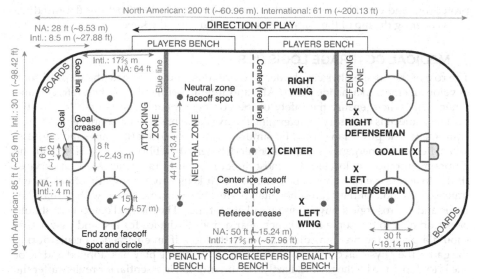

Figure 15.1 Ice rink layout with player positions, zones, and dimensions.
Source: Adapted from Ysangkok. Ice hockey layout [Image file]. Wikimedia Commons. https://com
mons.wikimedia.org/w/index.php?title=File:Ice_hockey_layout.svg&oldid=247510461. Published
June 30, 2006.

of puncture resistance plates, with padding for comfort and a tear-resistant nylon mesh outer covering. Hockey *shoulder pads* are composed of a padded vest with front and back panels and optional upper arm pads. *Elbow pads* cover the elbow joint and part of the upper and lower arm. Players' *gloves* are constructed with a very thin leather palm and fingers, while providing substantially more padding to the outside of the hands. *Lower limb pads* are knee-length oversized shorts, which include thigh, pelvic, hip, and sacral pads. They are often held up by a belt or suspenders. *Shin guards* are attached to knee pads which help protect the knee joint and tibia. The *jock* is a protective cup which is designed to protect the genitals in men. Similarly, *pelvic protectors* or *"jill-straps"* provide a hard shell protecting the female genitalia. *Hockey skates* have a rigid shell reinforced with metal mesh to prevent a skate blade from cutting through. Blades have a rounded heel and no toe picks. *Sticks* are made of wood or composite materials and come in various styles and lengths based on the size of the player. The *hockey puck* is a 3-in diameter, 1-in thick, 6-oz (170 g) vulcanized rubber disk.

Goalie Equipment: The *stick* has a larger blade as well as a wide, flat shaft. The *skates* have a larger blade radius, the boot is closer to the ice, and there is less ankle support. The *helmet* has a wire face mask with a throat protector. A *blocker* is worn on the stick hand and a *catch glove or "trapper"* is worn on the opposite hand. *Chest* and *arm protectors* are thickly padded in the front and incorporate forearm, elbow and biceps

>>> **Adaptive Sport Key Points: Sled (Sledge) Hockey**

Sled hockey is a sit-down version of ice hockey for players whose disability prevents them from skating. Players sit on double-bladed sleds and use two sticks. Each stick has a blade at one end and small picks at the other. Players use the sticks to pass, stickhandle and shoot the puck, and to propel their sleds. The rules are very similar to IIHF ice hockey rules.

protection, and extend down to protect the abdomen. Goalie *"legs"* are flat-faced leg pads covering the top of the skate, the player's shin, and the knees.

▣ MEDICAL COVERAGE LOGISTICS

The role of the on-site physician leader is to organize and coordinate the medical staff, develop an emergency action plan (EAP), and interact with both coaches, referees, and other staff to help ensure the safety of the competitors and spectators. Prior to the hockey game, it is necessary to determine the available medical personnel and medical equipment. The physician should be familiar with the ice rink (its name and address) and where the emergency exits, Automated External Defibrillators (AEDs) and the Zamboni entrance are located. The most direct route for Emergency Medical Services (EMS) to access the rink should be determined, it is usually through the Zamboni entrance. Make note of the nearest hospital, preferably a trauma center with both orthopedic and neurosurgical physicians on call at all times. The medical equipment should be set up next to the home team bench near a door to the ice for fast and easy access should a player require immediate medical attention. If an emergency occurs during the game, the physician cannot go out onto the ice until the play has stopped and he or she is told to do so by the referee. Lastly, documentation is essential for review after the event to evaluate utilization and plan for future events.

▣ MEDICAL EMERGENCIES AND MEDICAL BAG ESSENTIALS

It is important to be prepared for any and all medical emergencies that may arise. The collapsed or unconscious athlete is considered a medical emergency and may be due to concussion, cervical spine injury, asthma, or other underlying medical conditions. Catastrophic cervical spine injuries, although less common due to recent rule changes, are still a major source of severe injury in ice hockey and more common than in most other sports.[2] Arterial laceration from a skate blade is another potential emergency that requires immediate tourniquet proximal to the site of bleeding and pressure should be applied until EMS arrives. Nontraumatic deaths can be due to hypertrophic cardiomyopathy, cardiac arrhythmias, anaphylaxis, and asthma. Other musculoskeletal (MSK) emergencies include joint dislocations with neurovascular compromise and blunt thoracoabdominal trauma.

Medical Bag Essentials in Ice Hockey	
Medical Emergencies:	**Fractures and Dislocations:**
AED	Immobilizers and Slings
Tourniquet	Crutches
Cricothyrotomy kit	**Wound Care:**
14- and 16-gauge needles	Normal saline
Epi 1:1,000	Betadine swabs
Diphenhydramine or another antihistamine	Neosporin, mupirocin ointment
Albuterol inhaler	Moleskin
Head and Spine:	Elastic bandage
Concussion evaluation form	Tube stretch gauze
Stretcher & Spine board	Sterile gauzes
Cervical orthosis	Vaseline
Save a tooth kit	Steri-strips
	Suture tray
	Lidocaine 1%
	Skin stapler

EPIDEMIOLOGY

Hockey is a high-velocity sport with frequent player-on-player collisions as well as potential trauma from the boards, puck, or stick.[3] At all levels, most injuries occur to the head/face and shoulder and can result in concussions, contusions, or ligamentous injuries.[4] Injuries are more common in games than in practice and the rate of injuries increases as the players get older and with the introduction of checking.[4,5] Overall rates of injury are lower in women's hockey where checking is not allowed as compared to similar levels of play in men's hockey.[6,7] The knee is the most common lower limb injured and the shoulder/clavicle is the most commonly injured part of the upper limb.[8]

COMMON INJURIES

Head and Spine Injuries

Head and spine injuries include **concussions** which are defined as a pathophysiologic process affecting the brain and induced by traumatic forces, often an acceleration/deceleration event. Ice hockey has the second highest rate of concussion in the United States, after rugby and ahead of American football.[9] Concussions are the most common head, neck, and face injury in NCAA ice hockey.[10] Concussions occur most frequently in games rather than practice and are most commonly the result of player-on-player contact, often with secondary contact against the boards.[11] Initial assessment of the player with a suspected concussion should include airway, breathing, and circulation (ABCs). Examination of the cervical spine should be performed on all players with a suspected concussion. If deemed stable, the player should be removed from the game and not be allowed to return to play. Further cognitive testing to diagnose concussion in athletes who do not lose consciousness should include a concussion specific assessment using one of the available tools like the Sports Concussion Assessment Tool 5 (SCAT 5). Any sign of deterioration, focal neurological deficits, declining mental status, or pupillary changes should prompt immediate transfer to the emergency room. The player with a concussion will require close follow-up by a physician in order to evaluate symptom resolution and develop a stepwise return to play protocol.[12] **Cervical spine injury**, although uncommon, occurs more frequently in ice hockey as compared to all other sports.[8] Mechanism of injury is typically a hit from behind that pushes the player into the boards with a slightly flexed neck causing an axial load.[13] Players suspected of a cervical spine injury should be immobilized on the ice after assessing ABCs. Transfer to a spine board is done if enough trained personnel is available, using either the log roll maneuver with at least four people or the lift-and-slide technique with at least eight people depending on the athlete's size. The helmet and shoulder pads should be removed if the tools are available and the patient should be transferred to the nearest trauma center.[14] Players should not return to play until they are symptom free without neurological deficit.

Upper Limb Injuries

Upper limb injuries affect mostly the shoulder region. **Glenohumeral joint injuries** include **dislocations** and can result in **superior labrum anterior posterior (SLAP) tears** and/or **Hill-Sachs lesions**. In ice hockey, anterior dislocations commonly occur due to player-on-player contact causing a direct blow to the posterior shoulder or collision with the boards or ice that cause forceful external rotation and abduction of the shoulder. Players with a suspected dislocation can be evaluated immediately on the ice by placing a hand under the shoulder pad and palpating the lateral deltoid for fullness under the coracoid process anteriorly or a soft spot posteriorly.[15] The player should be removed from the game and a gentle reduction technique can be attempted in the locker room. If reduction cannot occur, the patient should be taken to the emergency room for radiographs and reduction under anesthesia. Once reduced, the player should be treated with ice, non-steroidal anti-inflammatory medications (NSAIDs), and a sling, followed by physical therapy. If apprehension persists or the player redislocates the shoulder, surgical stabilization may be required. **Acromioclavicular joint separation** is the most common joint injury in hockey.[15] Type I (no ligamentous tear) and type II (completed acromioclavicular ligament tear and partial coracoclavicular ligament tear) are treated nonoperatively. Type IV (avulsion of the coracoclavicular ligament with posterior displacement into the trapezius), Type V (coracoclavicular distance is >25 mm) and Type VI (clavicle inferiorly displaced behind biceps and brachioradialis tendons) require surgical intervention. Clinical indications for surgery in Type III separations (complete acromioclavicular and coracoclavicular ligament tears) include scapular dyskinesis despite rehabilitation, ongoing pain, or loss of function.[15] **Clavicular fractures** commonly occur in ice hockey from player-on-player contact or a player hitting the boards. They present with pain, guarding of the shoulder and, if displaced, deformity and tenting of the skin. Growth plates remain open in the clavicle until approximately 21 years of age; therefore, they should be treated as growth plate injuries in skeletally immature athletes.[15] Nondisplaced fractures can be treated with immobilization for 6 to 8 weeks with a figure-of-eight bandage or sling. Displaced fractures or fractures with significant shortening should be treated surgically. **Metacarpal fractures** commonly occur from contact with the puck, stick, boards, or due to fighting. Careful examination of the hands is warranted, looking for deformity and palpating for pain and crepitus. Nondisplaced fractures can be treated with splinting for 4 to 6 weeks, while displaced fractures may require surgery.

Lower Limb Injuries

Lower limb injuries are often acute in nature. **Adductor strains** are a common cause of groin pain in hockey players. This muscle group is particularly vulnerable as the adductors must "shift from powerful eccentric contraction to concentric contraction during the forward push off, the recovery phase of the skating stride, and cross-over skating."[16] Athletes with limited hockey-specific training in the off season are at greater risk of adductors strains.[15] They are usually self-limiting with conservative therapy including NSAIDs, avoiding exacerbating factors and appropriate hockey-specific warms-ups and stretching programs. **Femoroacetabular impingement (FAI)** is premature contact of the acetabulum with the femoral neck during range of motion. It is identified radiographically more often in hockey players than other athletes and nonathletes.[17] This is thought to be the result of repetitive loading of the hip while skating which leads to microtrauma and subsequent remodelling of the femoral head. Cam-type FAI is the most common type of impingement seen in hockey players.[18] Symptoms include anterior to posterior hip pain, often described as the "c-sign," as well as decreased range of motion and pain with flexion, adduction, and internal rotation (FADIR test). Diagnosis is confirmed with a radiograph, although an MRI may be helpful to rule out labral or chondral injury as well. If the player fails to improve with conservative management, arthroscopic repair has been shown to have good results in hockey players.[19] **Athletic pubalgia or "sports hernia"** is an injury to the abdominal wall at the fascial attachments of the rectus and adductors onto the pubis symphysis. In ice hockey, the unique "biomechanical demands of skating, shooting and passing may predispose athletes to a sports hernia."[15] Hockey players often complain of vague pain over the groin, although an inciting event can sometimes be described. Symptoms may worsen with coughing, Valsalva maneuver, and core activation. Nonoperative treatment, although not always effective, would include core stabilization exercises, postural training, and re-establishing the dynamic relation between the hip and pelvic muscles.[20] Conversely, surgical treatment has been favored over conservative management in NHL players.[15] *Medial collateral ligament (MCL) injuries* are the most commonly reported knee injury in hockey players.[3] Most MCL injuries occur due to player-on-player contact during a game causing a valgus stress on the knee.[21] Immediate examination of the knee is optimal as delay may limit the ability to notice subtle laxity due to edema, pain, and guarding. Grade I (0–5 mm) and Grade II (5–10 mm) are most often treated conservatively. Grade III (>10 mm) sprains are often treated operatively if they occur in conjunction with an anterior cruciate ligament (ACL) tear or the patient has failed nonoperative treatment. *High ankle sprains* affect the syndesmosis between the tibia and fibula and are the most common type of ankle sprain in hockey players as the rigid skate protects against lateral ankle sprains.[15] Compression of the tibia and fibula at the middle of the leg (squeeze test) often produces pain in a high ankle sprain. Nonoperative treatment includes immobilization with gradual progression to range of motion and strengthening and finally sports-specific exercises. If the player fails conservative treatment, has syndesmotic widening on stress radiographs or gross instability, the player may benefit from a surgical syndesmotic fixation. *Skate bite* is anterior ankle pain resulting from stiff new skates or old skates with an inflexible tongue.[3] With skating, the repeated friction of the tibialis anterior and extensor digitorum longus tendon can lead to tenosynovitis and pain. Manually breaking in the skate or placing a foam liner over the tongue of the skate can mitigate this.

Facial Injuries

Facial injuries *(lacerations, eye, and dental injuries)* commonly occur in ice hockey as a result of contact with the puck or stick.[22] The use of full-face mask helmets and mouth guards have significantly reduced the incidence of eye, dental, and facial injuries.[23] Eye injuries most commonly occur from contact with the hockey stick and can result in *scleral lesions, retina tear* and/or *retinal detachment*. In the case of a suspected eye injury, the player shoulder be removed from the game and be taken to an emergency room with an on-call ophthalmology service. *Facial injuries* should be cleaned and assessed in the locker room and determination should be made if the player requires further intervention. If bleeding can be stopped easily, patient may return to play with an appropriate dressing over the laceration. If bleeding cessation is not possible with pressure alone, consider steri-strips or suturing. If over a hairline or if aesthetics are not of concern, a skin stapler can be used to quickly close a laceration with easily opposed edges. In youth, referral to plastic surgery for suturing should be considered. With *loss of a tooth*, an attempt should be made to obtain the tooth. Pick the tooth up by the crown (never the root), clean it with saline, saliva, milk, or water and reimplant it into the socket if possible (once bleeding is controlled), ideally within 5 minutes of the injury. If reimplantation is not possible, store the tooth in milk, Hanks Balanced Salt Solution (save a tooth kit), or saline and have the player see a dentist immediately.

■ SUMMARY

Ice hockey is a high-velocity contact sport that can be played at all levels and ages. Understanding the game and the most common injuries is essential for rink-side coverage in order to properly assess, treat, and prevent injuries.

■ References

1. USA Hockey. 2019-2020 season final registration reports. https://cdn1.sportngin.com/attachments/document/2210-1687681/2019-20_USAH_Registration_Report_Final.pdf#_ga=2.238904581.464229911.1592880671-1933983345.1592880671. Published May 29, 2020.

2. Zupon AB, Kerr ZY, Dalton SL, et al. The epidemiology of back/neck/spine injuries in National Collegiate Athletic Association men's and women's hockey, 2009/2010 to 2014/2015. *Res Sports Med*. 2018;26(1):13-26. doi:10.1080/15438627.2017.1365295.

3. Laprade RF, Surowiec RK, Sochanska AN, et al. Epidemiology, identification, treatment and return to play of musculoskeletal-based ice hockey injuries. *Br J of Sports Med*. 2014;48:4-10. doi:10.1136/bjsports-2013-093020.

4. Lynall RC, Mihalik JP, Pierpoint LA, et al. The first decade of web-based sports injury surveillance: descriptive epidemiology of injuries in US high school boys' ice hockey (2008-2009 through 2013-2014) and National Collegiate Athletic Association men's and women's ice hockey (2004-2005 through 2013-2014). *J Athl Train*. 2018;53(12):1129-1142. doi:10.4085/1062-6050-176-17.

5. Anderson GR, Melugin HP, Stuart MJ. Epidemiology of injuries in ice hockey. *Sports Health*. 2019;11(6): 514-519. doi:10.1177/1941738119849105.

6. Agel J, Harvey EJ. A 7-year review of men's and women's ice hockey injuries in the NCAA. *Can J Surg*. 2010;53(5):319-323. https://www.ncbi.nlm.nih.gov/pmc/articles/PMC2947117.

7. Melvin PR, Souza S, Mead RN, et al. Epidemiology of upper extremity injuries in NCAA men's and women's ice hockey. *Am J Sports Med*. 2018;46(10):2521-2529. doi:10.1177/0363546518781338.

8. Tuominen M, Stuart MJ, Aubry M, et al. Injuries in World Junior Ice Hockey Championships between 2006 and 2015. *Br J Sports Med*. 2017;51(1):36-43. doi:10.1136/bjsports-2016-095992.

9. Pfsiter T, Pfister K, Hagel B, et al. The incidence of concussion in youth sports: a systematic review and meta-analysis. *Br J Sports Med*. 2016;50(5):292-297. doi:10.1136/bjsports-2015-094978.

10. Simmons MM, Swedler DI, Kerr ZY. Injury surveillance of head, neck and facial injuries in collegiate ice hockey players, 2009-2010 through 2013-2014 academic years. *J Athl Train*. 2017;52(8):776-784. doi:10.4085/1062-6050-52.4.03.

11. Kontos AP, Elbin RJ, Sufrinko A, et al. Incidence of concussion in youth ice hockey players. *Pediatrics*. 2016;137(2):e20151633. doi:10.1542/peds.2015-1633.

12. Harmon KG, Drezner J, Gammons M, et al. American Medical Society for Sports Medicine position statement: concussion in sport. *Clin J Sport Med*. 2013;23(1):1-18. doi:10.1136/bjsports-2012-091941.

13. Tator CH, Provvidenza C, Cassidy JD. Update and overview of spinal injuries in Canadian ice hockey, 1943 to 2011: the continuing need for injury prevention and education. *Clin J Sport Med*. 2016;26(3):232-238. doi:10.1097/JSM.0000000000000232.

14. National Athletic Trainers' Association. *Executive Summary of Appropriate Care of the Spine Injured Athlete Inter-Association Consensus*. St Louis, MO: NATA; 2015.

15. Mosenthal W, Kim M, Holzshu R, et al. Common ice hockey injuries and treatment: a current concepts review. *Curr Sports Med Rep*. 2017;16(5):357-362. doi:10.1249/JSR.0000000000000402.

16. Kuhn AW, Noonan BC, Kelly BT, et al. The hip in ice hockey: a current concepts review. *Arthroscopy*. 2016;32(9):1928-1938. doi:10.1016/j.arthro.2016.04.029.

17. Lerebours F, Robertson W, Neri B, et al. Prevalence of cam-type morphology in elite ice hockey players. *Am J Sports Med*. 2016;44:1024-1030. doi:10.1177/0363546515624671.

18. Ayeni OR, Banga K, Bhandari M, et al. Femoroacetabular impingement in elite ice hockey players. *Knee Surg Sports Traumatol Arthrosc*. 2014;22(4):920-925. doi:10.1007/s00167-013-2598-5.

19. Epstein DM, McHugh M, Yorio M, Neri B. Intra-articular hip injuries in National Hockey League players: a descriptive epidemiological study. *Am J Sports Med*. 2013;41(2):343-348. doi:10.1177/0363546512467612.

20. Larson CM, Pierce BR, Giveans MR. Treatment of athletes with symptomatic intra-articular hip pathology and athletic pubalgia/sports hernia: a case series. *Arthroscopy*. 2011;27(6):768-775. doi:10.1016/j.arthro.2011.01.018.

21. Grant JA, Bedi A, Kurz J, et al. Incidence and injury characteristics of medial ligament injuries in male collegiate ice hockey players. *Sports Health*. 2013;5(3):270-272. doi:10.1177/1941738112473053.

22. Rattai J, Levin L. Oral injuries related to ice hockey in the province of Alberta, Canada: trends over the last 15 years. *Dent Traumatol*. 2018;34(2):107-113. doi:10.1111/edt.12387.

23. Lawrence LA, Svider PF, Raza SN, et al. Hockey-related facial injuries: a population-based analysis. *Laryngoscope*. 2015;125(3):589-593. doi:10.1002/lary.24893.

Juan Galloza-Otero

HISTORY

Judo was created by Jigoro Kano in Japan in 1982. Initially a martial art, it is derived from jiu-jitsu. Judo removed the more dangerous techniques of jiu-jitsu with the intention to create a physical, intellectual and moral educational art. It officially became an Olympic sport in the Tokyo Games in 1964. In the Barcelona Olympic Games in 1992, both men and women were officially part of the tournament. In 1988 judo made its debut in the summer Paralympic Games in Seoul, Korea.

GOVERNING ORGANIZATIONS

- International: International Judo Federation (IJF)
- National: USA Judo
- Regional: PanAmerican Judo Confederation (PJC)
- Major professional leagues (organization): There is no official professional organization.

PARTICIPANTS

Judo is played internationally. Currently the International Judo Federation (IJF) is composed of 204 national federations and 5 continental unions estimating about 20 million participants worldwide.

RULES AND REGULATIONS

Judo fighting is composed of 2 types of techniques, throwing and grappling. The fighter can win by scoring an ippon (1 point) in 4 different ways, throwing an opponent on the back, controlling the opponent on the floor for 20 seconds, and gain a submission by armlock or strangling the opponent. The fighter can also win by scoring 2 waza-ari (1/2 point), which are gained by throwing the opponent on the side or controlling on the floor for 10–19 seconds. A fighter can also be disqualified from a fight if he commits 3 penalties. These are awarded for different reasons, such as stepping out of the mat area, grabbing the legs during a throw, or being passive and not attacking your opponent, among others. Each fight is 4 minutes long. A golden score time is allowed if the score is tied. Figure 1 is an example of a Judo tatami mat. **(A) Table judges:** Two referees, acting as judges, will be seated at the technical table and will be refereeing together with the referee. **(B) Medical Staff:** There should be at least one member of the medical staff next to the table judges constantly observing the match. There may be a team physician/trainer for each judoka or the lead physician covering the event. **(C) Contestants:** Judokas who will engage in the match. **(D) Referee:** The referee shall generally stay within the contest area. He shall conduct the contest and administer the decisions. **(E) Coaches:** A coach for each judoka will be seated opposite to the table judges.

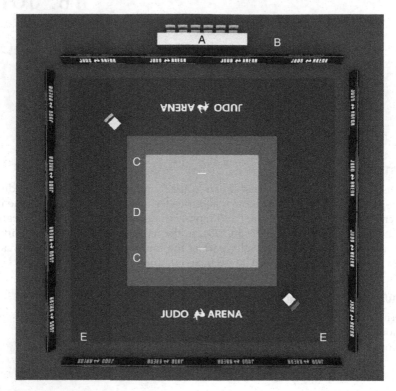

Figure 16.1 Judo tatami
Source: A. Luszczynski/Envato Market

■ EQUIPMENT

The *judogi* is the uniform used during judo competition. It is composed of a jacket, pants and belt. The jacket is made of hard cotton and is an essential part of grip fighting. The color of the jacket and pants may be white or blue to identify each judoka in the score board during a competition. The belt represents the experience level of the judoka and ranges from white (least experienced) to black (most experienced).

>>> **Adaptive Sport Key Points: Paralympic Judo**

Paralympic judo includes only athletes with visual impairment. It follows the same rules as judo, except the judokas start the fight already in a grip position. If the grip position is lost, the fight is stopped and they are placed again in the grip position.

■ MEDICAL COVERAGE LOGISTICS

The medical director must establish an emergency action plan (EAP), define roles, and identify communication lines. On the day of the event, it is important identify and introduce yourself to the emergency medical, support personnel, and referees. Venues can vary significantly, therefore identifying and clearing an emergency exit route is crucial prior to crowd arrival. Most events require having an ambulance with EMS personnel on site. Keep note of the nearest hospital with a trauma center and neurosurgical capabilities. The equipment should be set up by the mat (Figure 1), ideally with a medical provider assigned to monitor each individual judoka. If a medical evaluation needs to occur communicate with the referee.

MEDICAL EMERGENCIES AND MEDICAL BAG ESSENTIALS

The collapsed or unconscious athlete is considered a medical emergency and the proper channels should be activated. Commodio cordis can lead to cardiac arrest. Blunt abdominal trauma can cause internal bleeding requiring further evaluation and treatment. Judokas who are knocked out and unconscious or those reporting neck pain with neurologic symptoms from trauma should have the cervical spine immobilized. Nontraumatic deaths can be due to hypertrophic cardiomyopathy, cardiac arrhythmias, or asthma.

Medical Bag Essentials in Judo	
• **Medical Emergencies:**	• **Fractures and Dislocations:**
• AED	• Immobilizers and Slings
• Cricothyrotomy Kit	• Crutches
• 14-and 16-gauge needles	• **Wound Care:**
• Nitroglycerin (sublingual)	• Normal saline
• Aspirin	• Betadine swabs
• Epi 1:1,000	• Neosporin, mupirocin ointment
• Diphenhydramine or another antihistamine	• Moleskin
• Albuterol inhaler	• Elastic bandage
• **Head and Spine:**	• Tube stretch gauze
• Concussion evaluation form	• Sterile Gauzes
• Stretcher & Spine board	• Vaseline
• Cervical orthosis	• Steri-strips
• Save a tooth kit	• Suture tray
	• Lidocaine 1%

EPIDEMIOLOGY

Judo is a combat sport with a reported injury rate of about 1.18 injuries/athlete-year in some reports. The most commonly injured area are the hands and fingers, although these are sometimes considered a soft injuries and reporting varies between studies. They result from gripping which comprises most of the time spent during a fight. The knees and shoulders are the other most commonly injured areas as a result of throwing or being thrown.

COMMON INJURIES

Head and Spine Injuries

A way of scoring an ippon in judo is to perform a ***strangle hold***. This briefly cuts off the blood flow and oxygen to the brain and causes a brief loss of consciousness, confusion and memory dysfunction. Sometimes the athlete may experience seizure like movements while unconscious. The time of unconsciousness is usually brief (seconds). Not much scientific data is available on the extent of complications of these injuries. The athlete should be placed in a side-lying position while unconscious. Lifting the legs to promote blood flow to the brain may be applied. No specific return to play guidelines exists for strangle holds that produce loss of consciousness. According to the IJF refereeing rules, if a judoka loses consciousness while being submitted to a strangle hold, he or she is not allowed to continue the competition. It is the author's opinion that the fact that a strangle hold produces a *short-term anoxic brain injury*, the athlete should not return to play on the same day and a stepwise approach to return to play should be undertaken. *Concussions* occur in judo more commonly when being thrown (70%) due to a direct blow to the tatami. They are seen more commonly in younger judokas (<20 years) and who are relatively new to the sport (<3 years). This may be related to lack of falling skills. The judoka may or may not have loss of consciousness. Common symptoms are headache, dizziness and confusion. The possibility of a cervical spine injury should also be evaluated when evaluating a concussion. The judoka should be immediately removed from the match and should not return on the same day. Further evaluation by a medical professional and a stepwise protocol should be in place prior to returning to judo practice. *Cervical spine injuries* in judo are usually benign, mostly sprains or strains. Risk factors are lack of falling skills or head diving techniques which are now prohibited in the sport after newer rules and regulations. If a cervical spine injury is suspected, the physician may alert the referee to stop the fight. The judoka who is suspected to have a cervical spine injury should be immobilized onsite. The recommended technique to transfer the injured player with a suspected cervical spine injury is the lift and slide technique which requires 8 individuals: 1 at the head, 3 on each side and 1 controlling the spinal board. The other technique is the log roll and requires at least 4 providers: 1 controlling the head, 2 the body, and 1 the spinal board. Transfer to the nearest trauma hospital follows.

Upper Limb Injuries

Finger Dislocation is common, but often goes underreported. Usually the referee will stop the match and the judoka will reduce their own finger and continue fighting. The proximal interphalangeal joint (PIP) is the most common affected joint. Mostly occurs in medial to lateral or volar to dorsal direction. Acute management should check for possible fractures by looking for pain in the phalanx. If no fracture is suspected, then acute reduction should be done followed by buddy taping. The judoka can continue to fight if needed after taping. *Acromioclavicular (AC) Joint Injuries* are commonly seen in judo as a result of falling on the side of the shoulder while throwing or being thrown. The athlete will experience tenderness on the lateral shoulder at the AC joint and swelling or deformity may be seen from separation of the distal clavicle from the acromion. The judoka should be removed from the match and further evaluated with x-rays. Conservative management is recommended for grades I–II; recommendations vary for grade III injuries; while surgical treatment is recommended for grades IV–VI. *Shoulder Dislocations* occur anteriorly due to forced flexion, abduction and external rotation of the gleno-humeral joint. A neurovascular evaluation should be done in the distal limb to assess for neurovascular injury. Prompt reduction on-site is recommended to avoid further muscle spasms that will make reduction more difficult. The arm can be then immobilized with a sling and x-rays should be obtained. *Armlocks and Elbow dislocations* occur in judo as an inherent part of the sport. One of the ways of scoring an ippon is by performing an armlock. This is done by locking the elbow of the opponent between your legs and overextending the joint increasing the risk of an elbow dislocation. First do a neurovascular evaluation of the hand to assess for neurovascular injury. Performing x-rays before reduction is recommended due to high risk of fractures with this injury. Urgent reduction should be performed before x-rays if there is evidence of neurovascular compromise.

Lower Limb Injuries

Knee ligament injury is common in judo. The *anterior cruciate ligament (ACL) and medial collateral ligament (MCL)* are the most commonly injured. There are certain throwing techniques that require the attacker to lock the opponent's leg in an extended knee valgus position during the throw. These may predispose an additional risk for knee injuries. Acute management should include icing, evaluation for possible ACL injury before swelling and pain make examination more difficult. Further management will depend on the specific ligament injured. *Ankle sprains* can occur from the multiple changes in direction that occur during judo fight in addition to varus and plantar flexion foot position applied during throwing techniques. Acute management should include rest, icing, elevation. X-rays should be ordered if there is suspicion of possible fracture. *Metatarsophalangeal (MTP) Joint Sprain* can occur in judo in both extension and flexion since the sport is practiced barefoot. The 1st toe can get caught in the tatami and cause an injury in flexion or the athlete have a hyperextension injury when throwing or falling. Acute management should include icing and evaluation for possible fractures. Buddy taping may assist in pain control during practice. A rigid shoe insert can be used until pain free.

Other Injuries

If a judoka is *bleeding*, the referee will stop the match and allow a medical time-out of 1 minute to stop the bleeding. A judoka is allowed 2 medical time-outs during a match. If the bleeding cannot be controlled and a third medical time-out is needed, then the judoka will have a medical disqualification. *Epistaxis (Nosebleed)* results from blunt trauma to the nose. It is usually unilateral and more common during dry winter months. Contrary to common behavior by athletes, acute management should start by leaning forward to avoid blood passing to the pharynx. Order the athlete to do a soft blow of the affected nostril to clear clots and apply compression with fingers or cotton rolls. Vasoconstrictive agents such as oxymetazoline may be applied to a cotton roll to accelerate the process, but not during a match because the athlete may be disqualified. If the bleeding is well under control, the judoka may return to the fight. *Facial lacerations* in judo usually occur from accidental blunt trauma against the opponent (i.e. headbutt). First action should be to stop the bleeding. Clean with gauze and apply a tight wrap with elastic bandage or tape. Always do a neurological exam to assess if a concussion may have occurred. If the bleeding is well under control, the judoka may return to the fight. If not controlled then consider sutures. *Auricular Hematoma (Cauliflower Ear)* is a hematoma between perichondrium and auricular cartilage. It is caused by persistent trauma to the ear that causes cartilage death and fibrosis. The goal of management is to remove the hematoma and compress the underlying surfaces to promote healing. This can be done by aspirating the hematoma with an 18-G needle and then using magnetic compression bolsters to apply pressure. Also the auricular surfaces can be sutured with absorbable sutures. Similar to wrestling, *skin infections* can occur in judo. *Tinea corporis or ringworm* is the most common skin infection. It can be transmitted from contact with another athlete, the mattress or the judogi. Prevention is encouraged and judokas with ringworm should avoid returning to training or matches. Judogi sharing should be avoided to prevent spread of skin infections. Topical or oral antifungals can be used for treatment.

■ SUMMARY

Judo is a combat sport that has a wide variety of injuries. Proper understanding of the rules and regulations as well as the most common injuries that occur is essential for proper medical coverage of the sport.

▨ Further Reading

Green CM, Petrou MJ, Rolf CG, et al. Injuries among judokas during competition. *Scand J Med Sci Sports*. 2007;17(3):205-210.

IJF. International Judo Federation Refereeing Rules. Published 2018. https://www.ijf.org/documents. Accessed January 20, 2020.

IJF. International Judo Federation Sports and Organization Rules. https://www.ijf.org/documents. Published 2018. Accessed January 20, 2020.

Nishime RS. Sports Medicine Basics in the Judo Athlete (Part 1). USA Judo Sports Medicine Subcommittee. Accessed January 20, 2020.

Pocecco E, Ruedl G, Stankovic N, et al. Injuries in judo: a systematic literature review including suggestions for prevention. *Br J Sports Med*. 2013;47:1139-1143. doi:10.1136/bjsports-2013-092886

17. KARATE

Richard G. Chang and Lawrence G. Chang

▓ HISTORY

Karate is Japanese for "empty hand." It is an Okinawan close-combat martial art with origins from China and Korea. It is a martial art style, with various substyles—Shotokan, Goju-Ryu, Kyokushin, Shorin-Ryu, and Wado-Ryu—that focus mainly on striking and blocking, rather than grappling or throwing. A karate practitioner is known as "Karateka." Karate can be classified as a non-, light-, semi-, or full-contact sport. Under the World Karate Federation (WKF), formerly known as the World Union Karate Organization, karate has been a world sport since late 1960s–1970s. Every two years there is a world competition. From the 1970s to 1990s, injuries were prevalent in karate and there were safety concerns due to increased injury rates in competitive events. In the year 2000, WKF changed rules and regulations which included weight classes and point systems changes. These have improved safety in competitions. Karate will be featured for the first time in the upcoming 2020 Tokyo Summer Olympics.[1-5]

▓ GOVERNING ORGANIZATIONS

- International: World Karate Federation (WKF)
- National: USA Karate-Do Federation, National Collegiate Karate Association (NCKA), National Karate Institute

▓ PARTICIPANTS

Participants for kumite are grouped by age, gender (male/female), weight, and experience.

Age Divisions: Pupils, Cadets, Nonelites, Elites, Seniors, Masters
Experience Divisions: Beginner, Novice, Intermediate, Advanced, Elite
Individual versus team competitors

▓ RULES AND REGULATIONS

Karate Rules: divided into kata and kumite

Kata: a solo summary of set fighting techniques against an imaginary opponent(s).

Kumite: fight with an opponent. Punches and kicks are based on controlled and correct techniques executed without injury to the opponent. Poor execution of techniques and injury to opponent is a penalty and opponent receives a point. Revised Kumite Point System—three points (sanbon): Kicks to head and throwing; two points (nihon): Kicks to anywhere on back and trunk; one point (ippon): Punches to head and trunk. Blows to vital points, certain throwing techniques, and specific hand techniques to head are strictly forbidden. No groin or throat strikes are allowed. Participants using illegal behavior or moves or faking or intentional injuries are warned, given penalty points, or warrant suspension.[5-8]

▓ EQUIPMENT

Participants wear traditional *karate-gi uniform*; protective *head gear, gum shields, standardized gloves; forearm, shin,* and *instep padding*. Additionally, athletes may have *torso protection, chest protector (females),* or *groin guard*. Competition generally occurs on a *padded floor mat*.[6,7]

>>> **Adaptive Sport Key Points: Karate**

Individual kata are only performed. Three categories of adaptive athletes: wheelchair, visual, or intellectually impaired. Wheelchair athletes must have one of the seven impairments: impaired muscle power, impaired passive range of motion (PROM), limb deficiency, leg length difference, hypertonia, ataxia, or athetosis. Intellectually impaired athletes must meet three criteria to participate: IQ ≤75, adaptive behavior affecting skills in everyday life, and impairment before 18 years of age. All types of wheelchairs are allowed except for those with antitippers, electric drive support, and electric wheelchairs.[9]

▓ MEDICAL COVERAGE LOGISTICS

Pre-event preparation is imperative to improve safety measures, reduce risks to athletes during the event, and provide appropriate medical care. Medical providers should ensure that all equipment needs are met and know what supplies are available on-site and at local medical facilities. The medical team should arrive at least an hour early before the start of the event. It is critical to ensure that team members know the role they play in an emergency and review the Emergency Action Plan (EAP). The medical team should assess and manage the illnesses and injuries, determine if the patient requires treatment on-site or urgent/emergency transportation, and if the athlete may return to play. After the event, it is important to review injuries that occurred and follow up injured athletes. Lastly, there is the importance of the physician working with the referee and instructors in preventing injuries in potentially penalizing or stopping fights when further damage is possible or probable.[6,7]

▓ MEDICAL EMERGENCIES AND MEDICAL BAG ESSENTIALS

The collapsed or unconscious athlete is considered a medical emergency that requires activation of the proper channels of communication and protocols including basic life support (BLS)/advanced cardiac life support (ACLS). Although rarely reported, nontraumatic emergencies can include cardiac conditions like arrhythmias and hypertrophic cardiomyopathy (HCM), anaphylaxis, and asthma. Musculoskeletal injuries that may become medical emergencies include upper and lower limb fractures or dislocations with neurovascular compromise, traumatic brain injuries with or without spinal cord involvement, commodio cordis leading to cardiac arrest, and blunt thoracoabdominal trauma with possible internal bleeding.

▓ EPIDEMIOLOGY

Injury is common in karate, especially among the more active younger age group. Among youths less than 18 years old, in 12 months there is an injury risk of 5.6 per 100 athletes.[10] However, injury among younger athletes seems to have declined, especially among the women due to the addition of weight divisions.[6,7] Top level junior karate total injury rate was lower than higher classes due to an increase in weight categories

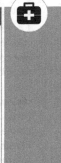

Medical Bag Essentials in Karate	
Medical Emergencies:	**Fractures and Dislocations:**
Automated External Defibrillator (AED)	Immobilizers and Slings
Cricothyrotomy kit	Crutches
14- and 16-gauge needles	**Wound Care:**
Nitroglycerin (sublingual)	
Aspirin	Normal saline
Epi 1:1,000	Betadine swabs
Diphenhydramine or another antihistamine	Neosporin, mupirocin ointment
Albuterol inhaler	Moleskin
Head and Spine:	Elastic bandage
	Tube stretch gauze
Concussion evaluation form	Sterile gauzes
Stretcher & Spine board	Vaseline
Cervical orthosis	Steri-strips
Save a tooth kit	Suture tray
	Lidocaine 1%
	Petroleum Jelly

from three to five.[7] Injuries were higher among lighter classes with men under 60 kg and women under 53 kg.[2] Higher injury risks occur more in karate competitions as opposed to training.[7]

Common mechanism of injury includes strikes, falls, throws, and jumps.[11] Face, head, and neck injuries were more common than lower limb injuries in competitions and tournaments, mostly secondary to strikes.[2,6,11]

▨ COMMON INJURIES

Head and Spine Injuries

The most common site of injury is strikes to the head due to higher points awarded for kicks to head.[6] Injuries include *lacerations, abrasions, contusions* to the head and neck. Periorbital swelling or bleeds are treated with closure of eye with steri-strip or suturing. Participants may develop visual deficits or severe blindness from head and neck single-blow injuries which warrants a full neurological workup and close follow up.[12] Participants may need to be sent to an emergency room with antibiotics for cellulitis and a CT scan to rule out cranial nerve deficits from sinusoidal abscess impinging on orbital nerves. *Nasal or zygomatic fractures* may occur as in boxers. Fractures can be reduced acutely and require follow-up. In any combat sport, there is always some risk of concussion. Protective head gear reduces head blow acceleration by 15%.[2] The advent of floor and head paddings has reduced the incidence of head injuries, lacerations, abrasions, and soft tissue injuries. Roundhouse kicks to the head or chin can potentially cause *blow out* and *skull fractures*. Spinning back kicks to neck can cause *cervical dislocations*, although rare.[3] Look for any signs of neurological deficits and mental status changes. A decision to suspend the athlete and stop return-to-play may be warranted if a concussion is suspected and the transfer to a trauma center is advised in the case of a possible spinal cord injury. An Emergency Medical Services (EMS) team should be ready and set up to take the patient to hospital for any medical emergency.

Lower Limb Injuries

Lower limb injuries are more common these days than *upper limbs* as the revised Karate rules reward greater points with kicks compared to hand strikes. *Hand injuries* are common and occur at the thumb and index finger. Blocking may cause *digital dislocations, sprains,* and *fractures.*[3] *Fractures of the neck of the second metacarpal* are very common. *Bennet's fracture, lateral collateral ligament avulsion fractures,* or *thumb dislocations* are common as well.[3] Standardized gloving can reduce head and hand injuries.[13] *Forearm* and *arm contusions* occur when blocking roundhouse kicks and may cause wrist drop due to *radial nerve injury.*[3] Arm padding may prevent nerve damage. *Meniscus injury* occurs when the femur rotates and compresses around the meniscus against the tibial bone in the grounded leg while the contralateral leg is conducting a roundhouse kick.[3] Low sweeps to the opponent may cause *superficial peroneal nerve injury, quadriceps contusion,* or *acute compartment syndrome.*[3] Quadriceps hematomas should be followed closely to prevent myositis ossificans.[3] Anterior compartment syndrome, although rare, may occur and requires surgical decompression.[3]

Practitioners may have *cuts, abrasions,* or *blisters.* Open wounds are rare. It is necessary to inspect these wounds as any associated hemorrhage should be thoroughly inspected. If open, they may be at risk for infections.

Abdominal Injuries

The abdominal region is at risk of blunt trauma. Direct blows from kicks to *spleen, liver, adrenals, kidneys, lungs, pancreas,* and *testicles* may induce organ rupture and bleeding, with pancreas being a common site of injury.[3,10] A thorough physical exam of abdomen, back, ribs, diaphragm, and breathing status is warranted. Any hematomas, soft tissue abnormalities, or pain should be inspected closely and palpated for tenderness; while fighting, participants should be examined for any functional decline during and after fight as this may indicate potential organ failure. Participants with suspicion for organ damage need to be sent to hospital to rule out rupture or any intraperitoneal bleeds. Use of padding to torso and groin can prevent/reduce such injuries.

▨ SUMMARY

Karate is a relatively safe combat sport as long as physicians, referees, instructors, tournament officials, and the athlete continue to collaborate and communicate as a team in order to optimize the athlete's performance, while reinforcing injury prevention techniques and strategies.

▨ References

1. Zetaruk MN, Violan MA, Zurakowski D, Micheli LJ. Karate injuries in children and adolescents. *Accid Anal Prev.* 2000;32:421-425. doi:10.1016/s0001-4575(99)00120-7.

2. Arriaza R, Leyes M. Injury profile in competitive karate: prospective analysis of three consecutive World Karate Championships. *Knee Surg Sports Traumatol Arthrosc.* 2005;13:603-607. doi:10.1007/s00167-004-0593-6.

3. McLatchie G. Karate and karate injuries. *Br J Sports Med.* 1981;15(1):84-86. doi:10.1136/bjsm.15.1.84.

4. Karate. Tokyo 2020. https://tokyo2020.org/en/games/sport/olympic/karate/.

5. Rules of Kumite Competition. USA National Karate-do Federation.https://www.teamusa.org/-/media/USA_Karate/Documents/Rules-Regulations/USA-KARATE-KUMITE-RULES-revised-January-1-2019.pdf?la=en&hash=8F14275D37D7A9103691F87C78AF3819D060A9BF. Revised January 1, 2019.

6. Macan J, Bundalo-Vrbanac D, Romić G. Effects of the new karate rules on the incidence and distribution of injuries. *Br J Sports Med.* 2006;40:326-330. doi:10.1136/bjsm.2005.022459.

7. Čierna D, Barrientos M, Agrasar C, Arriaza R. Epidemiology of injuries in juniors participating in top-level karate competition: a prospective cohort study. *Br J Sports Med*. 2018;52:730-734. doi:10.1136/bjsports-2017-097756.

8. Arriaza R, Čierna D, Regueiro P, et al. Low risk of concussion in top-level karate competition. *Br J Sports Med*. 2017;51:226-230. doi:10.1136/bjsports-2016-096574.

9. World Karate Federation. Para-karate kata competition rules. https://www.wkf.net/pdf/wkf-para-karate-rules.pdf. Published January 25, 2019.

10. Demorest RA, Koutres C. Youth participation and injury risk in martial arts. *Pediatrics*. 2016;138(6):1-9. doi:10.1542/peds.2016-3022.

11. McPherson M, Pickett W. Characteristics of martial arts injuries in a defined Canadian population: a descriptive epidemiological study. *BMC Public Health*. 2010;10:795. doi:10.1186/1471-2458-10-795.

12. Mars JS, Pimenedes D. Blinding choroidal rupture in a karateka. *Br J Sports Med*. 1995;29(4):273-274. doi:10.1136/bjsm.29.4.273.

13. Johannsen HV, Noerregaard FO. Prevention of injury in karate. *Br J Sports Med*. 1988;22(3):113-115. doi:10.1136/bjsm.22.3.113.

18. LACROSSE

Ariana Gluck

HISTORY

Lacrosse is considered one of the oldest team sports in North America and is based on games initially created by Native American communities as early as the 17th century. It is believed to be named by a Jesuit missionary named Jean de Brébeuf when he decided to write about it in his journals. It is believed that Brébeuf saw the Native Americans holding a stick that resembled a bishop's crozier, which is *crosse* in French.[1]

GOVERNING ORGANIZATIONS

- International: World Lacrosse
- National: US Lacrosse
- Major professional leagues: Major League Lacrosse (MLL), National Lacrosse League
- College: National Collegiate Athletic Association (NCAA)
- High School: National Federation of State High School Associations (NFHS)

PARTICIPANTS

Approximately 826,000 players participated in US Lacrosse as of 2017. These include athletes ranging from youth, high school, college, professional, and postcollege. Both men and women play the sport of lacrosse.[2]

RULES AND REGULATIONS

Lacrosse is played on a rectangular field with nets at opposing ends. The game begins with a face-off between two players on each team at midfield with the ball between them. Once the referee blows the whistle the two players try to gain possession of the ball. Once the ball is obtained, it is passed, caught, and carried in the netted stick until ultimately thrown in the opposing team's goal scoring one point. The winning team is the team that scored the most goals during the game. Men's lacrosse team consists of 10 players: three on defense, three on offense, three on midfield, and one goalie. Women's lacrosse team consists of 12 players: four on defense, four on offense, three on midfield, and one goalie. Specific rules regarding possession, movement, scoring, and contact vary widely depending on the league and level of sport and are gender specific. The regulation playing time is 60 minutes divided up into four quarters of 15 minutes each. There is a break between the second and third quarters, usually about 10 minutes long. Compared to women's lacrosse, men's lacrosse is a contact sport where body-checking is permitted, therefore necessitating more protective equipment.

■ EQUIPMENT

For Both Men's and Women's Lacrosse

The **crosse (lacrosse stick)** is historically made of wood; it is now more frequently synthetic material or a metal alloy with a shaped net pocket at the end. The crosse comes in a variety of lengths and styles that depend on the position played by the athlete. The **ball** is made of solid rubber. All lacrosse balls must meet National Operating Committee on Standards for Athletic Equipment (NOCSAE) standards. A **mouth guard** is mandatory for all players.

Men's Lacrosse

In men's lacrosse, in addition to the crosse, ball, and mouth piece, the following are required: A protective **helmet**, equipped with **face mask, chin pad,** and **a cupped four-point chin strap** fastened to all four hookups, must be worn by all players. All helmets and facemasks must be approved by NOCSAE. **Gloves, arm pads, protective cups** are mandatory for all players. **Shoulder pads** are mandatory for all players with the exception of the goalkeeper. **Rib pads** are optional. The goalkeeper is required to wear a **throat and chest protector**.

Women's Lacrosse

In women's lacrosse, in addition to the crosse, ball, and mouth guard, the following are required: All athletes must wear **eye protection** that meets ASTM international (formerly known as American Society for Testing and Materials) standard F3077 for women's adult/youth lacrosse. The goalkeeper must wear a **helmet with the face mask** (NOCSAE approved), **throat protector, padded gloves, mouth piece,** and **chest protector. High school level and below** must wear **padding on thighs and shins. Youth level** must wear some form of **abdominal and pelvic protection**.[4,5]

>>> **Adaptive Sport Key Points: Wheelchair Lacrosse**

Wheelchair Lacrosse is an adaptive version of traditional men's lacrosse and is full-contact. Teams are co-ed and consist of eight players (two defensemen, three midfielders, two attackmen, and one goalie), and grouped by classification rules based on equal level of ability. The game is played on a rectangular surface, 185 ft by 85 ft, usually on an indoor roller hockey rink or box lacrosse pad. A no-bounce indoor lacrosse ball is used. The game duration is four 15-minute quarters.[3]

■ MEDICAL COVERAGE LOGISTICS

The role of the on-site physician leader is to organize and coordinate the medical staff, develop an emergency action plan (EAP), and interact with the coaches and officials to help ensure the safety of the players and spectators. Prior to the game, it is important to identify available medical staff, support personnel, field map, and the available medical equipment. Sports medicine physicians and Emergency Medical Services (EMS) personnel, along with sports medicine fellows, residents, medical students, athletic trainers, or physical therapists can attend expected medical needs. Establishing an EAP is the most important task. Protocols and guidelines should include role definition of the medical staff, emergency transportation including personnel, routes, and adequate facilities with the capacity to evaluate and manage possible injuries, and an outline of the chain-of-command and communication standards. Contingency plans should be made for extreme temperature, humidity, and other weather conditions that may lead to game cancellation or postponement, or in game modifications like extra water breaks, especially at the youth level. Lastly, prior to the start of the competition, the medical team should confirm that players are wearing proper equipment. The referee will notify the head medical provider if an injured player needs to be evaluated on the field. Communication between individual members of the medical staff, coaches, referees, emergency medical staff, and local medical facilities is essential via two or more systems (e.g., hand-held radios and cell phones). Lastly, documentation is essential for review after the game/season to evaluate utilization and plan for future coverage.

▨ MEDICAL EMERGENCIES AND MEDICAL BAG ESSENTIALS

It is important to understand possible medical emergencies that you may encounter. The collapsed or unconscious athlete is considered a medical emergency and the EAP should be activated. Nontraumatic deaths can be due to hypertrophic cardiomyopathy, cardiac arrhythmias, heat-related illness such as heat stroke, anaphylaxis, and asthma. Commotio cordis is a life-threatening injury that can occur as a result of a blunt nonpenetrating impact of the ball over the cardiac silhouette at a critical time in the cardiac cycle, leading to cardiac arrest. If an athlete collapses after a sudden blow to the chest, the EAP should be activated, with early access to defibrillation.

Medical Bag Essentials in Lacrosse	
Medical Emergencies:	**Fractures and Dislocations:**
Automated External Defibrillator (AED)	Immobilizers and Slings
Tourniquet	Crutches
Cricothyrotomy kit	**Wound Care:**
14- and 16-gauge needles	Normal saline
Epi 1:1,000	Betadine swabs
Diphenhydramine or another antihistamine	Neosporin, mupirocin ointment
Albuterol inhaler	Moleskin
Rectal thermometer	Elastic bandage
Ice bath	Tube stretch gauze
Head and Spine:	Sterile gauzes
Concussion evaluation form	Vaseline
Stretcher & Spine board	Steri-strips
Cervical orthosis	Suture tray
Save a tooth kit	Lidocaine 1%
Protective equipment removal tools	

▨ EPIDEMIOLOGY

Men's lacrosse is a contact and collision sport, while women's lacrosse is considered a noncontact sport, where intentional body contact is prohibited; however, incidental contact does occur. The rates of injury in men's lacrosse varied from 0.095 to 12.98 per 1,000 athlete exposures. The game and practice injury rates increased with age from youth (0.55), to high school (0.5–1.4), and college (1.7–3.8) leagues. The most commonly injured body parts are the lower limbs, head, and shoulders. The rate of injury in women's lacrosse varied from 0.03 to 3.9 injuries per 100 athletes, and injury rates increased with age as well. Compared to their male counterparts, women sustain a higher percentage of head and facial injuries secondary to lack of full protective head gear.

Helmets are designed to prevent injury from the high velocity ball, fall, and incidental contact of a stick to the head.[6-8]

■ COMMON INJURIES

Head and Spine Injuries

Concussion is commonly seen in lacrosse at all levels with a higher incidence in men than women. Mechanism of injury includes direct trauma to the head or an acceleration/ deceleration force of the head due to trauma at another part of the body. Symptoms include confusion, dizziness, headaches, nausea, and, in severe cases, loss of consciousness. The player must be removed from the game/practice and a complete concussion evaluation performed that may include a Sport Concussion Assessment Tool (SCAT).[9,10] If no red flags are observed, then the player may remain on the sideline without his/ her equipment. Periodic assessment should follow until cleared to leave with a parent if under age. He or she will need to follow up with a sports medicine provider in 24 to 48 hours for further assessment. Second impact syndrome is a possible complication if a concussed brain suffers another impact before resolution of the initial injury and leads to cerebral hemorrhage and edema and can be fatal. **Cervical spine injury** is concerning in all contact and collision sports. Players who are found to be unconscious on the field or those reporting neck pain with neurologic symptoms from trauma during play should have the cervical spine immobilized. The recommended technique to transfer the injured player with a suspected cervical spine injury is the lift-and-slide technique that requires eight individuals: one at the head, three on each side and one controlling the spinal board. The other technique is the log roll and requires at least four providers: one controlling the head, two the body, and one the spinal board. Protective athletic equipment should be removed *prior* to transport to an emergency facility for an athlete–patient with suspected cervical spine instability. Equipment removal should be performed by at least three trained and experienced rescuers. If fewer than three people are present, the equipment should be removed at the earliest possible time after enough trained individuals arrive on the scene.[11] They should be transported to the ED for further evaluation.

Upper Limb Injuries

Upper limb injuries are acute due to direct trauma. **Acromioclavicular (AC) joint** injuries are commonly seen in lacrosse and result from a sprain or tear of the ligaments around the AC joint. The mechanism of injury can be due to direct trauma to the lateral shoulder, mainly with the arm close to the body as a result of a fall. Symptoms include tenderness over the AC joint and pain may radiate to the neck and shoulder. You may observe swelling, bruising, or a deformity of the AC joint such as a gap with displacement of the acromion from the clavicle. Players should be removed from play and obtain an x-ray of the shoulder. Depending on the severity of the injury, most will heal with conservative measures; however, some may require surgical intervention. Injuries to the hand include **goalkeeper's thumb** which occurs with forced abduction and hyperextension of the thumb metacarpophalangeal joint causing an injury to the thumb ulnar collateral ligament (UCL). Symptoms include pain made worse by placing the thumb in extension or abduction and swelling along the ulnar aspect of the thumb. Valgus stress testing may reveal a loss of integrity of the UCL. Players should be removed from play and obtain an x-ray of the thumb. If players have a bony fragment on the x-ray that is displaced greater than 2 mm, or involves greater than 25% of articular surface, then they should be referred for surgical intervention. Nondisplaced fractures can usually be treated with immobilization and protection. Mechanism of injury is usually from the impact of the ball on the thumb tip as the goalie attempts to save the shot on the goal.

Lower Limb Injuries

Anterior collateral ligament (ACL) injuries are common in lacrosse. The mechanism of injury is usually noncontact due to cutting and pivoting or landing with valgus stress of the knee. Symptoms may include pain, feeling an instant "pop," immediate swelling, and feeling of knee instability. Lack of a distinct endpoint suggests an ACL injury, and anterior tibial translation with Lachman's test suggests tear. Acute management includes removal from play and conservative measures such as rest, ice, compression, nonsteroidal anti-inflammatory drugs (NSAIDs). ACL injuries can be managed operatively or nonoperatively and depend upon the extent of the injury, patient characteristics, and activities. Physical therapy is important for nonoperative and postoperative management. **Muscle strains of the hamstrings, quadriceps,** and **adductors** are common. The mechanism of injury is due to trauma to the muscle belly or sudden eccentric contraction. Symptoms include tenderness over the area and players may have edema and ecchymosis as well. Management includes rest and return to play when the patient is asymptomatic. **Ankle sprains** are common in lacrosse. Mechanism of injury is typically due to noncontact cutting, dodging, or twisting activities. Lateral ankle sprains are the most common and mechanism of injury is inversion of a plantar-flexed foot, causing damage to the lateral ligament complex of the ankle. Management includes conservative treatment (rest, ice, NSAIDs), taping or bracing, and neuromuscular retraining.

■ SUMMARY

Lacrosse is a popular high-velocity sport with varying degrees of contact based on the league. The combination of speed, quick change of direction, and equipment make for a unique set of injury mechanisms and types. Understanding the game, positions, and most common injuries is essential for sideline coverage.

■ References

1. Adamski BK. Lacrosse. *The Canadian Encyclopedia.* https://www.thecanadianencyclopedia.ca/en/article/lacrosse. Published August 7, 2013. Updated July 31, 2018.

2. US Lacrosse. 2017 participation survey. https://www.uslacrosse.org/sites/default/files/public/documents/about-us-lacrosse/participation-survey-2017.pdf. Published 2017. Updated September 19, 2018

3. Wheelchair Lacrosse USA. WLUSA rules. http://www.wheelchairlacrosse.com/rules.

4. Scroggs W, Halpin Ty. 2019 and 2020 NCAA men's lacrosse rules and interpretations. http://www.ncaapublications.com/productdownloads/LC20.pdf. Published October 2018.

5. Smith SS, Seewald R. 2018 and 2019 NCAA women's lacrosse rules. http://www.ncaapublications.com/productdownloads/WLC19.pdf. Published December 2017.

6. Barber Foss KD, Le Cara E, McCambridge T, et al. Epidemiology of injuries in men's lacrosse: injury prevention implications for competition level, type of play, and player position. *Phys Sportsmed.* 2017;45(3):224-233. doi:10.1080/00913847.2017.1355209.

7. Barber Foss KD, Le Cara E, McCambridge T, et al. Epidemiology of injuries in women's lacrosse: implications for sport-, level-, and sex-specific injury prevention strategies. *Clin J Sport Med.* 2018;28(4):406-413. doi:10.1097/JSM.0000000000000458.

8. Putukian, M, Lincoln, AW, Crisco, JJ. Sports-specific issues in men's and women's lacrosse. *Curr Sports Med Rep.* 2014;13(5):334-340. doi:10.1249/JSR.0000000000000092.

9. Echemendia RJ, Meeuwisse W, McCrory P, et al. The Sport Concussion Assessment Tool 5th Edition (SCAT5). *Br J Sports Med.* 2017;51(11):848-850. doi:10.1136/bjsports-2017-097506.

10. Davis GA, Purcell L, Schneider KJ, et al. The Child Sport Concussion Assessment Tool 5th Edition (Child SCAT5): background and rationale. *Br J Sports Med.* 2017;51(11):859-861. doi:10.1136/bjsports-2017-097492.

11. National Athletic Trainers' Association. Appropriate care of the spine injured athlete. https://www.nata.org/blog/toddc/update-appropriate-care-spine-injured-athlete. Updated from 1998 document. Prof Rep. 2015.

19. MIXED MARTIAL ARTS

Richard G. Chang

■ HISTORY

Mixed martial arts is also referred to as "extreme cage fighting," "ultimate fighting," and "no holds barred" sports fighting. Historically, an early form of the sport existed in the ancient Greek Olympics, called "pankration" (Greek, "all powerful"). It was a freestyle combat sport, which combined elements of boxing and wrestling, that was first introduced in 648 BCE at the 33rd Olympiad. It often served as a final event for the ancient Olympics during this time.[1] However, the term "mixed martial arts" (MMA) did not become popularized until the 1990s when professional fighting organizations, such as Ultimate Fighting Championship (UFC) in the United States, sponsored events where fighters competed using a combination of various combat sports techniques, ranging from wrestling, Brazilian jiu-jitsu, judo, boxing, and Muay Thai kickboxing. Other martial arts, such as karate, kung-fu, capoeira, were also integrated depending upon the individual fighter. Prior to this, MMA was influenced and popularized by Brazilian combat sport, vale tudo (Portugese, "anything goes/everything allowed"), which allowed competitors to draw from a mix of striking, wrestling, grappling, and submission styles and skills.

■ GOVERNING ORGANIZATIONS

- International: The International Mixed Martial Arts Federation (IMMAF) and the World MMA Association (WMMAA)—both designed for regulation of amateur competitions
- National: Association of Boxing Commissions and Combative Sports (ABC) and sanctioned by each state's Athletic Commission body
- Major professional leagues:
  - *North America*: Ultimate Fighting Championship (UFC), Professional Fighters League (PFL), Bellator
  - *Asia*: ONE Championship, Rizin Fighting Federation (Rizin FF)

■ PARTICIPANTS

As per the IMMAF, it is estimated there are about 449 million followers of the sport globally. According to the 2014 Sports & Fitness Industry Association's (SFIA) survey of American persons aged 6 and above, there were 1,235,000 participants in MMA for competition and from 2012 to 2015, there has been a 72.3% increase in participation in the sport.[2]

■ RULES AND REGULATIONS

Competitors are mandated to follow the Unified Rules of MMA, which was first adopted by the New Jersey State Athletic Control Board and Nevada State Athletic Commission in September 2000. From then, all state and local municipal athletic commission bodies have adopted these rules. In July 2009, the ABC formally passed and adopted these rules, which all state commissions must follow.

The 10 Point Must System is the standard system of scoring a bout (similar to boxing). All bouts are evaluated and scored by three judges. The referee may not be one of the judges. Fighters are judged on effective striking, effective grappling, control of the ring/fighting area, and effective aggressiveness and defense. Scoring is based on a 10-point system where: 10-10 round is a draw between combatants, 10-9 round is a win by a close margin, 10-8 round is a win by a large margin, and 10-7 round is where combatant completely overwhelms the opponent. Each round lasts no more than 5 minutes, with a 1-minute rest period between rounds. Nontitle/nonchampionship bouts consist of three rounds, whereas title/championship bouts consist of five rounds. In amateur competitions, bouts consist of three, 3-minute rounds with a 1-minute rest period. Winning a bout is achieved by submission via physical or verbal tap out, knockout (KO), referee stops contest (RSC), technical knockout (TKO), decision by judges through scorecards, disqualification, forfeit technical draw, technical decision, or no decision.

A bout may be held in a ring of at least five ringed ropes, between 20 to 32 ft,[2] or a fenced area circular or octagonal, between 20 to 32 ft wide with two entrances (blue and red corner).

■ EQUIPMENT

Small open finger *gloves*: In general, 4-oz gloves are used in professional bouts, but up to 6-oz are allowed. A *mouth piece/mouth guard* is required for competition. The round cannot begin without a mouth piece. Competition is paused by the referee if the mouth piece is dislodged. *Headgear* is not permitted in both amateur and professional competitions. The respective regulatory Commission will determine if a contestant's head or facial hair will interfere with supervision and conduct of the bout. Fingernail length will also be inspected. If determined by the Commission, filing and clipping of long nails will be completed before the start of the event. *Bandages* made of soft gauze and surgeon's adhesive tape are allowed to wrap only the hands, knuckles, and wrists. This must be placed prior to the bout in the presence of the respective regulatory Commission and if warranted, in the presence of the manager or chief second of his or her opponent. Contestants may wear MMA (board shorts), biking shorts (vale tudo shorts), or kickboxing shorts approved by the State Commission. Traditional jiu-jitsu gis ("gis" for short), shirts, biking pants, shoes, jewelry, and piercings are prohibited. In amateur competitions, *shin guards* with insteps pads must be worn by all contestants. Male contestants must wear *groin protectors*. Female contestants must wear a *chest protector* approved by the Commission. As per Unified Rule, "no body grease, gels, balms, lotions oils, excessive water dumping, or other substances may be applied to the hair, face or body. However, *Vaseline or petroleum jelly* may be applied solely to the facial area at cage side or ringside in the presence of an inspector, referee, or a person designated by the regulatory commission."[3]

■ MEDICAL COVERAGE LOGISTICS

The medical director must establish an emergency action plan (EAP), define roles, and identify communication lines. On the day of the event, it is important to identify and introduce yourself to the emergency medical and support personnel. Venues can vary significantly, therefore identifying and clearing an emergency exit route is crucial prior to crowd arrival. Most events require having an ambulance with Emergency Medical Services (EMS) personnel on site. Keep note of the nearest hospital with a trauma center and neurosurgical capabilities. Communicate early with referees and inspectors at the event, as they will be your advocates to ensure fighter safety. The equipment should be set up at ringside, ideally with a medical provider assigned to monitor each individual fighter. Stay focused during the fight and watch for cues to see if a fighter is in trouble. Momentum changes, signs of exhaustion, and changes in style or strengths are all important aspects to determine if a fighter is having issues. Action moves fast, so minimize distractions from the crowds, fans, and coaches; utilize security to minimize any distractions. If medical evaluation needs to occur, communicate with the referee. Know which decisions can be determined from the ringside and which decisions need to be made from inside the ring. Bear in mind that as soon as a physician steps onto the octagon, the bout is over. If you determine that you must stop a fight, be confident but remain reasonable.

■ MEDICAL EMERGENCIES AND MEDICAL BAG ESSENTIALS

Although MMA is a combat sport, true medical emergencies occur infrequently. Acute traumatic brain injury and second impact syndrome are the most emergent injuries that need to be addressed immediately. Second impact syndrome is a possible complication if a concussed brain suffers another impact before resolution of the initial injury and leads to cerebral hemorrhage and edema that can be fatal. The collapsed or unconscious athlete is considered a medical emergency and the proper channels should be activated. Commodio cordis can lead to cardiac arrest. Blunt abdominal trauma can cause internal bleeding requiring further evaluation and treatment. Fighters who are knocked out and unconscious or those reporting neck pain with neurologic symptoms from trauma should have the cervical spine immobilized. Nontraumatic deaths are rare due to pre-event screening, but can be due to hypertrophic cardiomyopathy, cardiac arrhythmias, or asthma.

Medical Bag Essentials in MMA	
Medical Emergencies:	**Fractures and Dislocations:**
Automated External Defibrillator (AED)	Immobilizers and Slings
Cricothyrotomy kit	Crutches
14- and 16-gauge needles	**Wound Care:**
Nitroglycerin (sublingual)	Normal saline
Aspirin	Betadine swabs
Epi 1:1,000	Neosporin, mupirocin ointment
Diphenhydramine or another antihistamine	Moleskin
Albuterol inhaler	Elastic bandage
Head and Spine:	Tube stretch gauze
Concussion evaluation form	Sterile gauzes
Stretcher & Spine board	Vaseline
Cervical orthosis	Steri-strips
Save a tooth kit	Suture tray
	Lidocaine 1%
	Petroleum Jelly

■ EPIDEMIOLOGY

Although there are no large, quality, longitudinal epidemiological studies of either amateur or professional MMA athletic injuries, studies suggest an average injury rate of 246.4/1,000 Athletic Encounters (AE) in male fighters,[4] and 101.9/1,000 AE in female amateur and professional MMA fighters.[5] When comparing professional to amateur fighters, the average rate of injury was 135.5/1,000 AE versus 71.0/1,000 AE. Reasons for stopping matches were KO/TKO, 173.9/1,000 AE for males and 175.9/1,000 AE for females; submission 228.6/1,000 AE; and referee's decision 98.2/1,000 AE. When compared to other combat sports, there appeared to be a greater injury incidence (228.7 per 1,000 athlete exposures). However, the injury pattern was similar to professional boxing. The most commonly injured region was the head/neck, followed by the wrist/hand. The most frequent reported injuries were lacerations, fracture, and concussions. Losers and fighters ending in a decision with a KO or TKO were identified at greater risk for injury.[6]

■ COMMON INJURIES

Head and Spine Injuries

Concussions will generally occur due to KOs from strikes and blows to the head. A rapid neurologic and cognitive assessment must be performed at multiple time points (ringside and postbout) to ensure a fighter's health and safety. Most combatants recover within seconds, but will display some form of posttraumatic amnesia (e.g., will not recall how the round ended). Any fighter who remains unresponsive, unconscious, confused, combative, has unsteady gait, and/or reports persistent headache, nausea, vision changes, with associated vomiting and/or neck pain will need to be transferred immediately via EMS to the nearest level-1 trauma hospital for imaging and ready access to neurosurgical services. **Facial and scalp lacerations** are important to be wary of, especially if located in areas that interfere and obscure vision (e.g., lacrimal border and tarsal plate of the eyelid) and/or areas which may further tear (the vermilion border of the lip of the fighter). If a deep laceration is found in these zones, the ringside physician should consider ending the bout. **Oral, ocular, ear/nose/throat traumas** are a common occurrence in this sport. More visible injuries such as **"cauliflower" ear (auricular hematomas),** which are also seen in wrestlers, may be managed by simple aspiration and suturing, but more advanced cases which occlude the auricular canal or affect hearing, require surgical treatment. Other potentially life-threatening injuries include airway compression and/or if there is an unstable nasal fracture, a deeper zygomatic fracture is suspected. Unstable nasal bridge fractures, persistent epistaxis involving blood in the oropharynx despite compression, blunt trauma to the anterior or posterior neck due to a chokehold are all conditions a ring/cageside physician must evaluate and rule out at the time of injury and postbout. Prompt emergency supportive care and rapid transfer to a nearest level-1 trauma center is key in fighters with compromised cardiopulmonary statuses. **Cervical spine injuries** must be taken into consideration always whenever the fighter sustains a KO and his or her face contacts the mat/ring/fence (with risk for second impact syndrome) and/or when the fighter undergoes a chokehold injury.[7] A focused cognitive, skin, vascular, and neuromusculoskeletal exam that may include Sport Concussion Assessment Tool (SCAT) exam is vital to ensure the fighter has not sustained a significant whiplash injury, cervical radiculopathy, fracture, or in rare cases, a vertebral artery dissection, in addition to a concussion. With a loss due to a rear naked chokehold (chokehold placed with fighter posterior to opponent), the larynx, respiratory, and neurocognitive status will need to be assessed immediately and postfight, whereas with a loss due to a guillotine chokehold (chokehold placed anterior to opponent), a similar assessment will need to be completed. However, since this is a vascular chokehold, examination of any significant headache and neck pain, of skin for any ecchymoses, of facial symmetry, and of range of motion will also need to be carefully completed.

Upper Limb Injuries

Hand fractures, contusions, and sprains to the fingers and wrist are common upper limb injuries. Although there are no large studies looking at hand/wrist injuries in MMA fighters, it is expected that when fighters use techniques originating from boxing and grappling, then similar injuries such as metacarpal fractures, interphalangeal and thumb subluxation/dislocation injuries, and acute wrist sprains and tendinopathies may occur. Management is generally conservative with cool compresses, rest, and possibly bracing/splinting. In cases where a fracture is suspected that affects the ability of the combatant to fight safely, then the decision to end the bout should be advised. Initial management includes pain control, bracing, and to have at least plain films completed.[8] **Elbow sprains** and **subluxation/dislocation injuries** may occur if a fighter does not tap out during an armbar lock (elbow is placed in hyperextension). A neurovascular exam is important to ensure that the fighter has full strength, full range of motion with no laxity, sensation, and circulation of the limb. The ringside physician should watch for any focal compression neuropathies such as ulnar neuropathic symptoms. Management includes relative rest and referral to physical therapy. **Shoulder injuries** may occur similar to boxing. Injuries to the **rotator cuff, labrum, acromioclavicular and sternoclavicular joint sprains** and **fractures** are all possible due to the repetitive stress of using the affected shoulder when striking and/or when defending oneself. Acute management may involve reduction, immobilization with a sling, and pain control in cases of dislocation/subluxation at the glenohumeral joint. Any fractures, such as those involving the clavicle and proximal humerus, will need to be sent to the nearest level-1 trauma center and be seen by orthopedics.

Lower Limb Injuries

In contrast to boxing, lower limb injuries in MMA are common. Due to repetitive stresses, symptomatic **femoracetabular impingement** and **labral tears** may occur, as well as injuries to the knee due to kicking or joint locks **(meniscal, collateral ligament sprains/ tears)**. Management involves pain control and possible bracing if there is instability noted. **Ankle dislocation/subluxation** may occur if a fighter is placed in an ankle/heel lock. **Injury to the peroneal nerve** at the fibular head is possible due to sidekicks to the lower limb. Management and workup may include electrodiagnostics, bracing, and physical therapy.

Other Injuries

Blunt chest trauma can occur with strikes to the chest wall and/or during grappling. Injuries to the ribs are the most common and examination is necessary if there is significant tenderness or deformity noted that interferes with respiration. **Blunt abdominal trauma** due to striking or a kick to the right upper quadrant ("liver shot"), left upper quadrant, or posterior torso warrants careful examination of the abdomen and trunk. If a fighter still reports persistent pain or hematuria is noted after a short period of rest, hydration, and cool compresses during the postbout examination, then the fighter should be transferred to the hospital for further investigation with at least an abdominal CT to rule out a hepatic/splenic and/or renal injury, respectively. **Genital injuries** can occur due to an accidental blow or strike below the waistline (please refer to Chapter 11 *Boxing* for further management).

■ SUMMARY

MMA is a combat sport that will continue to grow in popularity and participation among multiple age groups. Being readily familiar with the rules and most common injuries and their associated mechanisms is important for ring/cageside physician coverage.

■ References

1. Buse GJ. No holds barred sport fighting: a 10 year review of mixed martial arts competition. *Br J Sports Med.* 2006;40:169-172. doi:10.1136/bjsm.2005.021295.

2. Lefton T. Fitness, sports in flux: paddle boarding, MMA show growth. https://www.sportsbusinessdaily .com/Journal/Issues/2016/08/29/Research-and-Ratings/Participation.aspx. Updated August 29, 2016.

3. Mixed martial arts unified rules of conduct. New Jersey State Athletic Control Board. https://www.nj.gov/ lps/sacb/docs/martial.html. Updated September 5, 2002.

4. Thomas RE, Thomas BC. Systematic review of injuries in mixed martial arts. *Phys Sportsmed.* 2018;46(2): 155-167. doi:10.1080/00913847.2018.1430451.

5. McClain R, Wassermen J, Mayfield C, et al. Injury profile of mixed martial arts competitors. *Clin J Sport Med.* 2014;24(6):497-501. doi:10.1097/JSM.0000000000000078.

6. Lystad RP, Gregory K, Wilson J. The epidemiology of injuries in mixed martial arts: a systematic review and meta-analysis. *Orthop J Sports Med.* 2014;2(1):2325967113518492. doi:10.1177/2325967113518492.

7. Kochhar T, Back D, Mann B, et al. Risk of cervical injuries in mixed martial arts. *Br J Sports Med.* 2005;39: 444-447. doi:10.1136/bjsm.2004.011270.

8. Pomerantz ML. Hand and wrist injuries in mixed martial arts. In: Luchetti R, Pegoli L, Bain G, eds. *Hand and Wrist Injuries in Combat Sports.* Cham, Switzerland: Springer; 2018:63-76.

■ Further Reading

Committee report on unified rules for MMA. https://www.abcboxing.com/committee-report-on-unified-rules -for-mma. Updated July 7, 2019.

Kelly M. *Fight Medicine: Diagnosis and Treatment of Combat Sports Injuries for Boxing, Wrestling, and Mixed Martial Arts.* Boulder, CO: Paladin Press; 2008.

Mixed martial arts (competition) participation report 2017. https://www.sfia.org/reports/553_Mixed-Martial -Arts-%28Competition%29-Participation-Report-2017.

20. RUGBY

Daniel P. Spunberg, Tiffany M. Lau, Vincent Lee, and Courtney Pinto

■ HISTORY

The sport of rugby was created in 1823 by William Webb Ellis. During a soccer match in the town of Rugby, England, Ellis used his hands to pick up the soccer ball and run it towards the opposition's goal. Since then, "Rugby Football" has evolved into a sport millions of people play and watch worldwide.[1,2]

■ GOVERNING ORGANIZATIONS

- International: World Rugby
- National: USA Rugby (formerly known as the United States of America Rugby Football Union)
- Major Professional Leagues: Major League Rugby, Women's Premier League
- College: USA Rugby
- High School: USA Rugby (Club), National Federation of State High School Associations (NFHS)

■ PARTICIPANTS

As of 2018, about 120,000 athletes participate in rugby football throughout the United States, including roughly 30,000 females and almost 90,000 males.[2] Additionally, the number of American high schools with NFHS-certified rugby teams more than doubled from 40 to 83 schools between the years 2012 and 2018.[3]

■ RULES AND REGULATIONS

In Rugby 15s, there are two 15-person teams in play. The offense has 80 minutes to advance the ball over the opponents' goal line, touching it to the ground to score a "try." Gameplay is continuous even after players are tackled on the field. The ball can be passed only backwards or sideways with no blocking allowed; kicking is the only method to move the ball forward. Phases known as "lineouts," "mauls," "rucks," and "scrums" are used to retain or take possession of the ball. A team may score by either a try, conversion, penalty, or drop goal. Total game time is 80 minutes split into two 40-minute halves with a 10-minute half time break. Rugby 7s has two 7-person teams that are in play and the rules reflect that of 15s with minor differences. Total game time is 14 minutes split into two 7-minute halves with a 2-minute half time break.

■ EQUIPMENT

Studs and **cleats** must conform with World of Rugby Specifications and must be no longer than 22 mm and without burring or sharp edges. **Shin guards** may be worn under socks and made of nonrigid fabric, no thicker than 0.5 cm when compressed. **Mouth guard** should not have any part extended outside the mouth. **Mitts** can cover only up to the outer joint of fingers and thumb and down to the wrist and must be made of stretch-type material with grip material made of soft rubber/synthetic compounds no greater than 1 mm in depth. **Shoulder pads** should be made of soft and thin material that can cover only shoulders and collar bone with a thickness no greater than 1 cm when uncompressed and density no greater than 45 kg/m.[3] **Headgear** should be made of soft and thin material with a thickness no greater than 1 cm when uncompressed and density no greater than 45 kg/m.[3] Women may wear **chest pads** made of soft and thin material with a thickness no greater than 1 cm when uncompressed and density no greater than 45 kg/m.[3] **Rugby ball** is elliptical in profile, typically made of either leather or synthetic material. The dimensions required are 28 to 30 cm long and 58 to 62 cm in circumference at the widest point.

》》》 Adaptive Sport Key Points: Rugby

The International Wheelchair Rugby Federation (IWRF) monitors the sport. Athletes who participate in wheelchair rugby are required to possess some form of disability, specifically with a loss of function in the upper and lower limbs. Wheelchair rugby is played by two teams of 12 players. Only four players from each team may be on the court at any time. Total game time is 32 minutes split into four 8-minute quarters. There is various adaptive equipment including manual custom-made sports wheelchairs, and the ball is a regulation volleyball typically of a "soft-touch" design.[3]

▥ MEDICAL COVERAGE LOGISTICS

The role of the on-site physician leader is to organize and coordinate the medical staff, develop an emergency action plan (EAP), and interact with the coaches and officials to help ensure the safety of the players and spectators. Prior to the game, it is important to identify available medical staff, support personnel, field map, and the available medical equipment. Sports medicine physicians and Emergency Medical Services (EMS) personnel, along with sports medicine fellows, residents, medical students, athletic trainers, or physical therapists can attend expected medical needs. Establishing an EAP is the most important task. Protocols and guidelines should include role definition of the medical staff, emergency transportation including personnel, routes, and adequate facilities with the capacity to evaluate and manage head and spine injuries, and an outline of the chain-of-command and communication standards. Contingency plans should be made for extreme temperature, humidity, and other weather conditions that may lead to game cancellation or postponement, or in game modifications like extra water breaks, especially at the youth level. Lastly, prior to the start of the competition, the medical team should confirm that players are wearing proper equipment. During the game the medical team and equipment is set up on the home team's sideline. The referee will notify the head medical provider if an injured player needs to be evaluated on the field. Communication between individual members of the medical staff, coaches, referees, emergency medical staff, and local medical facilities is essential via two or more systems (e.g., hand-held radios and cell phones). Lastly, documentation is essential for review after the game/season to evaluate utilization and plan for future coverage.

MEDICAL EMERGENCIES AND MEDICAL BAG ESSENTIALS

Medical Bag Essentials in Rugby	
Medical Emergencies:	**Fractures and Dislocations:**
Automated External Defibrillator (AED)	Immobilizers and Slings
Tourniquet	Crutches
Cricothyrotomy kit	**Wound Care:**
14- and 16-gauge needles	Normal saline
Epi 1:1,000	Betadine swabs
Diphenhydramine or another antihistamine	Neosporin, mupirocin ointment
Albuterol inhaler	Moleskin
Rectal thermometer	Elastic bandage
Ice bath	Tube stretch gauze
Head and Spine:	Sterile gauzes
Concussion evaluation form	Vaseline
Stretcher & Spine board	Steri-strips
Cervical orthosis	Suture tray
Save a tooth kit	Lidocaine 1%

The collapsed or unconscious athlete is considered a medical emergency that requires activation of the proper channels of communication and protocols including basic life support (BLS)/advanced cardiac life support (ACLS). Although rarely reported, nontraumatic emergencies can include cardiac conditions like arrhythmias and hypertrophic cardiomyopathy (HCM), anaphylaxis, asthma, and heat-related illness, specifically heat stroke. Musculoskeletal injuries that may become medical emergencies include, upper and lower limb fractures or dislocations with neurovascular compromise, traumatic brain injuries with or without spinal cord involvement, and blunt thoracoabdominal trauma with possible internal bleeding.

EPIDEMIOLOGY

There is a higher incidence of injuries and more severe injuries in rugby 7s than in rugby 15s. This may be related to the faster game pace and that there are fewer players on the field at any given time.[4] The most commonly injured body areas in rugby 7s are the lower (58.3%) and upper (21.4%) limbs.[4] The most common injuries are ligamentous knee injuries, shoulder dislocations, and ankle sprains. Concussions also occur at a significantly higher frequency and severity in Rugby 7s (8.3 concussions/1,000 player-match-hours) as compared to Rugby 15s (4.5 concussions/1,000 player-match-hours), due primarily to tackling in rugby 7s and collisions in rugby 15s.[5] Shoulder injuries are common and occur as a result of either direct player-to-player impact or contact with the ground and are also the most common area injured in wheelchair rugby.[6]

COMMON INJURIES

Head and Spine Injuries

Rugby, as is true of other contact sports, is associated with a high potential for **concussions**. This is due to the speed and contact inherent to the sport. Symptoms include confusion, dizziness, headaches, nausea, and, in severe cases, loss of consciousness. Remove the player from play and conduct a neurological exam including a Sport

Concussion Assessment Tool (SCAT) test. If no red flags are observed, then the player may remain on the sideline without his or her equipment. Periodic assessment should follow until cleared to leave with a parent if under age. The athlete will need to follow up with a sports medicine provider in 24 to 48 hours for further assessment. Second impact syndrome is a possible complication if a concussed brain suffers another impact before resolution of the initial injury. **Cervical spine injuries** can result in quadriplegia or even death. Many of the cervical spine injuries that are reported in rugby play occur from a buckling of the spinal column. According to recent data, injuries are more likely to occur during the "tackle" as compared to the "scrum." The lower cervical spine is more often affected than the upper cervical spine. Rare incidences of Jefferson fractures (fracture of the C1 vertebrae) have been documented; however, cervical injuries are more common in the lower vertebral levels, particularly at the C4/5 and C5/6 motion segment. Of all, **facet dislocations** are the most commonly observed cervical spine injuries. Trauma to the spinal cord can occur in conjunction with fractures or dislocations. The recommended technique to transfer the injured player with a suspected cervical spine injury is the lift-and-slide technique which requires eight individuals: one at the head, three on each side, and one controlling the spinal board. The other technique is the log roll and requires at least four providers: one controlling the head, two the body, and one the spinal board. They should be transported to the ED for further evaluation.

Upper Limb Injuries

A **Shoulder dislocation** can be caused by a blow to an abducted, externally rotated, and extended arm. Anterior dislocation is most common. The acromion appears prominent in thin individuals and there is typically a loss of the normal rounded appearance of the shoulder. **Bony injuries** include those to the glenoid labrum, known as a "Bankart lesion," and to the humeral head, known as a "Hills-Sachs lesion," often associated with glenohumeral joint (GHJ) dislocations and may require surgical management if the athlete wants to continue a collision sport. **Rotator cuff tears** occur as a result of falling on an outstretched arm or by lifting something heavy with a jerking motion. Acute tears can cause intense pain felt as a snapping sensation with immediate weakness in the arm. Players should be removed from play and x-ray of the shoulder, MRI and/or ultrasound of the shoulder should be obtained. Partial tears can be treated conservatively with physical therapy and nonsteroidal anti-inflammatory drugs (NSAIDs). Complete tears may require surgical intervention. **Acromioclavicular (AC) joint injury** results from a sprain or tear of the ligaments around the AC joint. The mechanism of injury can be due to direct trauma to the lateral shoulder or due to falling on the point of the shoulder during a tackle. Symptoms include tenderness over the AC joint, and on exam, one may feel a gap with displacement of the acromion from the clavicle. When there is suspicion for this injury, players should be removed from play and an x-ray of the shoulder should be obtained. Most AC joint injuries will heal with conservative measures; however, some injuries may require surgical intervention depending on injury severity. **Hand fractures** include **Bennett's fractures** (fracture of the first metacarpal which extends into the carpometacarpal joint), **metacarpal fractures**, and **fracture/dislocations of the proximal interphalangeal (PIP) joint** are commonly seen. In most cases, the hand fractures will heal with nonsurgical management; however, in certain instances, hand fractures will require surgery to realign and stabilize the fracture fragments. Any open fracture will require emergent surgery.

Lower Limb Injuries

Lower limb injuries are more common. **Contusions** and **hematomas of the lower limb** occur due to blunt trauma. Treatment includes rest, ice (20–30 minutes following the injury), elevation, light compression wrapping, and acetaminophen for pain relief. *Anterior cruciate ligament (ACL) injuries* occur more frequently in the female rugby athlete. Classic signs and symptoms of an ACL tear include a report of a "pop," deep knee pain, and swelling. Increased laxity in the forward translation of the tibia or a lack of an "end point" on Lachman's test may indicate a tear in the ACL. Definitive diagnosis requires MRI. Surgical treatment in a high-level collision/contact athlete is often surgical. *Meniscal injuries* are caused by forceful twisting or rotation of the knee. These injuries are associated with pain localizing to the medial or lateral aspect of the knee, locking or clicking of the knee, and/or delayed or intermittent swelling. MRI is needed for diagnosis; these injuries can be managed operatively or nonoperatively depending on the severity. *Ankle sprains* are caused by inversion of the ankle in a plantarflexed or dorsiflexed foot. The anterior talofibular ligament (ATFL) and the calcaneofibular ligament (CFL) are the two ligaments most frequently injured. Symptoms include pain with weight-bearing or inability to bear weight, swelling, ecchymoses, and recurrent instability. On physical exam there may be focal tenderness and swelling over the involved ligament(s). Radiographs may be needed to rule out a fracture; otherwise initial management includes protection, rest, ice, compression and elevation (PRICE), followed by neuromuscular, proprioceptive, and strengthening training before return to sport.

SUMMARY

Rugby is a contact sport that can be played in many forms. The nature of the high-velocity movement and continuous game play in the sport places the rugby athlete at a heightened susceptibility for significant and/or severe injuries. As a clinician during sideline coverage, it is crucial to be able to recognize when players warrant removal from play, thereby preventing the development of more devastating injuries.

References

1. World Rugby. World rugby handbook. https://www.world.rugby/handbook. Published June 6, 2017.

2. USA Rugby. Rugby 101: how the sport works. https://www.usarugby.org/rugby101.

3. National Federation of State High School Associations. Participation statistics. https://members.nfhs.org/participation_statistics.

4. Toohey LA, Drew MK, Finch CF, et al. A 2-year prospective study of injury epidemiology in elite Australian rugby sevens: exploration of incidence rates, severity, injury type, and subsequent injury in men and women. *Am J Sports Med*. 2019;47(6):1302-1311. doi:10.1177/0363546518825380.

5. Fuller CW, Taylor A, Raftery M. Epidemiology of concussion in men's elite Rugby-7s (Sevens World Series) and Rugby-15s (Rugby World Cup, Junior World Championship and Rugby Trophy, Pacific Nations Cup and English Premiership). *Br J Sports Med*. 2015;49(7):478-483. doi:10.1136/bjsports-2013-093381.

6. Soo Hoo JA, Latzka E, Harrast MA. A descriptive study of self-reported injury in non-elite adaptive athletes. *PM R*. 2018. doi:10.1016/j.pmrj.2018.08.386.

Further Reading

International Wheelchair Rugby Federation. Introduction to wheelchair rugby. https://www.iwrf.com/?page=about_our_sport. Published 2012.

Kaplan KM, Goodwillie A, Strauss EJ, Rosen JE. Rugby injuries: a review of concepts and current literature. *Bull NYU Hosp Jt Dis*. 2008;66(2):86-93. http://hjdbulletin.org/files/archive/pdfs/414.pdf.

21. WATER POLO

Francisco De la Rosa

HISTORY

Water polo originated in Britain in the 1870s, fashioned after rugby, and further developed in Scotland in the 1890s adopting football-style rules. Water polo was played with a hard ball manufactured in India called a "pulu," which was pronounced "polo," which influenced the name of the game.[1,2]

GOVERNING ORGANIZATIONS

- International: Fédération Internationale de Natation (FINA)
- National: USA Water Polo (USAWP)
- Major Water polo leagues: FINA World Water Polo league
- College: National Collegiate Athletic Association (NCAA)
- High School: National Federation of State High School Associations (NFHS)

PARTICIPANTS

According to USAWP, nationwide membership jumped 25% in the last 5 years, from 35,750 in 2011 to 44,773 in 2016.[3] High school water polo participation is also growing nationwide. The NFHS reported that women's high school water polo grew 7.9%, while men's water polo increased 5.5% during the 5 years from 2011 to 2016. During this period, mainstream high school sports such as football, soccer, wrestling, field hockey, indoor volleyball, and basketball registered declines in varsity participation.[3]

RULES AND REGULATIONS

The duration of the game is 32 minutes of game time divided into four 8-minute periods with 2 minutes break between quarters and 5 minutes at half time. Each team consists of a maximum of 13 players: 11 field players and two goalkeepers. There are seven players, one of whom is the goalkeeper playing at a time for each team. The objective of the game is to score more goals than the opposite team during the game.

EQUIPMENT

The **water polo cap** has a chin strap and plastic cups over ears, called "ear guards." They should be worn at any time (water and bench). A swim cap is the only item to be worn below a water polo cap. **Mouth guards** are custom made for each player; they are mandatory in college and high school, but FINA does not require them. Players should wear nontransparent, one-piece competitive **swimsuits**. Suits shall completely cover the buttocks and breasts in females. The girls' suits shall have a solid high back with broad straps (style optional for goalkeepers). Before taking part in a game, all players must remove any articles likely to cause injury, including, but not limited to jewelry, medical or religious medals, watches, and swim goggles. Sharp fingernails and toenails must

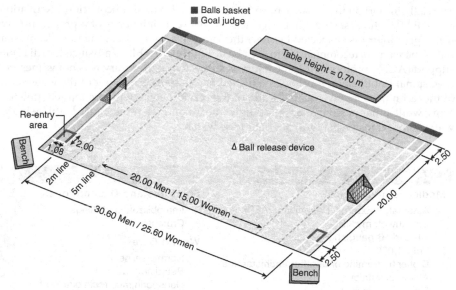

Figure 21.1 Water polo pool for Olympic games.

be trimmed. The referee may direct the player to remove items deemed to likely cause injury, including the trimming of nails.[4]

>>> **Adaptive Sport Key Points: Water Polo**

At this time there is no official Paralympic or Special Olympics rules or participation for water polo. World Water Polo Referees and Italian Paralympic Sports Federation recognizes it as a promotional sport. Teams are composed of 10 to 13 male or female athletes (at least 12 years old), at least five athletes with a disability (athletes with physical disability or athletes with intellectual relationship disability). In the water there should always be at least three athletes with a disability.[5]

▣ MEDICAL COVERAGE LOGISTICS

Prior to competition, confirm available healthcare personnel including physicians, certified lifeguard, and emergency medical technicians (EMTs). It is recommended to have an ambulance with EMT personnel on site for quick transport to the nearest trauma center. An Emergency Action Plan (EAP) should be available and reviewed with all personnel prior to the event day and rechecked on event day making sure no changes need to be made to best ensure efficient and appropriate care when necessary. Medical personnel should be familiar with and trained in water rescue and spine boarding. The medical provider with other support staff should establish an open line of communication with coaches, referees and other staff. FINA regulations require that the water temperature should be 26°C plus or minus 1°C (25°C–27°C = 77°F–80.6°F). Injuries or events should be documented for record keeping and future event planning.

▣ MEDICAL EMERGENCIES AND MEDICAL BAG ESSENTIALS

Water polo is unique because the physician or trainer must rely on other players and/ or lifeguards to bring the injured athlete to the pool side for evaluation; assistance is especially important in cases where an injured player becomes unconscious. Activation of the EAP is the first step. Time is critical to ensure maintenance of a proper airway. If no spine injury is suspected because the injury was witnessed, then quick transfer out of the water is recommended to start basic life support (BLS)/advanced cardiac life support (ACLS) protocols. If spine injury is suspected or the injury was not witnessed, then spinal stabilization must be established before transferring out of the water. One of the techniques involves stabilization of the cervical spine with the injured athlete's arms, while other personnel bring the spine board and strap the injured athlete in the water before transferring him/her out of the water.

Medical Bag Essentials in Water Polo	
Medical Emergencies:	**Fractures and Dislocations:**
Automated External Defibrillator (AED)	Immobilizers and Slings
Cricothyrotomy kit	Crutches
14- and 16-gauge needles	**Wound Care:**
Epi 1:1,000	Normal saline
Diphenhydramine or another antihistamine	Betadine swabs
Albuterol inhaler	Neosporin, mupirocin ointment
Floatation devices	Moleskin
Head and Spine:	Elastic bandage
Concussion evaluation form	Tube stretch gauze
Stretcher & Spine board	Sterile gauzes
Cervical orthosis	Vaseline
Save a tooth kit	Steri-strips
	Suture tray
	Lidocaine 1%

▥ EPIDEMIOLOGY

Water polo is a very physical contact sport. Head and face injuries are most common, along with upper limbs, especially shoulder and hand. More than 57% of all injuries, and 90% of the 10 most severe injuries, were reported to have occurred due to contact with another player. Water polo has higher rates of contact injuries than the other aquatic disciplines of swimming, diving, synchro, and open-water swimming. Almost three-quarters of the injuries were not expected to result in time-loss from sport, and 83.8% of time-loss injuries were classified as "mild." The incidence of match injuries was on average 56.2 injuries per 1,000 match hours. The rate of time-loss injuries was almost five times higher in matches than in training.[2]

▥ COMMON INJURIES

Head and Spine Injuries

The most frequent *head injuries* include *contusions* (31.3%) and *lacerations* (36.5%).[2] *Concussions* are thought to be under-reported due to fear of being pulled out of the game. Meanwhile, face lacerations are common in water polo games. Bleeding should be addressed immediately, as the referee will take the player out. As soon as the player is no longer bleeding, he or she may return to the game. Direct contact with another player carries sufficient force to fracture the thinner bones of the face. *Fractures of the facial bones* represent severe head and face injuries, and immediate medical evaluation and x-ray assessment are necessary. In all facial or head injuries, players must be closely monitored for signs of disorientation, poor balance, and co-ordination. Also, the patient must be awakened at regular intervals during the night for the first 24 hours. If a concussion is diagnosed, then a graduated return to sport protocol is initiated. The most frequent **eye injuries** in water polo can be roughly divided into three main categories. **Corneal abrasions** occur as a result of a scratch from either a fingernail or foreign body. Treatment is antibiotic eye drops and pad-ding of the eye. **Hyphema** is bleeding into the anterior chamber of the eye as a result from ruptured iris vessels. It may be visible on slit lamp examination. The aim of the treatment is to prevent further bleeding, which may in turn result in uncontrollable glaucoma or blood staining of the cornea. The patient needs to rest in bed while the hemorrhage clears, usually 3 to 5 days. **Blow-out fracture of the orbit** is the result from a direct trauma caused by a fist or a ball. Compression of the globe and orbital con-tents produces a fracture in the weakest part of the orbit, the orbital floor. Contents of the orbit may herniate through the defect. The patient typically presents with a periorbital hematoma, protruding or sunken eye, double vision on upward gaze, and numbness of the cheek. A detailed examination of the eye must be performed to exclude intraocular injuries. Surgery may be required to release the trapped muscle and repair the bony defect.[6] **Traumatic perforation of the tympanic membrane** is un-fortunately a fairly common injury in water polo. The injury is the result of a slap on the side of the head with a cupped palm. This causes a dramatic rise in pressure in the canal. The increased pressure causes rupturing and development of a hole in the tympanic membrane. In most of the cases, this injury will heal without any signifi-cant impairment, but during the healing phase, players should be kept out of water, or use a molded earplug and a bathing cap.[6] Although the International Dental Fed-eration classifies water polo as a medium risk sport for dental injury, with frequent body contact the risk is high. Despite this, FINA does not require the use of a mouth guard, with only 7.7% of athletes reported wearing a mouth guard, but nearly 50% of those athletes reported witnessing a dental injury in water polo, with 21% reported having suffered a tooth injury while playing water polo, the most common being **tooth fracture**.[7,8] The broken portion of the tooth must be placed in milk or save-a-tooth solution and dentist evaluation must be made within 24 hours. The athlete may finish the game. Special consideration is taken for an avulsed toot. Emergency treatment is required which consists of reimplantation if possible and transfer to a dentist immediately.

Repetitive cervical spine rotation required for breathing in freestyle swimming often produces **neck pain**. A relatively common injury that can be extremely painful for the player is acute wry neck or **torticollis**. It is characterized by a sudden onset of sharp neck pain with deformity and limitation of movement. It occurs either after a sudden, quick movement or upon awakening. A **stinger** can occur after a direct blow from an opponent player or acute acceleration/deceleration. It is characterized by moderate to severe arm pain with or without motor-sensory. Neck pain may or may not be a feature. The pain is aggravated by the movements of the cervical spine. There may be associated sensory symptoms. In older athletes or those who had previously suffered trauma to the neck, **cervical facet arthropathy** can be present. **Low back pain** is a common symptom in water polo players because the amount of rotational forc-es is significant during throwing and passing the ball. Any of the pain-producing structures of the lumbar spine may cause low back pain, but the **facet syndrome** and **radiculopathy** are the most common causes. These may include abnormalities of the ligaments of the intervertebral joints, muscles, and fascia, as well as neural structures. In the acute phase, the most appropriate treatment is rest in a position of maximum comfort with administration of analgesics, followed by physiotherapy to stabilize the spine. Spinal interventions can be considered in refectory cases and surgery may be required if neurological signs persist or worsen or bowel or bladder symptoms are present.

Upper Limb Injuries

Water polo players are at risk of **traumatic dislocations of the glenohumeral and the acromioclavicular joints** from contact with opponent players or the ball. Both injuries usually occur to the throwing arm during the act of shooting or passing the ball, when the player has the arm in cocking position. The force may be great enough to rupture the anterior capsule and glenohumeral ligament complex (Bankart lesion), resulting in anteroinferior subluxation or dislocation. Posterior dislocation is less frequent. Closed reduction of acute shoulder dislocation is a treatment of choice and follow-up imaging to assess for proper relocation and secondary injuries.[7] Injuries to the elbow, wrist, and hand are less frequent than the head/face and shoulder. **Ulnar collateral ligament injuries** ("gamekeeper's thumb"), **osteochondritis dissecans of the capitellum, de Quervain's tenosynovitis, and lacerations or dislocations of the interphalangeal and metacarpophalangeal joints, and fractures of the phalanges and metacarpal bones** are the most common elbow, wrist, and hand injuries in water polo.[6,7] Evaluation should be performed, and depending on injury severity, a decision whether to tape or immobilize the joint must be made. FINA does not allow players to compete with any taping.

Lower Limb Injuries

Lower limb injuries are less common, but still important to consider, with contusions and sprains as the most common injury types. Water polo is unique in the use of the eggbeater kick to help athletes tread water and propel themselves out of the water as required for both offense when shooting as well as a defensive posture to block shots or passes. Expert water polo players can produce a considerable amount of explosive force over a very short time (161 ms) to propel themselves about 1 m above the water. It seems intuitive that this large amount of repetitive force may lead to hip/knee/foot pain, similar to breaststroke swimmers, but the authors were not able to find any published data on this topic in water polo. Prevention and treatment should focus on proper eggbeater technique and adequate warm-up of the legs before play.[7]

Abdominal and Groin Injuries

Abdominal and groin injuries can occur in water polo as a result of underwater grappling and kicking. This is difficult to police during matches because the referees are located out of the water on the pool deck and therefore underwater activities are often not seen. Grappling injuries may include **trauma to intra-abdominal organs (e.g., spleen), genitals (men), and breasts (women).**

▒ SUMMARY

Water polo is a game that combines strength and resistance along with speed, precision, and team play. As a contact sport, traumatic injuries are frequent, and it demands special attention due to its unique aquatic environment.

▒ References

1. Fédération Internationale de Natation. Water polo: origins. http://www.fina.org/content/origins-2.

2. Mountjoy M, Miller J, Junge A. Analysis of water polo injuries during 8904 player matches at FINA World Championships and Olympic games to make the sport safer. *Br J Sports Med.* 2019;53(1):25-31. doi:10.1136/bjsports-2018-099349.

3. Rieder D. Water polo one of fastest-growing sports in U.S., according to NFHS. https://www.swimming worldmagazine.com/news/water-polo-one-of-fastest-growing-sports-in-u-s-according-to-nfhs. Published January 31, 2017.

4. 2018-20 NFHS water polo uniform rules. https://www.nfhs.org/media/1020368/2018-20-nfhs-water-polo -uniform-rules.pdf. Published August 1, 2019.

5. Paralympic water polo in Italy. http://wwpra.org/wwr-news/newsid510/67. Published June 23, 2017.

6. Franić M, Ivković A, Rudić R. Injuries in water polo. *Croat Med J.* 2007;48(3):281-288. https://www.ncbi .nlm.nih.gov/pmc/articles/PMC2080536.

7. Spittler J, Keeling J. Water polo injuries and training methods. *Curr Sports Med Rep.* 2016;15(6):410-416. doi:10.1249/JSR.0000000000000305.

8. Hersberger S, Krastl G, Kühl S, Filippi A. Dental injuries in water polo, a survey of players in Switzerland. *Dental Traumatol.* 2012;28(4):287-290. doi:10.1111/j.1600-9657.2011.01083.x.

Further Reading

ABC aquatic lifeguards: spinal backboarding procedure - shallow water. https://www.youtube.com/watch?v= De6z2gCKptk. Published February 17, 2014.

Fédération Internationale de Natation. Part X: FINA facilities rules 2017–2021. https://www.fina.org/sites/ default/files/2017_2021_facilities_06102017_full_medium.pdf.

22. WRESTLING

Michael R. Baria and Bryant Walrod

■ HISTORY

Records of wrestling have been found in ancient Sumerian and Egyptian cultures. At the inception of the modern Olympic Games, wrestling was contested in Greco-Roman only, with freestyle introduced in 1904. One-hundred years later, women's freestyle was introduced into the Olympic program.

■ GOVERNING ORGANIZATIONS

- International: United World Wrestling (UWW)
- National: USA Wrestling (USAW)
- Collegiate: National Collegiate Athletic Association (NCAA)
- High School: National Federation of State High School Associations (NFSHSA)

■ PARTICIPANTS

In a 2017–18 survey of high school athletes, wrestling was the seventh most popular boys' sport with 245,564 participants nationally. Girls' high school wrestling grew by 13.5%, for a total of 16,562 athletes. There were 76 Division I NCAA Teams in 2018–19, with three teams to be added. Women's college wrestling achieved a milestone with the NCAA recommending it receive "emerging sport" status in 2019. If accepted, women's wrestling will attain full NCAA championship status.

■ RULES AND REGULATIONS

There are two main positions in all wrestling styles: a) Neutral: athletes are on their feet and attempt to gain control of their opponents by forcing them to the mat; b) Par terre: both wrestlers are on the mat. The wrestler in the "top" position attempts to turn and pin the opponent, while the "bottom" wrestler defends.

Olympic Styles

Greco-Roman (men only): Technique is limited to upper body only. The athlete may use only the arms to attack the opponent's torso/upper body. No use of or contact with the lower body is permitted. Therefore, high-amplitude throws are more common and increase injury risk.

Freestyle (men and women): Arms and legs can be used to attack any portion of the opponent (tackling, tripping, throwing, etc).

In both styles, par terre is limited to a few seconds. If scoring does not occur quickly, the official will bring both athletes back to their feet to resume the neutral position. There are two 3-minute periods.

Folkstyle/Scholastic: Practiced exclusively in the United States (youth through NCAA). Similar to freestyle except par terre position can continue throughout the period, regardless of scoring. Periods: In high school, there are three 2-minute periods. In the NCAA, the first period is 3 minutes, followed by two 2-minute periods.

EQUIPMENT

All levels of folkstyle wrestling require headgear for auricular hematoma prevention. Headgear is not mandatory internationally and must be approved by UWW.

> ### ⟫ Adaptive Sport Key Points: Wrestling
>
> Currently it is not a Paralympic sport after a short presence in 1980 and 1984. Categories were based on weight class and type of disability. The rules were similar to able-body wrestling. Only men could participate.

MEDICAL COVERAGE LOGISTICS

The role of the medical director and/or on-site physician leader is to organize and coordinate the medical staff, develop an emergency action plan (EAP), and interact with the event director to help ensure the safety of the competitors and spectators. Prior to the competition, it is important to identify available medical staff, support personnel, venue map, and the available medical equipment. Protocols and guidelines should include role definition of the medical staff, emergency transportation including personnel, routes and adequate facilities, preferably a trauma center with capacity to manage brain and cervical spine injuries, and an outline of the chain-of-command and communication standards. Some wrestling events have several matches occurring on multiple mats.[1] It is important to have medical personnel assigned to each mat. Injury time varies by level of competition. At the high school level a total of 2 minutes of injury time and 5 minutes of "blood time" to stop bleeding is allowed while collegiate rules allow for 90 seconds of injury time, and "blood time" is at the discretion of the referee. In freestyle and Greco-Roman wrestling, both injury time and "blood time" are at the discretion of the head physician at the competition.[1] Lastly, documentation is essential for review after the event to evaluate utilization and plan for future events.

MEDICAL EMERGENCIES AND MEDICAL BAG ESSENTIALS

The collapsed or unconscious athlete is considered a medical emergency that requires activation of the proper channels of communication and protocols including basic life support (BLS)/advanced cardiac life support (ACLS). Although rarely reported, nontraumatic emergencies can include anaphylaxis, asthma, heat-related illness, specifically heat stroke, cardiac arrhythmias, and hypertrophic cardiomyopathy. Musculoskeletal injuries that may become medical emergencies include, facial, upper and lower limb fractures or dislocations with neurovascular compromise, traumatic brain injuries with or without spinal cord involvement, and blunt thoracoabdominal trauma with possible internal bleeding.

EPIDEMIOLOGY

At the collegiate level, injury rate is estimated at 19.6 per 1,000 exposures. Over a 9-year surveillance period, 96% of division I college wrestlers sustained either a musculoskeletal or concussive injury or a dermatologic lesion.[2] High school injury rates are lower at 2.33 per 1,000 exposures.[3] High school wrestling has the second highest injury rate behind football.[3,4] Knee and shoulder injuries are most common, typically from an opponent applying a torque/twisting force at the joint.[4]

Medical Bag Essentials in Wrestling	
Medical Emergencies:	**Wound/Laceration/Skin Care:**
Automated External Defibrillator (AED)	Normal saline
Nitroglycerin (sublingual)	Betadine swabs
Aspirin	Neosporin, mupirocin ointment
Epi 1:1,000	Moleskin
Diphenhydramine or another antihistamine	Elastic bandage
Albuterol inhaler	Tube stretch gauze
Rectal thermometer	Sterile gauzes
Ice bucket	Vaseline
14- and 16-gauge needles	Steri-strips
	Suture tray
Head and Spine:	Lidocaine 1%
Concussion evaluation form	Nasal pack
Stretcher & Spine board	Silver nitrate
Cervical orthosis	**Others:**
Cricothyrotomy kit	Acetaminophen
Safe a tooth kit	Glucose tabs
Fractures and Dislocations:	
Immobilizers, Crutches. Slings	

■ COMMON INJURIES

Precompetition Medical Issues

Skin Infections and Return to Training and Competition[5]: Skin infections are common given prolonged skin-to-skin contact. All wrestlers undergo independent, precompetition skin examinations and, if failed, result in disqualification. Routine skin examinations by medical personnel should be performed regularly throughout the season to begin immediate treatment. Staphylococcus and streptococcus are common bacterial infections, which manifest as impetigo, cellulitis, folliculitis, and abscesses. Required treatment: 72 hours of appropriate antibiotic therapy and 48 hours of no new lesions. Herpes gladiatorum (herpes simplex virus I) is a painful and/or pruritic vesicular lesion, typically on the face or upper limbs. Required treatment: 5 days of antiviral therapy (longer for a primary outbreak with systemic symptoms) and 3 days of no new lesions. Tinea (ringworm) presents as a flaky ring with central clearing on the scalp, face, or limbs. Required treatment: a) Limb lesions: 3 days of oral or topical treatment, b) Scalp/facial lesions: 2 weeks of oral treatment.

Weight cycling/cutting[6]: Weight cutting is ubiquitous in the sport. Rationale includes: a) minimizing body fat/maximizing muscle mass to confer a competitive advantage and b) making starting line-up if multiple athletes are clustered around a single weight class. In order to reduce weight leading up to weigh-ins, many dehydrate by exercising in layered clothes, using saunas or sauna suits, or taking diuretics. Medical staff should pay close attention to all athletes leading up to competition. If they exhibit "red flags" of dehydration or rhabdomyolysis (altered mental status, hematuria, cardiovascular compromise) the weight cut must be stopped, and the athlete should begin immediate rehydration and be transported for further evaluation. Oral rehydration should be used unless the athlete cannot tolerate oral intake.

In Competition Injuries

Facial lacerations/nasal epistaxis: Bleeding requires match stoppage until hemostasis is achieved. If control is not achieved in a very short time (no more than 5 minutes, cumulative, depending on competition level), the athlete is forced to forfeit. Therefore, knowledge of hemostatic techniques is imperative. Lacerations on the bridge of nose, under the chin, or over the orbital bone should be treated with careful application of silver nitrate and covered with an occlusive dressing. Lacerations above the eye should also be treated with silver nitrate and wrapped with athletic tape. Definitive suturing should be deferred until after the match. If suturing is performed between matches, vertical mattress sutures provide strong approximation and should be covered. Prophylactic antibiotics are not required unless there was clear exposure of laceration to an opponent with an active skin infection. **Nasal epistaxis** should be packed with dental cotton rolls coated in petroleum jelly. Examination for a septal hematoma should be performed after competition, as this requires specialist evaluation within 2 days to avoid complications such as cartilage necrosis. **Auricular hematomas**: Shearing forces across the ear cause hematoma formation between the perichondrium and cartilage layers. It is painful and if not treated leads to fibrotic scarring and permanent deformity (cauliflower ear). Severe deformities can block the external auditory canal and impair hearing. The hematoma can be aspirated through a large bore needle or through a small incision (in line with the helix). Postaspiration compression must be performed to prevent reaccumulation and is best achieved by using a mattress suture technique to fix dental cotton roles to the anterior and posterior ear. **Facial fractures** commonly result from direct trauma. While some have low morbidity (nasal fractures), others have significant consequences (orbital blow-out fracture) and must be recognized. **Nasal fracture** results in a visible deformity. Closed reduction can be performed once concomitant injuries are ruled out (septal hematoma, orbital fracture, etc). The wrestler may return to competition (use of protective facemask is permitted). Follow-up with otolaryngologist should occur soon after competition. **Orbital fracture** presents as eye pain, diplopia or impaired extraocular movements (sign of extraocular muscle entrapment). Athlete should be removed from competition immediately and evaluated emergently, as extraocular muscle entrapment rapidly causes muscle necrosis and permanent visual impairment (chronic diplopia). Athletes with a suspected orbital fracture should be explicitly instructed not to blow their nose, as this will push blood and mucous through the fracture and could lead to significant swelling and infectious complications.[7]

Spine Injuries

Cervical spine injuries include **radiculitis/radiculopathy** or **Brachial plexus neurapraxia ("stingers")**. Transient neurologic dysfunction includes paresthesias, pain, and weakness in a unilateral upper limb. It is due to direct axial loads to the cervical spine or an opponent pulling on head/neck. Same day return to sport is permitted if symptoms resolve, strength normalizes, and cervical spine is cleared. Persistent deficits (>24–48 hours) or recurrent symptoms warrant further work up, beginning with cervical spine MRI to evaluate for compressive lesions. Patients with bilateral upper limb symptoms must be treated as a cervical spinal cord injury. The cervical spine must be immobilized and transported to the trauma center for further work up (including a cervical spine MRI).

Upper Limb Injuries

Upper limb injuries are mostly traumatic in nature. **Joint dislocations (shoulder/elbow):** Mechanisms of injury include; a) fall on outstretched hand when bracing a fall, or b) torsional force applied by opponent. Athlete will feel joint dislocate and deformity is obvious. Examination must first rule out a neurovascular injury. One to two attempts at immediate reduction using simple traction can be attempted. If these attempts fail, reduction under anesthesia in a hospital setting is warranted. Postreduction films are required to evaluate for concomitant injuries such as Hill-Sachs lesions, bony Bankart lesions, and coronoid fractures. Shoulder dislocations have a high rate of redislocation in wrestling, so athletes should be monitored for chronic instability which would necessitate a surgical referral. *Ulnar collateral ligament (UCL) tears* typically occur from a valgus force with resultant medial pain. In competition, protective equipment (tape/hinged brace with soft cover) is permitted. In contrast to overuse UCL injuries seen in baseball, acute UCL injuries in wrestling have a favorable prognosis. Most wrestlers with acute UCL injuries can return to sport with a period of rest, rehabilitation, and bracing. Persistent pain or instability should prompt evaluation with a MRI and surgical consultation.

Lower Limb Injuries

Lower limb injuries involve mostly the knee. *Meniscus tears* are the most common knee injury due to torsional/rotational and hyperflexion forces. Athletes may experience an acute mechanism with an obvious pop or locked knee with subsequent effusion. Repetitive hyperflexion moments (in routine offensive techniques) can lead to degenerative tears. Given the long-term consequences of meniscus tears, MRI and surgical consultation are recommended before continuing competition. *Posterolateral (PLC) corner/lateral collateral ligament (LCL) injuries* occur when an opponent applies a varus force at the knee, typically using the head or shoulder as a fulcrum on the medial knee. Wrestlers feel a pop or posterolateral/lateral pain. Both injuries should undergo MRI. PLC injuries warrant surgical consultation given the risk of chronic instability. Isolated LCL tears have an excellent prognosis and can be treated with a period of protection and functional rehabilitation. *Anterior cruciate ligament (ACL) injuries* are less common in wrestling because of the relative lack of cut-pivot movements. Some athletes will elect for surgical reconstruction, but wrestling is not an ACL-dependent sport so definitive management can be deferred until the conclusion of the season. *Prepatellar bursitis* results from: a) repetitive trauma (traumatic/hemorrhagic bursitis) or b) infection due to increased exposure to bacterial pathogens (septic bursitis, usually from staphylococcus). All cases should be assumed septic until proven otherwise. Aspiration and culture are mandatory for all cases. Injection with doxycycline can be performed at the time of aspiration to begin treatment of either entity (antibiotic for septic cases, acts as sclerosant in traumatic cases). Steroid injections should be avoided in all cases, as they lead to immunosuppression and could increase risk of conversion to septic bursitis. Septic bursitis should be sent to the Emergency Room for intravenous antibiotics and potential wash-out. For traumatic bursitis, recurrent cases should be referred to a knee surgeon.

▦ SUMMARY

Wrestling coverage poses the unique challenge of possible athlete disqualification secondary to dermatologic issues as well as neuromuscular injuries. A sports clinician should always be available at a wrestling event independent of the competition level.

▦ References

1. Kiningham R, Monseau A. Caring for wrestlers. *Curr Sports Med Rep.* 2015;14(5):404-412. doi:10.1249/JSR.0000000000000193.

2. Otero JE, Graves CM, Bollier MJ. Injuries in collegiate wrestlers at an elite division I NCAA wrestling program: an epidemiological study. *Iowa Orthop J.* 2017;37:65-70. https://medicine.uiowa.edu/orthopedics/sites/medicine.uiowa.edu.orthopedics/files/wysiwyg_uploads/2017%20-%20Volume%2037_0.pdf.

3. Yard EE, Collins CL, Dick RW, Comstock RD. An epidemiologic comparison of high school and college wrestling injuries. *Am J Sports Med.* 2008;36(1):57-64. doi:10.1177/0363546507307507.

4. Hewett TE, Pasque C, Heyl R, Wroble R. Wrestling injuries. *Med Sport Sci.* 2005;48:152-178. doi:10.1159/000084288.

5. Peterson AR, Nash E, Anderson BJ. Infectious disease in contact sports. *Sports Health.* 2019;11(1):47-58. doi:10.1177/1941738118789954.

6. Davis SE, Dwyer GB, Reed K, et al. Preliminary investigation: the impact of the NCAA wrestling weight certification program on weight cutting. *J Strength Cond Res.* 2002;16(2):305-307. doi:10.1519/1533-4287(2002)016<0305:pitiot>2.0.co;2.

7. Shuttleworth GN, David DB, Potts MJ, et al. Orbital trauma. Do not blow your nose. *BMJ.* 1999;318(7190):1054-1055. doi:10.1136/bmj.318.7190.1054.

▧ Further Reading

Kenter K, Behr CT, Warren RF, et al. Acute elbow injuries in the National Football League. *J Shoulder Elbow Surg.* 2000;9(1):1-5. doi:10.1016/S1058-2746(00)80023-3.

COVERAGE ESSENTIALS FOR LIMITED-CONTACT SPORTS

23. BASEBALL

Jason L. Zaremski

HISTORY

Baseball's origins begin in the 18th century when a combination of Rounders (a game reportedly played in early colonists) and Cricket were brought to the United States. The game slowly morphed into Baseball. In 1845 the New York Knickerbocker Baseball Club was founded with Alexander Joy Cartwright establishing a new set of rules the resemble baseball as we know it today.[1] As of 1871, the National Association of Professional Base Ball Players professional league was founded. Then, in 1876, the National League was created with the American league following in 1901. The world series began in 1903 and became an annual event, except for 1994, since 1905. Baseball became an Olympic sport in 1992 before being dropped after the 2008 games. It has been readded to the Olympics as of the 2020 games. Little League baseball (and softball), founded in 1939 by Carl Stotz, can include children from ages 4 to 16. The Little League world series has been played annually in Williamsport, Pennsylvania since 1947. As of 2000, Little League Baseball has more than 200,000 teams in all 50 states and more than 80 countries around the globe.[2]

GOVERNING ORGANIZATIONS

- International: The World Baseball Softball Confederation
- National (Professionally): Major League Baseball and Minor League Baseball
- College: National Collegiate Athletic Association (NCAA), National Association of Intercollegiate Athletics (NAIA), and National Junior College Athletic Association (NJCAA)
- High School: National Federation of State High School Associations
- Little League: Little League Baseball and Softball

PARTICIPANTS

Little league had more than 2.4 million participants,[3] nearly 500,000 at the high school (HS) level,[4] approximately 36,000 in college,[5] and more than 15.6 million ages 6 and up recreationally.[6] There are 30 major league teams (25 players per team) and 256 minor league teams (25–35 players per team based on level) in the United States.[7]

RULES AND REGULATIONS

The goal of baseball is to score more runs than the opposition. A Little League game is six innings up to age 12, seven innings ages 13 to 18, HS seven innings, and College, Minor and Major Leagues is nine innings. It is played on a diamond-shaped infield field with a fan shape extension to the outfield. A pitching mound is at the middle of the infield, 46 ft up to age 12 and 60 ft 6 in HS and older, from home plate. The distance between the bases is 50 ft in Tee ball, 60 ft up to age 12, and 90 ft HS and older. There are two teams, each with nine players playing at one time. The team in the field has a pitcher, catcher, first baseman, second baseman, shortstop, third baseman, and three outfielders at left field, center field, and right field, plus the batter from the opposing team.

■ EQUIPMENT

Baseball rules with respect to equipment vary to some degree based on age of the players and each association's rules. A *baseball* shall weight between 5 to 5 ¼ oz and have a circumference of 9 to 9 ¼ in. The *baseball bat* measurements vary by level of play and wood or nonwood bats must "not have exposed rivets, pins, rough or sharp edges, or any form of exterior fastener or attachment(s) that would present a potential hazard."[8] *Baseball cleats* cannot have pointed spikes similar to golf or track shoes. *Baseball gloves* size restrictions apply by position and level of play. All players must wear some form of *helmet* protection when batting. All players must wear a double ear flap helmet except for major league baseball players who may wear a single ear flap helmet. All baseball catchers wear a *head protector, mask with a throat protector, chest or body protector,* and *baseball shin guards*. In addition, males must wear a *protective cup*. As of January 1st, 2020, all HS catchers will be required to wear a chest protector, helmet and mask combination which includes having full ear protection with dual ear flaps that meets the National Operating Committee on Standards for Athletic Equipment (NOCSAE) standard at the time of manufacture.[9]

> **》》》 Adaptive Sport Key Points: Baseball**
>
> Established in 1989, the Little League Baseball Challenger Division is an adaptive baseball program for individuals with physical and intellectual challenges. Individuals— between ages 4 and 18 or up to age 22 if still enrolled in school—with an intellectual or physical challenge may participate. The Senior League Challenger Division is an adaptive baseball program that accommodates players ages 15 and up. There is no maximum age for the Senior League Challenger Division.[10]

■ MEDICAL COVERAGE LOGISTICS

Prior to each game, the sports medicine team should review the emergency action plan, check the battery in the Automated External Defibrillator (AED), and introduce themselves to the umpires as well as the opposition's sports medicine staff and (if present) emergency medical services team. While timing varies, this should be performed at least 30 minutes prior to first pitch, but ideally before the start of batting practice, if possible. Roles of the sports medicine providers should be reviewed before the start of the game. All umpires should be made aware of who should be contacted if an injured player, coach, or umpire needs evaluation.

■ MEDICAL EMERGENCIES AND MEDICAL BAG ESSENTIALS

Possible medical emergencies that one might encounter in a baseball game include a collapsed or unconscious athlete if hit by a thrown or batted ball to the head; chest injury and/or cardiac injury secondary to possible commotio cordis; acute joint injury resulting in fracture, instability, or dislocation. Heat-related injuries are less common in baseball but one should be prepared, particularly with baseball catchers, to treat athletes for potential heat illness.

Medical Bag Essentials in Baseball	
Medical Emergencies:	**Wound Care:**
AED	Normal saline
14- and 16-gauge needles	Betadine/Alcohol swabs
Epi 1:1,000	Neosporin, mupirocin ointment
Albuterol inhaler	Gauzes
	Steri-strips
Head and Spine:	Suture tray
Concussion evaluation form	Lidocaine 1%
Eye kit	Gloves
	Wound irrigation kit
Fractures and Dislocations:	
Immobilizers and Slings	
Crutches	

■ EPIDEMIOLOGY

Head injuries, mild traumatic brain injury (MTBI) or concussions, for all professional baseball players have been noted to be 0.42 per 1,000 athlete exposures (AEs) with an average of 9 days of lost time from sport.[11] Additionally, there was an increased representation of catchers sustaining injuries as opposed to other positions. As one would expect, injuries to the dominant upper limb in baseball are very common. At the professional level, 39% of injuries involve the upper limb with 39% occurring in pitchers.[12] At the HS level, the incidence rate for shoulder injury is 1.39/10,000 AEs with a greater likelihood of injury during games versus practice. Similar to the professional level, the majority of upper limb injuries were sustained by pitchers with the mechanism chronic overuse.[13] Injury risk factors include playing pitcher and catcher in the same game, pitching while fatigued, not adhering to pitch count regulations, throwing more than 8 months per year, pitching on consecutive days, excessive throwing when not pitching (e.g., playing catcher or participation in another throwing sport), use of a radar gun, and playing on multiple teams.[14] The overall elbow injury rate at the HS level is 0.86/1,000 AEs with nearly 57% of all injuries sustained by pitchers. The likelihood of sustaining an elbow injury during a game was significantly greater than during practice and considered chronic due to overuse, similar to shoulder injuries in the same age group. Of pitchers, 64.6% returned to play within 21 days; however, more than 11% of elbow injuries resulted in medical disqualification, more than double when compared to shoulder injuries. Ninety-six percent of elbow injuries were treated nonoperatively.[13] What this information suggests is that while ulnar collateral ligament (UCL) injuries have the potential to be serious, a majority of elbow injuries and UCL injuries may be managed nonoperatively and do not require surgical intervention.[12] Core musculature including the lumbar paraspinals and the abdominal oblique muscles are at high risk of injury due to the rotational aspect of the sport of baseball with constant acceleration and deceleration movements. While throwing injuries are very common in overhead throwing athletes, the most common injury in baseball players is a hamstring strain.[12] Sliding can result in ankle injuries nearly 14% of the time at the professional level, though this number increases to nearly 24% when the slide was feet first and is the most common location of injury during a feet-first slide; the location of the injury most commonly sustained was at second base.[15]

▪ COMMON INJURIES

Head and Spine Injuries

For **concussions** in any sport, and regardless of level of play, providers must be up to date on the appropriate treatment. This includes immediate removal from play and a full neurological assessment including a Sport Concussion Assessment Tool (SCAT) test should be administered. Periodic assessment following injury should be performed until the athlete is stable and cleared to go home or in the case of the under aged athlete allowed to leave with his/her parents. Further evaluation with a sports medicine provider and/or concussion specialist will be required for further assessment in the next 1 to 2 days.

Upper Limb Injuries

Rotator cuff (RC) tendon injury (tendinopathy/tear) is the second most common injury at the professional level and biceps tendinopathy is the fourth most common.[12] Pain and weakness are common symptoms with RC injury. A physical examination may detect isolated weakness and/or decreased range of motion. As with most throwing-related injuries, rest from throwing is initially recommended until the player is asymptomatic. A rehabilitation program should be initiated to incorporate strengthening of the scapular and RC muscles as well as improving mechanics of throwing and range of motion (ROM) of the spine. As with all throwing-related injuries, return to competition is recommended once the athlete is asymptomatic and has completed a functional throwing program without pain. ***Internal impingement***, a result of contact between the posterosuperior glenoid and the greater tuberosity in positions of overhead throwing (hyperabduction and external rotation), can become symptomatic when repeated overhead throwing results in a RC injury and/or a posterior-superior labral injury. There is controversy as to whether anterior instability of the glenohumeral joint is a culprit for this syndrome. However, ***internal Impingement*** is likely a combination of posterior shoulder capsular contracture, scapular dyskinesis, resulting in a reduced glenohumeral internal rotation deficit (GIRD).[16] Removal from play and a focused rehabilitation program aimed at identifying kinetic chain defects, such as reduced ROM, should be initiated.[17] ***Labral tears*** are common in overhead-throwing athletes such as baseball players, particularly in older throwers. They may involve the long head of the biceps tendon. A variation of a labral tear is the superior labrum anterior posterior (SLAP) tear, which stands for superior labral extending from the anterior to posterior portion. As with most throwing injuries, the mechanism of injury is due to repetitive overhead motion, such as throwing, injuring the glenohumeral joint. Symptoms typically include deep pain in the shoulder and weakness. Management includes removal from play and, depending on severity of injury, rest from throwing, a rehabilitation program with focus on correcting scapular kinetics and posterior capsular stretching. A return to throw program may be implemented. If nonoperative management fails, then surgical referral may be indicated. ***Proximal humeral epiphysiolysis, aka Little League Shoulder***, is a common injury in baseball players aged 11 to early teenage years. Pain in the shoulder with throwing is the most common symptom. In addition to clinical examination, radiographs with a contralateral (nondominant) image for physeal comparison is used to confirm a diagnosis. Treatment includes initially rest from throwing for 6 to 12 weeks, then a nonthrowing rehabilitation program, and then a return to throw and pitch program.[18] ***UCL injury*** and resulting UCL surgical reconstructions (UCLr) have been increasing in the past two decades.[19] Typically, UCL injury begins with mild pain in the medial aspect of the elbow. Pain may continue to increase if the athlete continues to throw through pain. Additionally, it is common for an athlete who sustains a UCL tear to admit to prior elbow throwing injuries when he or she was younger. Diagnosis may be confirmed with MRI-Arthrogram and or ultrasonography. A complete UCL rupture will require a surgical referral, whereas a low-grade sprain or partial tear may attempt nonoperative management. High-grade partial tears are controversial in terms of operative versus nonoperative management. **Little League Elbow** commonly refers to **medial epiphyseal apophysitis** and typically is due to overuse valgus stress on the joint. Location of pain is typically medial and pain is exacerbated with throwing. A physical examination will reveal pain with palpation to the medial epicondyle and possibly reduced extension of the elbow. Immediate management includes removal from play and restriction from throwing. Pain control, an initial nonthrowing rehabilitation program, and then a return to throw program once asymptomatic is the typical treatment algorithm. Sliding is a common mechanism for injury in baseball players. As of result of sliding more than 25% of injuries sustained involved the **hands or fingers** and more than 31% of those injuries required surgery.

Lower Limb Injuries

Given the necessity of flexibility and core musculature, forces around the low back put baseball players at risk for **low back injury**. The third most common injury sustained at the professional level is a **paralumbar muscle strain**.[12] Functional screening assessing for dynamic strength deficits as well as poor dynamic control may alert the sports medicine team to muscle weakness contributing to poor mechanics. The fifth most common injury sustained at the professional level is an **oblique strain** and the average time missed at the professional level is more than 22 days per injury.[12] Batting was the most common mechanism for injury with pitching second (approximately 46% vs. 35%, respectively).[20] Sports medicine providers should be aware that the location of the abdominal injury was most likely occurring on the leading side, whether the mechanism was batting, pitching, or playing defense. Treatment is nonoperative.

　　Hamstring strains may present with tenderness, ecchymosis, and swelling over the affected area. Initial treatment may include rest and swelling control. When possible, a rehabilitation program should be initiated. Once the patient is asymptomatic, he or she may return to play. Consideration of an off-season eccentric rehabilitation program should be part of baseball players workout routines for a reduction in hamstring injuries. **Ankle Injuries** are common as well. Depending on the severity of injury (e.g., a sprain vs. a fracture), treatment may include usage of a walking device (e.g., a walking boot vs. ankle brace), a rehabilitation program to restore proprioception, control swelling and pain, and strengthening should commence immediately. If radiography is indicated, potential bony injuries may necessitate a surgical referral.

■ SUMMARY

Baseball is an extremely popular game, played by individuals of all ages and at different levels of competition. Sports medicine team members involved in the care of these athletes and their teams must be aware of the game rules, regulations, common injuries, and potential sideline emergency situations in order to be a successful baseball sports medicine provider.

■ References

1. History Channel. Who invented baseball? https://www.history.com/news/who-invented-baseball. Published March 27, 2013. Updated March 28, 2019.

2. Little League. History of Little League. https://www.littleleague.org/who-we-are/history.

3. Little League. Little League® baseball and softball pleased to see overall interest in sport increase, according to SFIA report. https://www.littleleague.org/news/little-league-baseball-softball-pleased-see-overall-inter est-sport-increase-according-sfia-report. Published June 6, 2017.

4. National Federation of State High School Associations. Participation statistics. http://www.nfhs.org /ParticipationStatistics/PDF/2017-18%20High%20School%20Athletics%20Participation%20Survey.pdf.

5. Estimated probability of competing in college athletics. http://www.ncaa.org/about/resources/research /estimated-probability-competing-college-athletics. Published March 2, 2015. Updated April 8, 2020.

6. Number of participants in the United States from 2006 to 2017 (in millions). Statista. https://www.statista .com/statistics/191626/participants-in-baseball-in-the-us-since-2006.

7. Frequently asked questions: the business of MiLB. MiLB.com. http://www.milb.com/milb/info/faq .jsp?mc=business.

8. Major League Baseball. Official baseball rules 2018 edition. http://mlb.mlb.com/documents/0/8/0/268272080 /2018_Official_Baseball_Rules.pdf.

9. Miller M. High school baseball rules changes focus on player safety. https://www.nfhs.org/articles/high -school-baseball-rules-changes-focus-on-player-safety. Published April 24, 2018.

10. Little League. Little League Challenger. https://www.littleleague.org/play-little-league/challenger.

11. Green GA, Pollack KM, D'Angelo J, et al. Mild traumatic brain injury in major and minor league baseball players. *Am J Sports Med*. 2015;43(5):1118-1126. doi:10.1177/0363546514568089.

12. Camp CL, Dines JS, van der List JP, et al. Summative report on time out of play for major and minor league baseball: an analysis of 49,955 injuries from 2011 through 2016. *Am J Sports Med*. 2018;46(7):1727-1732. doi:10.1177/0363546518765158.

13. Saper MG, Pierpoint LA, Liu W, et al. Epidemiology of shoulder and elbow injuries among United States high school baseball players: school years 2005-2006 through 2014-2015. *Am J Sports Med*. 2018;46(1):37-43. doi:10.1177/0363546517734172.

14. Hibberd EE, Oyama S, Myers JB. Rate of upper extremity injury in high school baseball pitchers who played catcher as a secondary position. *J Athl Train*. 2018;53(5):510-513. doi:10.4085/1062-6050-322-16.

15. Camp CL, Curriero FC, Pollack KM, et al. The epidemiology and effect of sliding injuries in major and minor league baseball players. *Am J Sports Med*. 2017;45(10):2372-2378. doi:10.1177/0363546517704835.

16. Spiegl UJ, Warth RJ, Millett PJ. Symptomatic internal impingement of the shoulder in overhead athletes. *Sports Med Arthrosc Rev*. 2014;22(2):120-129. doi:10.1097/JSA.0000000000000017.

17. Kibler WB, Wilkes T, Sciascia A. Mechanics and pathomechanics in the overhead athlete. *Clin Sports Med*. 2013;32(4):637-651. doi:10.1016/j.csm.2013.07.003.

18. Zaremski JL, Krabak BJ. Shoulder injuries in the skeletally immature baseball pitcher and recommendations for the prevention of injury. *PM R*. 2012;4(7):509-516. doi:10.1016/j.pmrj.2012.04.005.

19. Mahure SA, Mollon B, Shamah SD, et al. Disproportionate trends in ulnar collateral ligament reconstruction: projections through 2025 and a literature review. *J Shoulder Elb Surg Am Shoulder Elb Surg Al*. 2016;25(6):1005-1012. doi:10.1016/j.jse.2016.02.036.

20. Camp CL, Conte S, Cohen SB, et al. Epidemiology and impact of abdominal oblique injuries in major and minor league baseball. *Orthop J Sports Med*. 2017;5(3):2325967117694025. doi:10.1177/2325967117694025.

24. CHEERLEADING

Richard A. Fontánez-Nieves and Belmarie Rodríguez-Santiago

■ HISTORY

The use of organized chants during sporting events to motivate the crowd was practiced in different parts of the world since the 1800s. However, some claim that cheerleading was originated on November 2nd, 1898 by Johnny Campbell when he entered the field during a college football game at the University of Minnesota to lead the crowd with cheers and chants, becoming the first cheerleader in history.[1] In the following decades the concept spread throughout the United States incorporating the use of signs, megaphones, "pom-poms," arm motions, dance moves, partner stunts, pyramids, air tosses, and tumbling skills to enhance the crowd interaction. Cheerleading has evolved dramatically for over 100 years becoming a physically demanding sport practiced worldwide. Currently there is a variety of competitive and recreational formats ranging from sideline performances to entertain the crowd and support other athletes during sporting events, to year-round competitive cheerleading.[1,2]

■ GOVERNING ORGANIZATIONS

- International: International All-Star Federation (IASF), International Cheer Union (ICU), International Federation of Cheerleading (IFC)
- National: National Cheerleaders Association (NCA), US All Star Federation (USASF), Universal Cheerleaders Association (UCA), USA Federation for Sport Cheering (USA Cheer), United Spirit Association (USA)

■ PARTICIPANTS

Cheerleading is practiced worldwide, and its participants are divided into multiple modalities of cheerleading (e.g., all-star, recreational, scholastic, national teams, master, special abilities, and paracheer/adaptive abilities) which in turn are divided into categories based on age, number of team members, gender distribution, and skill level. Approximately 3.6 million athletes practice cheerleading in the United States with approximately 400,000 students participating in high school teams, predominantly females (96%).[1-3]

■ RULES AND REGULATIONS

Cheerleading is usually practiced on foam mattresses or spring floor with a competition area of 42 by 54 ft or 42 by 42 ft, depending on the division and category. Routine time is usually 2 minutes and 30 seconds. Some cheerleading modalities also involve a 30-second cheer as part of their routines. During competitions each routine is evaluated by a group of judges who will give a score to the routine composition, performance, building creativity, and to each routine component including stunts, pyramids, tosses, standing and running tumbling, jumps, and dance (if applicable). Deductions to the total score are applied in the case of bubbles, falls, inappropriate behavior, and violations to the safety rules or performance boundaries. Rules, regulations, scoring, and deductions system may vary between competition organizations, categories, and cheerleading divisions.[4]

■ EQUIPMENT

Soft-soled athletic *shoes* are required for practices and competitions, as well as the appropriate practice or competition *surface* as described above. *Braces* can be used for competition and do not require any additional padding if unaltered from the manufacturer's original design. If any alteration needs to be made, the brace must be covered with closed cell padding at least 0.05- inch thick if the participant is involved in partner stunts, pyramids, or tosses. The use of solid orthotics such as plaster cast or walking boot must not be used by any athlete involved in partner stunts, pyramids, or tosses. The rules are limited regarding the use of face masks or eye protectors during practice or competitions; however, their use should be encouraged for athletes at risk of recurrent injuries.

>>> **Adaptive Sport Key Points: Abilities/Para Cheer**

Adaptive Abilities Teams include each age division and level from beginners (L0) to advanced (L4) with no basket tosses allowed. They are divided into two principal divisions, Unified and Traditional. The Unified Division teams consist of 1% to 99% athletes with disabilities per team and the Traditional Division teams consist of 100% athletes with disabilities per team. Percentages and divisions are established by the competition organizer prior to the event as well as the pertinent adaptive abilities rule modifications. Time of routine and competition area are the same for adaptive cheer, but no penalty exists for stepping out of the performance floor area. Eligible impairment types include impaired muscle power, impaired passive range of motion, limb deficiency, leg length difference, short stature, hypertonia, ataxia, athetosis, visual impairment, intellectual impairment, and hearing impairment.[5]

■ MEDICAL COVERAGE LOGISTICS

It is recommended to arrive 1 hour prior to the start of the event to introduce yourself to the organizing staff, coaches, judges, and emergency medical technician (EMT) personnel, and to check the available equipment especially the Automated External Defibrillator (AED), and review the emergency action plan (EAP) with the medical team as well as the rules for medical intervention for the event. Review the best route to the nearest hospital with trauma center capabilities that include on call neurosurgery. It is recommended to have medical equipment and staff at both the warm-up site and competition sites, close to the performance area. At least two channels of communication (radio and cell phones) among the medical team and organizing personnel should be established. Lastly, documentation of medical encounters is essential for future planning.

■ MEDICAL EMERGENCIES AND MEDICAL BAG ESSENTIALS

Cheerleading has a relatively low injury rate in comparison to other sports, but when injuries occur, they tend to be more severe.[6] In older age groups, the injury rates are greater and more catastrophic and injuries tend to occur due to more complex routines and greater height-based stunts and tosses.[6] Medical emergencies in cheerleading that might lead to death or severe injury can be divided into traumatic and nontraumatic.

Nontraumatic emergencies include metabolic, cardiac, and respiratory causes such as arrhythmias, asthma, heat stroke, hypoglycemia, and anaphylaxis. Traumatic emergencies tend to occur due to direct impact against the performing surface or other person. These can include concussion, traumatic brain injury, spinal cord injury, fractures, dislocations, and internal organ damage such as splenic rupture, lung injury, and commotio cordis. The most common stunts performed during catastrophic injuries were pyramids and basket tosses.[7]

Medical Bag Essentials in Cheerleading	
Medical Emergencies:	**Fractures and Dislocations:**
AED	Immobilizers and Slings
Tourniquet	Crutches
Cricothyrotomy kit	**Wound Care:**
14- and 16-gauge needles	Normal saline
Epi 1:1,000	Betadine swabs
Diphenhydramine or another antihistamine	Neosporin, mupirocin ointment
Albuterol inhaler	Moleskin
Rectal thermometer	Elastic bandage
Ice bath	Tube stretch gauze
Head and Spine:	Sterile gauzes
Concussion evaluation form	Vaseline
Stretcher & Spine board	Steri-strips
Cervical orthosis	Suture tray
Save a tooth kit	Lidocaine 1%
	Skin stapler

■ EPIDEMIOLOGY

Due to the lack of recognition of cheerleading as a sport by many state athletic associations, the epidemiologic literature of athletic injuries in cheerleading is scarce. Some studies have reported an injury rate of 0.71 injuries per every 1,000 athletic exposures in high school cheerleading in the United States. Sprains and strains are the most common types of injuries sustained in cheerleading (53%), especially in the lower limbs, followed by abrasions, contusions or hematomas (13%–18%), fractures and dislocations (10%–16%), lacerations or punctures (4%), and concussions or head injuries (3.5%–4%). Upper limb injuries are more prevalent in younger cheerleaders, who tend to suffer more fractures. In general, the most commonly injured joint is the ankle, followed by the wrist/hand, knee, head/neck, and trunk. The most common mechanism of injury is falling against another person or the ground while attempting a stunt, pyramid, basket toss, or tumbling. The injury rates are comparable between competition and practice and between flyers and bases/spotters, although some argue that bases are at higher risk.[2,3,6-8]

■ COMMON INJURIES

Head and Spine Injuries

Head and spine injuries are among the most severe injuries that can occur in cheerleading. **Concussion** rates in cheerleading are low in comparison with other female high school sports in the United States. However, a recent increase in concussion rate has been attributed to growing concussion awareness and increased difficulty in routines. The most common cause is a direct trauma to the head due to a fall. Symptoms include headaches, dizziness, confusion, nausea, balance problems. Severe cases may present with loss of consciousness. The athlete must be removed from training or competition and a concussion-specific assessment, like the Sport Concussion Assessment Tool (SCAT), should be completed. If no severe headache, changes in mental status, neurological deterioration, vomiting, or other red flag sign or symptom is noted, then the athlete may remain on the sideline for serial neurologic assessment until cleared to leave, with a parent if he or she is a minor. Close follow-up in 24 to 48 hours with a sports medicine provider is ideal to guide a step-wise return to sports and to prevent the second impact syndrome which can be fatal. *Spinal cord injuries (SCI)* are commonly caused by falling from pyramids and basket tosses, resulting in blunt trauma, vertebral fractures, or subluxations leading to local ischemia, hemorrhage, or edema in the spinal cord. Signs and symptoms can include paralysis, sensory impairment, loss of deep tendon reflexes, and sphincter tone, depending on the level and severity of the injury. Players who are found to be unconscious or those reporting neck pain with neurologic symptoms from trauma during play should have the cervical spine immobilized and be transferred to a trauma center for further evaluation. The recommended technique to transfer the injured player with a suspected cervical spine injury is the lift-and-slide technique which requires eight individuals: one at the head, three on each side and one controlling the spinal board. The other technique is the log roll and requires at least four providers: one controlling the head, two the body, and one the spinal board. *Lower back sprain or strain* are common in flyers who repeatedly land on their feet from a stunt or tumbling after extreme trunk flexion, extension, and twisting movements. Bases and spotters are also at risk because they are continuously holding a cheerleader above the head, compressing the spine, or catching a flyer in a cradle. Usually they present with localized pressure-like or stabbing pain with passive or active range of motion (ROM) and should be managed with relative rest, oral anti-inflammatory and muscle relaxants, and physical therapy followed by gradual asymptomatic return to sport. If there is no significant improvement in 1 to 2 weeks, radiologic imaging can be considered to rule out fractures, spondylosis/spondylolysis, and intervertebral disc disease.

Upper Limb Injuries

Upper limb injuries include *fractures* which are not as common as other types of injuries but landing on nonimpact-absorbing surfaces such as asphalt or concrete can increase their likelihood. Prepubertal or early pubertal cheerleaders are at greater risk of bone fractures, especially in the upper limb while falling on an outstretched hand. They may present with severe pain with palpation and ROM of the affected area. Deformity can be present, depending on the severity of the injury. If a fracture is suspected, the integrity of the neurovascular structures should be assessed. The involved structures should be splinted in a comfortable and safe position and should be evaluated radiographically to determine the appropriate course of treatment. *Wrist sprains* can involve any of the ligaments of the wrist which is usually injured during a fall on an outstretched hand or due to the repetitive upper limb weight-bearing activity during tumbling, propelling their own bodies to the air, tossing and catching other athletes, and supporting the weight of one or more cheerleaders overhead during stunts or pyramids. Repetitive wrist-forced hyperextension and weight-bearing activity may lead to other chronic pathologies such as *dorsal impingement* or *triangular fibrocartilage complex injury* that present with localized pain with movement and palpation. Ligament instability may be present, depending on the severity of the injury. Initially it should be managed with protection, rest, ice, compression, and elevation (PRICE). Oral analgesics or anti-inflammatory medication can be considered if no contraindication. If no significant improvement with conservative measures within 2 weeks, consider imaging studies to rule out a fracture or other bony injury. *Jersey and mallet finger* injuries are common in cheerleading, especially in bases while grabbing and twisting the flyers' feet during stunts and pyramids involving rapid and complex transitions. Mallet finger is a flexion injury of the distal interphalangeal (DIP) joint causing trauma to the extensor tendon resulting in difficulty to fully extend the DIP joint. Radiographs are indicated to rule out a fracture and the involved DIP joint should be splinted in mild hyperextension for 6 weeks. Jersey finger is an avulsion injury of the flexor digitorum profundus due to forced extension of a flexed finger resulting in inability to flex the DIP joint. Imaging studies should be done, along with a surgical referral.

Lower Limb Injuries

Acute injuries are common in the lower limbs. *Hamstring strains* can occur to any cheerleader due to eccentric contraction of the hamstring muscle during tumbling or with a forced hamstring stretching during stunts, jumps, or aerial elements such as "toe-touch," "heel stretch," and "bow-and-arrow." Strains tend to occur in the myotendinous junction and present with pain during hamstring contraction and passive stretching. A muscle gap or hematoma may be seen depending on the severity of the injury. Management involves rest, multimodal physical therapy, and a step-wise asymptomatic return to play. *Anterior cruciate ligament (ACL) tears* can occur upon landing from a stunt or tumbling with extended knee and trunk with increased knee valgus moment, presenting with severe pain, sudden knee effusion, limited range of motion (ROM), and positive Lachman's, Anterior Drawer and Lateral Pivot Shift tests. Initial management involves PRICE, oral analgesic or anti-inflammatory medication, and prompt radiologic evaluation to confirm the diagnosis and consider surgical evaluation for ligament reconstruction preceded by prehabilitation and followed by a multimodal step-wise rehabilitation and return to sports protocol. *Ankle sprains* are the most common injury in cheerleading among all ages. They occur while landing with inverted and plantar-flexed ankles, and present with swelling, discoloration, tenderness to palpation, and limited ROM due to pain in the affected ligaments. Physical exam may reveal positive anterior drawer and talar tilt tests. Radiographic images are recommended to rule out fracture if the physical examination reveals tenderness of the posterior lateral malleolus, navicular bone, base of fifth metatarsal, or unable to walk four steps. Radiographs of the fibula should be also be included to rule out a high-ankle sprain, interosseous membrane injury, and Maisonneuve fracture if the physical exam reveals positive squeeze test, pain with ankle external rotation, or painful fibular head.

■ SUMMARY

Cheerleading is a moderate contact sport with growing popularity in the United States and practiced worldwide by athletes of all ages and categories. It is practiced in a variety of competitive and recreational modalities including Special Abilities and Paracheer/Adaptive Abilities. It has a relatively low injury rate in comparison to other sports, but when injuries occur, they tend to be more severe.

■ References

1. International Cheer Union. History of the sport of cheer. http://cheerunion.org.ismmedia.com/ISM3/std-content/repos/Top/docs/ICU_History_2018.pdf. Published March 14, 2018.

2. LaBella CR, Mjaanes J. Policy statement: cheerleading injuries: epidemiology and recommendations for prevention. *Pediatrics*. 2012;130:966-971. doi:10.1542/peds.2012-2480.

3. Currie DW, Fields SK, Patterson MJ, Comstock RD. Cheerleading injuries in United States high schools. *Pediatrics*. 2016;137(1):e20152447. doi:10.1542/peds.2015-2447.

4. IASF. IASF cheer scoring. http://www.iasfworlds.com/cheer-page/#Cheer-Scoring.

5. International Cheer Union. Adaptive abilities divisions (ParaCheer). https://cheerunion.org.ismmedia .com/ISM3/std-content/repos/Top/ParaCheer/ICU_Paraheer_Rules_2017.pdf.

6. Mueller FO. Cheerleading injuries and safety. *J Athl Train*. 2009;44(6):565-566. doi:10.4085/1062-6050-44.6.565.

7. Jones G, Kazzam M. Cheerleading injuries. *Sports Med Update Arch*. 2017;(3):3-7. https://www.sportsmed .org/aossmimis/members/downloads/SMU/2017Fall.pdf.

8. Shields BJ, Smith GA. Epidemiology of strain/sprain injuries among cheerleaders in the United States. *Am J Emerg Med*. 2011;29:1003-1012. doi:10.1016/j.ajem.2010.05.014.

Gautam Anand

HISTORY

Cricket may have originated as a children's game in southeast England in the mid-1500s. During the rise of the British Empire, it spread to English colonies across the world. The late 1800s saw the beginning of international play.[1]

GOVERNING ORGANIZATIONS

- International: International Cricket Council (ICC)
- National: Afghanistan Cricket Board, Cricket Australia, Bangladesh Cricket Board, England and Wales Cricket Board, Board of Control for Cricket in India, Cricket Ireland, New Zealand Cricket, Pakistan Cricket Board, Cricket South Africa, Sri Lanka Cricket, Cricket West Indies, Zimbabwe Cricket

PARTICIPANTS

There were 105 nations having membership in the ICC as of 2017. Although it is played worldwide, it is most popular in the Indian subcontinent, Australia, Great Britain, South Africa, and the West Indies. It is played by nearly 2 million people in these countries.[1,2]

RULES AND REGULATIONS

As its most basic premise, the game involves players using a bat and ball. Each team consists of 11 players. One team starts as the batters, while the other team consists of the "bowler" (pitcher) and fielders. At the center of the field, the bowler hurls a hard ball in an overhead fashion at the batter. The batter stands in front of posts in the ground called "wickets," and he intends to hit the hurled ball away from the wickets to score runs. On the other hand, the bowler tries to hit the wickets or at least prevent the batter from hitting the ball. When the ball is hit in the air and caught by a fielder without touching the ground, the batter is out. Once all 11 batters have been eliminated, the two teams switch roles. The team with the greatest number of runs wins the match. The match is split into two innings played by each team. However, there is no set time for a match to end, similar to baseball.

EQUIPMENT

A **safety helmet** is especially imperative for the batter and wicket keeper. **Knee and tibial pads** are worn by the batter and wicket keeper. Batters can also wear additional padding including but not limited to **arm pads, thigh pads, rib protectors,** and **shoulder pads**. **Batting gloves** are worn by the batter. Male players can wear a **protective cup** inside the underwear to protect the genitals.

MEDICAL COVERAGE LOGISTICS

Identify appropriate medical staff, support, and equipment before the match starts. Review the Emergency Action Plan (EAP) and introduce the medical team to the referees, coaches, and support personnel. Protocols and guidelines should include role definition of the medical staff, emergency transportation including personnel, routes, and adequate facilities with the capacity to evaluate and manage possible injuries, and an outline of the chain-of-command and communication standards. It may be beneficial to dedicate a medical response team for the batters and a separate team for the bowlers and fielders since injuries differ depending on the player's position. Contingency plans should be made for extreme temperature, humidity, and other weather conditions that may involve match cancellation.

MEDICAL EMERGENCIES AND MEDICAL BAG ESSENTIALS

The medical provider should be keenly aware of potential emergencies in cricket. Although less common with the advent of improved helmets, craniofacial injuries from the hard cricket ball (a solid sphere composed of compressed leather around a cork core wound with tight string) can still be devastating, especially in the form of an extra- or intracranial hemorrhage. Also, chest injury and/or cardiac injury secondary to possible commotio cordis can be seen, as well as acute joint injury resulting in fracture, instability, or dislocation with neurovascular compromise. Nontraumatic causes of death are similar to other sports, including heat stroke, hypertrophic cardiomyopathy, anaphylaxis, and cardiac arrhythmias.

Medical Bag Essentials in Cricket	
Medical Emergencies:	**Wound/Laceration/Skin Care:**

Automated External Defibrillator (AED)
  Nitroglycerin (sublingual)
  Aspirin
  Epi 1:1,000
  Diphenhydramine or another antihistamine
  Albuterol inhaler
  Rectal thermometer
  Ice bucket
	Normal saline
	  Betadine swabs
	  Neosporin, mupirocin ointment
	  Moleskin
	  Elastic bandage
	  Tube stretch gauze
	  Sterile gauzes
	  Vaseline
	  Steri-strips

Head and Spine:	Suture tray Lidocaine 1%

Concussion evaluation form
  Stretcher & Spine board
  Cervical orthosis
	Others:

Fractures and Dislocations:	Acetaminophen Glucose tabs
Immobilizers and Slings Crutches	Waterproof SPF 50 sunscreen

EPIDEMIOLOGY

Injuries are highly prevalent in cricket. The back is most commonly affected for all cricketers, particularly the low back. This can start from a young age, as 17% to 33% of schoolboys and high school players suffer from back injuries.[3] However, depending on the player's designated position, different body parts may be at risk, including the shoulder joint, elbow, hand, and lower limb. Of injuries suffered by cricket bowlers,

12% to 40% affect the shoulder joint, and 23% to 36% of professional cricketers have experienced shoulder pain for at least one season.[2]

Cricket injuries can be categorized as direct or indirect. Direct occur from impact with the ball, bat, or field. Indirect are from overuse and repetitive motions. Bowlers suffer the highest injury rate, followed by batters.

▪ COMMON INJURIES

Head and Spine Injuries

Spine and head injuries include **craniofacial injuries** and **low back injuries.** Batsmen are the most vulnerable to a craniofacial injury usually resulting from direct blunt trauma of the incoming cricket ball. This injury can take several forms, including **zygomatic fracture, nasal fracture, eye injury, skull fracture, concussion,** and **extra- or intracranial hemorrhage.** Symptoms include vision deficit, headache, syncope, gait instability, hearing loss, and more. The management depends on the specific injury, and long-term follow-up with an otolaryngologist or neurologist may be indicated.[4,5] A common trunk pathology is a **tear of the internal oblique muscle**, which happens when a bowler pulls his nonbowling arm down from maximum elevation with lateral trunk flexion. This is known as "bowler's side strain." Chronically, the tips of the lowest ribs can hypertrophy and impinge during the delivery stride. This leads to pain in the midaxillary line. Rest, taping, rehabilitation, and modifying bowling technique are the mainstays of treatment. Steroid injections have not been proven to help.[5] Back injuries can be devastating for a cricket player's career. Besides **lumbar muscle strain**, they include **lumbar disc degeneration,** and **spondylolysis**. The injury comes from repetitive stress of lateral flexion with rotation during the bowling stride. Disc degeneration is seen mainly at L4-L5 and L5-S1. Despite this, bowlers may be asymptomatic and continue to play. Spondylolysis patients have progressive low back pain, but an acute fracture can also occur.

Upper Limb Injuries

Upper limb injuries include acute/traumatic and overuse injuries. Shoulder pathology usually is secondary to overhead motion overuse with repetition. Bowlers and fielders are particularly prone to it. Bowlers who emphasize spin on their deliveries rotate the shoulder internally while circumducting the arm. This motion can cause **shoulder impingement**, a condition in which the rotator cuff muscles are inflamed. **Biceps tendinopathy, superior labral tears, acromioclavicular (AC) joint injury,** and **dislocated shoulder** are other common shoulder injuries. Treatment includes rest of the affected joint, anti-inflammatory medications, and physiotherapy. If symptoms are refractory to these therapies, steroid injection can be effective at decreasing inflammation. Besides long-term rehabilitation, the patient may need follow-up with an orthopedic surgeon for potential arthroscopic surgical intervention.[2,4,5] Incorrect batting technique or using inappropriate equipment can lead to **lateral epicondylopathy** in batters. The batter feels pain in the lateral elbow joint. Physiotherapy and rehabilitation are typically adequate for elbow injuries, but in cases of chronic extensor carpi radialis brevis tendinopathy, surgical repair could be indicated.[5,6] Hand injuries usually take the form of a superficial hematoma from **blunt trauma** or **distal interphalangeal joint dislocation**. Taping together the fourth and fifth fingers may help prevent injury, and only around 11% of cricket players need surgery.[5]

Lower Limb Injuries

Lower limb injuries affect the thigh, knee, foot, and ankle. **Muscle strains and tears in the quadriceps and hamstrings** can be seen in any position on the field. Bowlers are classically affected, particularly with torque on the knee joint during the landing stride. *Patellar tendinopathy* is secondary to overuse. Other diseases include *chondral degeneration* and *medial tibial* or *femoral stress fractures*. Treatment is conservative, focusing on pain control modalities and interventions as well as correction of biomechanical deficits and incorrect sports specific technique. Acute injury is often the mechanism in a forefoot injury, but hindfoot suffers from more chronic pathology such as overuse and lateral ankle instability. Bowlers may be prone to *posterior ankle impingement syndrome*, which encompasses *flexor hallucis tendinopathy, peroneal tenosynovitis, ankle synovitis*, and more. The bowler has pain in the hindfoot with dorsiflexion during front-foot landing in the stride. Treatment focuses on physiotherapy, rehabilitation, and anti-inflammation, but consequential bone spurs may need surgical resection.

■ SUMMARY

Cricket is a limited-contact sport. While it may not be as popular across the world as other sports, knowing the injury patterns of direct blunt trauma and repetitive overuse is vital to diagnosing and treating those who do play the game.

■ References

1. Terry D. The seventeenth century game of cricket: a reconstruction of the game. *Sports Historian*. 2000;20: 33-43. doi:10.1080/17460260009445828.

2. Zaremski JL, Wasser JG, Vincent HK. Mechanisms and treatments for shoulder injuries in overhead throwing athletes. *Curr Sports Med Rep*. 2017;16(3):179-188. doi:10.1249/JSR.0000000000000361.

3. Stretch R. The seasonal incidence and nature of injuries in schoolboy cricketers. *S Afr Med J*. 1995;85(11): 1182-1184. http://archive.samj.org.za/1995%20VOL%2085%20Jan-Dec/Articles/11%20November/1.15%20 THE%20SEASONAL%20INCIDENCE%20AND%20NATURE%20OF%20INJURIES%20IN%20SCHOOL BOY%20CRIKETERS,%20Richard%20A%20.Stretch.pdf.

4. Miller J. Cricket injuries. https://physioworks.com.au/sports-physio/cricket-injuries/.

5. Pardiwala DN, Rao NN, Varshney AV. Injuries in cricket. *Sports Health*. 2018;10(3):217-222. doi:10.1177/1941738117732318.

6. Brukner P, Khan K. *Brukner and Khan's Clinical Sports Medicine: Injuries*. 5th ed. North Ryde, NSW, Australia: McGraw-Hill; 2017.

26. DIVING

Nathaniel S. Jones

■ HISTORY

The Tomba del Tuffatore (Tomb of the Diver) circa 470 BCE, contains an early painting depicting a young man diving into waves, but it was only in 1883, in Great Britain, that modern competitive diving was born.[1,2] In 1904, springboard diving became an Olympic sport with platform diving being added in 1908 during the London Olympic games. Our present-day diving style became popular only in the 1920s, in Germany and Sweden, where "fancy diving" was performed by gymnasts performing acrobatics over water.[3]

■ GOVERNING ORGANIZATIONS

- International: Fédération Internationale de Natation (FINA)
- National: USA Diving
- College: National Collegiate Athletic Association (NCAA)
- High School: National Federation of State High School Associations (NFHS)

■ PARTICIPANTS

Competitive diving athlete participation numbers for the NCAA and the NFHS are reported in conjunction with swimming athlete participants. Therefore, a reliable national participant number cannot be currently delineated. The most recent number figure from the FINA 2013 World Championships had 21 high-diving and 228 diving athletes out of 2,223 water sport athletes.[4]

■ RULES AND REGULATIONS

The objective is to score more points in a series of dives than the opposition. A panel of five or more judges evaluates five to six dives using five different elements to come up with a score between 0 and 10. The lowest and highest scores are thrown out and then remaining scores are multiplied by dive degree of difficulty, ranging between 1.2 to 4.1. The five different elements which include starting position, the approach, takeoff, flight, and entry are judged on technique and grace. Dives must not be repeated and must come from each of the following categories: forward, back, reverse, inward, twisting and arm stand (platform only). Dives are performed from 1 m and 3 m springboards, and a 10 m platform into a 25 m pool with a minimum depth of 5 m.

■ MEDICAL COVERAGE LOGISTICS

Prior to competition, confirm available healthcare personnel including physicians, athletic trainers, and emergency medical technicians (EMTs). It is recommended to have an ambulance with EMT personnel on site for quick transport to the nearest trauma center. An Emergency Action Plan (EAP) should be available and reviewed with all personnel prior to event day and rechecked on event day making sure no changes

need to be made to best ensure efficient and appropriate care is provided when necessary. Medical personnel should be familiar with and trained in water rescue and spine
boarding. The medical provider with other support staff should establish an open line
of communication with coaches, referees, and other staff.

■ MEDICAL EMERGENCIES AND MEDICAL BAG ESSENTIALS

Only few fatal head injuries in diving have been reported, occurring during a three
and a half summersault tuck dive attempt from a 10-m platform.[5] As in other sporting
events, it is of vital importance to activate the EAP during a medical emergency. Other
serious injuries including cervical spine injuries, pulmonary contusions, and spontaneous pneumothoraxes can occur due to quick deceleration during entry into water,
usually associated with a dive gone wrong.

Medical Bag Essentials in Diving	
Medical Emergencies:	**Wound Care:**
Automated External Defibrillator (AED)	Normal saline
Tourniquet	Betadine swabs
Cricothyrotomy kit	Neosporin, mupirocin ointment
14- and 16-gauge needles	Moleskin
Epi 1:1,000	Elastic bandage
Diphenhydramine or another antihistamine	Tube stretch gauze
Albuterol inhaler	Sterile gauzes
Head and Spine:	Vaseline
Concussion evaluation form	Steri-strips
Stretcher & Spine board	Suture tray
Cervical orthosis	Lidocaine 1%
Fractures and Dislocations:	
Immobilizers and Slings	
Crutches	

■ EPIDEMIOLOGY

The typical ages for an elite caliber diver range between 14 to mid-20s, with the average
age now more commonly found to be in the 20s.[7–14] Divers can average 200 dives per
week with sometimes performing 100 dives during an intense practice. During these
dives, divers are exposed to high-velocity and high-energy forces that can lead to injury when dives go wrong or with repeated exposure to such forces. A 10 m platform
diver can reach a velocity up to 16.4 m/s (36.8 mph) before entering the water with
quick deceleration to 20.51 mph on impact with water, with a force of about 400 kg N.
That is to say that at water surface impact a diver can reach between 2.0 g to 2.4 g. A
1-m spring board dive reaches an average peak velocity of 8.4 m/s (18.75 mph).[9] Upon
water impact, velocity is decreased by greater than 50% within 1 second.[8] Diving injury
incidence reporting is not consistent for diving and many times is included as part of
the swim injury data, but most recent data suggests an injury rate of 1.94 injuries per
1,000 athlete exposures (AEs) for males and 2.49 injuries per 100 AEs for females with
more injuries occurring in practice. Many of the injuries seen in diving can be attributed to the large forces applied to the body upon entry into the water and repetitiveness
of these dives in practice and competition. Risk of injury to the wrist may be reduced
with a step-wise increase in number of dives and height with taping of wrist offering
modest benefit.

■ COMMON INJURIES

Head and Spine Injuries

Divers are at risk of **concussion** from direct head contact with board or platform but also from water entry impact, especially in the setting of a dive gone wrong. A diver's vestibular systems are always challenged during a dive due to changes in linear acceleration and rotation and water impact with rapid deceleration. Some forward rotating dives take the diver through 1,260 degrees of rotation and more recently many divers go through 1,620 degrees of rotation with certain dives. Therefore, it can be a challenge to differentiate between a concussion or vestibular dysfunction when vestibular symptoms are reported, because they can occur in both injuries. Frequent checks and follow-up over 48 to 72 hours are advised. **Scalp laceration** can occur from direct trauma to the board or platform and are more commonly seen with reverse and inward dives. **Corneal epithelial injuries** can be seen commonly from repetitive microtrauma, but usually resolve with rest, while **tympanic membrane perforations** occur from directly landing on the ear. Much of the literature on **cervical spine injuries** is based on data from recreational, nonorganized diving associated with lack of experience, shallow water, inadequate supervision, and many times alcohol ingestion. In the competitive diving setting, cervical hyperflexion injuries occur when divers enter the water with a flexed neck; the impact of entry causes hyperflexion of the neck injuring the anterior spine. Divers report symptoms of pain, paresthesias, and radicular symptoms. To protect the cervical spine, proper technique with the neck positioned in neutral sitting between the two arms is recommended (Figure 26.1).

    Lumbar spine injuries are not only the most common reason for retirement from the sport but are among the most common injuries, with studies reporting an incidence of

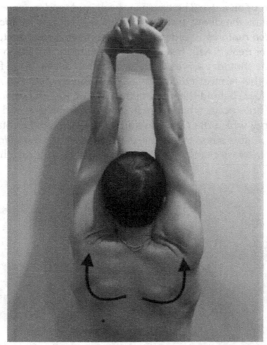

Figure 26.1 Arrows demonstrating appropriate placement of glenoid fossa under humeral head providing optimum support prior to entry with head and neck stabilized between arms.

38.4% to 89%. There is a 45% chance of having back pain within a year after the age of 13, which is a period of spine growth changes and increased vulnerability to injury. During take-off and entry, the anterior segments (vertebral body, vertebral end plate and intervertebral disc) are vulnerable to increases in loads; the posterior segments (facet joints, pars interarticularis) commonly are injured with forces applied during extension. One possible etiology for the back pain occurs when divers attempt to correct malrotation with a "save" underwater in order to attain a splashless entry. During a "save" the diver increases the arching in the lumbar spine to attain a more vertical orientation. A breakdown in the kinetic chain at the shoulder, with poor form and reduced shoulder flexion, leads many times to trunk hyperextension. Pain is the principal symptom and is usually insidious in nature. A high index of suspicion is important to have for early recognition. Treatment includes prolonged rest, physical therapy, and training modification.

Upper Limb Injuries

Only a minority of **wrist injuries** occur from trauma, such as hitting the board; most occur due to hitting the water repetitively. Repetitive microtrauma can lead to injuries such as **carpal bone contusions, triangular fibrocartilage complex (TFCC) tears, extensor pollicis longus ruptures** and **stress fractures of the wrist**. Hand positioning for entry is important in order to create the least amount of splash; the flat-hand grab is the most common technique as it provides a larger contact surface area and in turn dissipation of forces (Figure 26.2).

Divers are more susceptible to **scaphoid impaction syndrome**, which presents with pain at the snuff box region of the wrist, from repetitive hyperextension stresses of the board and entry phase. Treatment includes prolonged rest and rehabilitation, but if conservative measures are exhausted, surgery should be considered. The elbow is locked in extension upon entry. The triceps muscle and tendon experience great stress as they try to maintain the elbow in extension placing it at risk for **triceps tendinopathy, muscle strain, tendon ruptures** in older divers, **olecranon stress fracture** from overuse. Overuse injuries are treated with rest, and a rehabilitation program that is guided by pain symptoms. The shoulder serves as an endpoint of deceleration forces upon water entry impact, and this is most efficiently accomplished when the abducted scapula places the glenoid fossa behind the humeral head allowing for better absorption of axial load impact. Injuries occur when there is scapular abduction and there is impaired dissipation of energy which then stresses soft tissue such as the rotator cuff, labrum, and ligaments. Repetitive stress to such structures can lead to **shoulder instability** and, in some instances, increase chances of glenohumeral subluxation. Shoulder instability

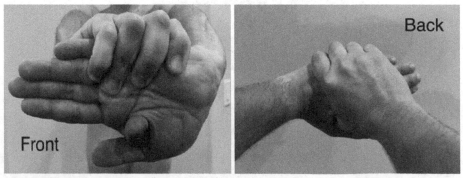

Figure 26.2 Flat-hand grab technique use to create a rip entry (minimal splash).

is a clinical diagnosis and is typically treated first with extensive shoulder strengthening and stabilization rehabilitation. On the one hand, a stable shoulder is vital for a diver's water entry, but a lack of shoulder flexibility tends to place stress on other structures, such as the spine, in order to make up for the lack of flexibility. Technique, form, and strength are vital in order to maintain the kinetic chain and avoid pathology such as **shoulder instability, labral tears,** and **shoulder impingement**. Aside from presence of pain, a consistent pattern of breakdown in form can be observed and lead to suspicion of underlying shoulder injury. Both MRI and ultrasound can be used to assess extent of injury in addition to a thorough neck and shoulder exam. Many times, rest, rehabilitation, and technique and form adjustment can lead to successful return to sport.

Lower Limb Injuries

Although high divers land feet first, all other divers enter the water hand first. Lower limb injuries still occur with dry-land training and also with the take-off phase of the dive. Timing of take-off phase is vital because when the timing is off, injuries such as **osteochondral lesions and knee and ankle sprains** occur. Diagnosis and treatment is similar to that of any other sport. More commonly overuse injuries from poor form or high volume of practice dives lead to such injuries as: **patellar** and **quadriceps tendinopathy, patellofemoral pain syndrome, Achilles** and **posterior tibialis tendinopathy**. These overuse injuries are diagnosed with physical exam and sometimes ultrasound. Treatment entails rest and rehabilitation. High divers who dive from 20-m (women) or 27-m (men) platforms by entering the water feet first are at higher risk of **ligamentous knee injuries** and **lower limb fractures**.

Pulmonary Injuries

Pulmonary contusions can be an alarming injury which occur from the rupture of pulmonary blood vessels and a resultant hemoptysis secondary to landing flat, most commonly from a 10 m platform dive. Symptoms include shortness of breath, cough, and hemoptysis. Fortunately, recovery is rapid with most returning over a period of a few days. Use of a bubbler in the water during practice to decrease surface tension can mitigate some of the risk for a pulmonary contusion.

Psychological Issues

Anxiety and psychological stress secondary to individual pressure to perform is very common and can be amplified by complexities of learning and performing dives. It is helpful to address this prior to learning more difficult dives. In addition, the emphasis placed on body type for performance and appearance can lead to anxiety, and places divers at higher risk for **eating behaviors** and **disordered eating**.

■ SUMMARY

In general diving is a safe sport. Nevertheless, proper preparation by the medical team covering an event is crucial since acute injuries can be life threatening. Due to the repetitive nature of the sport overuse injury is common leading to decrease in performance.

■ References

1. Rubin BD. The basics of competitive diving and its injuries. *Clin Sports Med*. 1999;18:293-303. doi:10.1016/S0278-5919(05)70145-9

2. Anderson SJ, Rubin BD. The evaluation and treatment of injuries in competitive divers. In: Buschbacher B, Braddom RL, eds. *Sports Medicine & Rehabilitation: A Sport Specific Approach*. Philadelphia, PA: Hanley & Belfus; 1994:111-122.

3. Badman BL, Rechtine GR. Spinal injury considerations in the competitive diver: a case report and review of the literature. *Spine J*. 2004;4:584-590. doi:10.1016/j.spinee.2004.03.002.

4. Mountjoy ML, Junge A, Benjamen S, et al. Competing with injuries: injuries prior to and during the 15th FINA World Championships 2013 (aquatics). *Br J Sports Med*. 2015;49:37-43. doi:10.1136/bjsports-2014-093991.

5. Rubin BD. Injuries in competitive diving. *Sports Med Digest*. 1987;9:1.

6. Carter RL. Competitive diving. In: Fu FH, Stone DA, eds. *Sports Injuries: Mechanisms, Prevention and Treatment*. 2nd ed. Philadelphia, PA: Lippincott Williams and Wilkins; 2001:352-371.

7. Kerr ZY, Baugh C, Hibberd E, et al. Epidemiology of National Collegiate Athletic Association men's and women's swimming and diving injuries from 2009/2010 to 2013/2014. *Br J Sports Med*. 2015;49:465-471. doi:10.1136/bjsports-2014-094423.

8. Day C, Stolz U, Mehan TJ, et al. Diving-related injuries in children <20 years old treated in emergency departments in the United States: 1990-2006. Pediatrics. 2008;122:e388. doi:10.1542/peds.2008-0024.

9. Narita T, Kaenoka K, Takemura M, et al. Injury incidence in Japanese elite junior divers. *Jpn J Sci Swimming Water Exerc*. 2011;14:1-6. doi:10.2479/swex.14.1.

10. Korres DS, Benetos IS, Themistocleous GS, et al. Diving injuries of the cervical spine in amateur divers. *Spine J*. 2006;6:44-49. doi:10.1016/j.spinee.2005.06.013.

11. Krejci L, Relek P. Ocular changes in competitive divers. *Cesk Oftalmol*. 1982;38:96-99.

12. Narita T, Kaneoka K, Takemura M, et al. Critical factors for the prevention of low back pain in elite junior divers. *Br J Sports Med*. 2014;48:919-923. doi:10.1136/bjsports-2012-091875.

13. Haase SC. Management of upper extremity injury in divers. *Hand Clin*. 2017;33(1):73-80. doi:10.1016/j.hcl.2016.08.017.

14. Chan JS-E, Wee JC, Ponampalam R, Wong E. Pulmonary contusion and traumatic pneumatoceles in a platform diver with hemoptysis. *J Emerg Med*. 2017;52(2):205-207. doi:10.1016/j.jemermed.2016.07.092.

27. EQUESTRIAN

Adrian McGoldrick and Michael Turner

HISTORY

There are records of horse racing dating back to the 5th century BCE, with polo mentioned a century earlier. Australia has the largest number of registered racecourses in the world (360), followed by France with 250. There are just over 100 racecourses in the United States and the first horse race took place in 1665 at Long Island, New York. Since horses were first domesticated, the number of equestrian sports has multiplied to over 100 different disciplines including the Olympic sports (dressage, eventing, and show-jumping), racing, English riding, Western riding, Arabian horse racing, stock handling, rodeo, harness racing, trotting, team events (pato and polo), tent pegging, skijoring, pony racing, gymkhana, endurance, reining, quarter horse racing, and so on. This chapter will focus on the sport that is most commonly associated with horses, thoroughbred horse racing.

GOVERNING ORGANIZATIONS

- International: International Federation of Horseracing Authorities (IFHA), International Federation for Equestrian Sports (FEI), Federation of International Polo (FIP)
- National: Most countries have central governance of horse racing to regulate the sport and ensure probity in a sport that is associated with betting/wagering. France (France Galop), Great Britain (British Horseracing Authority [BHA]), Ireland (Irish Horseracing Regulatory Board [IHRB]), Australia (Australian Racing Board).
- The is no central governance in U.S. racing and different regulations are in force in each state. These may also vary from racecourse to racecourse.

PARTICIPANTS

Jockeys normally start race riding at the age of 16 (by obtaining a license from the regulator). They serve a period of apprenticeship when they start, anything up to 5 years, and are usually referred to as "Apprentice (or Conditional) Jockeys" during this time. Jump jockeys retire around the age of 40 but Flat jockeys can go on to 60 and older. There are weight limitations in all forms of racing, and this varies from country to country. Flat jockeys tend to weigh around 110 lbs (50 kg), and jump jockeys weigh around 140 lbs (63.7 kgs). Jockeys are weighed before and after every race and this weight includes the weight of their clothing, boots, and the saddle. In Europe, Flat jockeys ride in around 600 races/year and Jump jockeys ride an average of 300 races/year. In the United States, jockeys may ride 1,000 to 1,500 races/year and earn more than $250 million during their careers.

RULES AND REGULATIONS

Horse racing is divided into Flat racing (also called "Track racing" which takes place on grass/turf, dirt, and all-weather/synthetic surfaces), and Jump racing (racing over obstacles, e.g., hurdle fences and steeplechase fences). In racing, distances are often measured in furlongs and 1 furlong is 660 ft (0.20 kms); 8 furlongs equal 1 mile (5 furlongs = 1 km). Flat racing takes place over distances of 5 furlongs (0.625 miles, 1.0 kms) to 2.75 miles (4.4 km) and Jump racing takes place over distances of 2.0 miles (3.2 kms) to 4.3 miles (6.9 km). Jump racing requires horses to jump over either hurdles (3.5 ft high [106 cm]) or steeplechase fences (4.5 ft high [137 cm]). There is no racing over a mixture of hurdles and steeplechase fences. The number of horses in a thoroughbred race ranges from one (a one-horse race) to 40 (the Grand National).

Integrity

Horseracing and the betting industry are closely linked, and wagering has been an integral part of the sport since its inception. The need to ensure that the sport is free from drug use/abuse is paramount for both horses and jockeys (doping), as is the need to ensure that jockeys are not influenced to breach the rules of the sport (bribing). In Europe, jockeys are banned from placing bets on racing and the use of mobile phones (by jockeys on race days) is heavily restricted and monitored. In Japan, jockeys are totally isolated before every race meeting and are required to stay in a guarded, residential facility (attached to the racecourse) for 24 hours before the day of racing. During this period, they are not allowed to have contact with anyone on the outside.

■ EQUIPMENT

In Europe, jockeys must wear **helmets** and **safety vests** manufactured to an appropriate standard (the current European Union equestrian helmet standard). **Goggles** and **gum shields** are optional. There are no uniform requirements in the United States regarding the use of safety equipment.

》》 Adaptive Sport Key Points: Para Equestrian

Although this chapter focuses on horse racing, there is Paralympic Equestrian. Equestrian first appeared on the Paralympic program at the 1984 Games held in Stoke Mandeville and New York, and have been featured at every Games since Atlanta 1996. Male and female riders with any type of physical or vision impairment compete together in dressage events. Dressage is the epitome of beauty and style. The program comprises an individual event; a team event involving three members, set to music; and a freestyle event in which riders with the top scores from individual events can choose their own routine and set it to their own choice of music. Riders are awarded points by a panel of five judges for accuracy of gait and how well the rider and horse work as one.

■ MEDICAL COVERAGE LOGISTICS

Injuries in horse racing are not incidental; they are inevitable and medical staff should be appropriately trained and qualified before undertaking duties on a racecourse. Regular acute trauma training and prehospital care training is strongly recommended (at least every 3 years). Medical coverage at racetracks varies enormously around the globe but gaining immediate access to fallen riders is a priority. The role of the on-site physician leader is to organize and coordinate the medical staff, and develop an emergency action plan (EAP) to help ensure the safety of the competitors and spectators. Prior to the race, it is necessary to determine the available medical personnel, medical equipment, and race support staff. At least two channels of communication (radio and cell phones) among the medical team and organizing personnel should be established. In Europe, many countries require a minimum of two ambulances, with appropriately trained staff (to follow the riders around the track), and one to two mobile doctors in support.

In New Zealand and Japan, qualified paramedics provide acute support but in New Zealand there are no doctors on site, while in Japan the doctor is static in the medical room. Every racecourse has a medical facility/medical room to assess and stabilize injured jockeys and diagnostic equipment (x-ray) is available in some jurisdictions (Japan). Communication with the nearest trauma center should be done prior to race day.

■ MEDICAL EMERGENCIES AND MEDICAL BAG ESSENTIALS

Horse racing produces numerous fractures, dislocations, spinal cord, and head injuries. Clavicle fractures are common, but fractures of the femur or pelvis are not rare. Major trauma to the chest and abdomen can produce a pneumothorax, haemothorax, or a rupture of the spleen, viscera, or liver. Dislocation of the shoulder, skull fractures, and spinal cord injuries (SCI) should be anticipated. Nontraumatic deaths can be due to hypertrophic cardiomyopathy, cardiac arrhythmias, anaphylaxis, and asthma.

Medical Bag Essentials in Horseracing	
Medical Emergencies:	**Fractures and Dislocations:**
Automated External Defibrillator (AED)	Immobilizers and Slings
Tourniquet	Crutches
Cricothyrotomy kit	**Wound Care:**
14- and 16-gauge needles	Normal saline
Epi 1:1,000	Betadine swabs
Diphenhydramine or another antihistamine	Neosporin, mupirocin ointment
Albuterol inhaler	Moleskin
Rectal thermometer	Elastic bandage
Ice bath	Tube stretch gauze
Head and Spine:	Sterile gauzes
Concussion evaluation form	Vaseline
Stretcher & Spine board	Steri-strips
Cervical orthosis	Suture tray
	Lidocaine 1%

■ EPIDEMIOLOGY

Horses weigh 1,000 to 1,200 lbs (450–550 kg) and travel at speeds of 20 to 40 mph (32–64 km/hour). Jockeys are seated 6 ft (183 cms) above ground level, with their heads approximately 8.5 ft (260 cms) above the ground (higher when jumping over fences). Concussion rates in horseracing are the highest in the recorded literature. Flat jockeys fall every 250 rides (concussion rate 17.1/1,000 participant hours), jump jockeys fall every 16 rides (concussion rate 25.0/1,000 participant hours) and amateur jockeys fall every eight rides (concussion rate 95.2/1,000 participant hours). In Flat racing, 0.41% of rides result in a fall and 40% of falls result in an injury. In Jump racing, 6.1% of rides result in a fall and 17% of falls result in an injury. Fatality rates are of the order 460 to 900 per100 million rides (approximately one death every 250,000 rides in European flat racing and one death every 110,000 rides in Jump racing). Comparable fatality rates per100 million participant days in other sports are: more than 780 in mountaineering; more than 640 in air sports; 146 in motor sports; 67.5 in water sports; 15.7 in rugby union; and 3.8 in football (soccer). In addition to the trauma caused by falling off, horses can inflict injuries by biting, pulling, kicking, hitting the rider in the face with a sudden movement of the head, standing on or rolling over the jockey. Soft tissue injuries (these may include a ruptured anterior cruciate ligament [ACL] or bruised kidney) make up 75% to 80% of all injuries, while fractures make up 10% to 18%, dislocations 1% to 4%, and concussions 8%.

■ COMMON INJURIES

Head and Spine Injuries

Head and spine injuries are among the most severe injuries that can occur in horseracing. **Concussion** rates are very high secondary to falls. Skull fracture incidence has decreased with helmet use. Symptoms include headaches, dizziness, confusion, nausea, and balance problems. Severe cases may present with loss of consciousness. The athlete must be removed from training or competition and a concussion specific assessment, like the Sport Concussion Assessment Tool (SCAT), should be completed. If no severe headache, changes in mental status, neurological deterioration, vomiting, or other red flag sign or symptom is noted, then the jockey may remain on the venue for serial neurologic assessment until cleared to leave. Close follow up in 24 to 48 hours with a sports medicine provider is ideal to guide a step-wise return to sports and to prevent the second impact syndrome (SCI) which can be fatal. **SCIs** are commonly caused by falling as well, resulting in blunt trauma, vertebral fractures, or subluxations leading to local ischemia, hemorrhage, or edema in the spinal cord. Signs and symptoms can include paralysis, sensory impairment, loss of deep tendon reflexes, and sphincter tone, depending on the level and severity of the injury. Jockeys who are found to be unconscious or those reporting neck pain with neurologic symptoms from trauma during play should have the cervical spine immobilized and be transferred to a trauma center for further evaluation. The recommended technique to transfer the injured individual with a suspected cervical spine injury is the lift-and-slide technique which requires eight individuals: one at the head, three on each side and one controlling the spinal board. The other technique is the log roll and requires at least four providers: one controlling the head, two the body, and one the spinal board.

Upper and Lower Limb Injuries

Fractures may involve the **clavicle, pelvis, femur,** or **tibia** and **fibula**. Neurovascular assessment must be performed to identify athletes that need to be transferred to a trauma center for further evaluation and treatment. Otherwise, close and stable fractures can be reduced, splinted, and followed with radiographies. **Shoulder dislocation** can occur after a fall as well. Reduction can be performed on site with follow-up radiographs to assess for bony injury and adequate reduction.

■ SUMMARY

Horseracing is an immensely popular global sport with television audiences of over 100 million for major events: Kentucky Derby, Grand National, Melbourne Cup, Dubai World Cup, Prix De L'Arc de Triomphe. Attendance at major meetings may be over 150,000 (Kentucky Derby) and horse racing is set to be a billion-dollar industry in the United States by 2026.

The Pegasus World Cup (Florida, USA) is currently the richest race in the world with a prize fund of $12 million, ahead of the Dubai World Cup and the Everest (Sydney, Australia) both at $10 million. It is a very high-risk sport that involves a heavy, mobile, and unpredictable hazard (the horse) that poses a major threat to all the jockeys who take part. Medical staff in attendance need to be prepared for major trauma and have the training and resources to manage life-threatening injuries.

■ Further Reading

Balendra G, Turner M, McCrory P. Career-ending injuries to professional jockeys in British horse racing (1991-2005). *Br J Sports Med*. 2008;42(1):22-24. doi:10.1136/bjsm.2007.038950.

Balendra G, Turner M, McCrory P, Halley W. Injuries in amateur horse racing (point to point racing) in Great Britain and Ireland during 1993-2006. *Br J Sports Med*. 2007;41(3):162-166. doi:10.1136/bjsm.2006.033894.

Bixby-Hammett DM. Accidents in equestrian sports. *Am Fam Physician*. 1987;36(3):209-214.

Bixby-Hammett DM, Brooks WH. Common injuries in horseback riding. A review. *Sports Med*. 1990;9(1):36-47. doi: 10.2165/00007256-199009010-00004.

Equestrian. https://tokyo2020.org/en/games/sport/paralympic/equestrian/. Published 2020.

Hitchens PL, Blizzard CL, Jones G, et al. The incidence of race-day jockey falls in Australia, 2002-2006. *Med J Aust*. 2009;190(2):83-86. doi:10.5694/j.1326-5377.2009.tb02284.x.

McCrory P, Turner M, LeMasson B, et al. An analysis of injuries resulting from professional horse racing in France during 1991-2001: a comparison with injuries resulting from professional horse racing in Great Britain during 1992-2001. *Br J Sports Med*. 2006;40(7):614-618. doi:10.1136/bjsm.2006.028449.

Press JM, Davis PD, Wiesner SL, et al. The national jockey injury study: an analysis of injuries to professional horse-racing jockeys. *Clin J Sport Med*. 1995;5(4):236-240. https://journals.lww.com/cjsportsmed/abstract/1995/10000/the_national_jockey_injury_study__an_analysis_of.5.aspx.

Rueda MA, Halley WL, Gilchrist MD. Fall and injury incidence rates of jockeys while racing in Ireland, France and Britain. *Injury*. 2010;41(5):533-539. doi:10.1016/j.injury.2009.05.009.

Waller AE, Daniels JL, Weaver NL, Robinson P. Jockey injuries in the United States. *JAMA*. 2000;283(10):1326-1328. doi:10.1001/jama.283.10.1326.

28. FENCING

■ HISTORY

The use of the sword for combat has existed for centuries as a means for survival, but first seen as a sport in ancient Egypt. It was popularized during the Middle Ages in Europe for tournament combat and toward the end of the 19th century the weapons of epee, sabre, and foil were recognized. Foil and sabre for men were first presented in the 1896 Olympic Games in Athens followed by epee in the 1900 games. For women, foil was introduced in 1924, epee in 1996, and sabre in the 21st century.[1]

■ GOVERNING ORGANIZATIONS
- International: International Fencing Association (FIE)
- National: United States Fencing Association (USFA)
- College: National Collegiate Athletic Association (NCAA)

■ PARTICIPANTS

Fencing is considered niche sport with about 23,000 competitive fencers in the United States in 2017. The majority of these fencers are within the 12 to 17 years of age category and the ratio of men to women in competitive fencing is 68.4% to 31.6%.[2] Club fencing is gaining increasing popularity in players of all ages.

■ RULES AND REGULATIONS

Modern fencing includes three weapons: foil, épée, and sabre and each has its own rules and regulations. In **foil**, the target is the torso only (includes the back, neck, and groin) and must be contacted by the tip of the sword for a valid point. If the tip makes contact elsewhere (off target hit), then the play is stopped. If both fencers score at the same time, then the referee decides who gets the point. The **epee** is the heaviest of the three and the entire body can be the target. Scoring is with the tip of the sword as in foil, but there is nothing that is considered off target unless the ground is hit. Unlike the other two, both fencers are awarded points for simultaneous hits. In **saber**, the torso, head, and arm (with the exception of the weapon hand) are valid targets and unlike the other two, the tip and blade can be used for scoring. As in foil, there is the possibility for off target contact; however, this would not stop the play. Depending on the competition, bouts can last up to five touches within 3 minutes or 15 touches within 9 minutes. Competition takes place on a long, narrow strip known as a **"piste"** that can be 1.5 to 2 m (4.9–6.6 ft) wide and 14 m (46 ft) long. Stepping off the strip is a point for the opponent. **Medical time outs** can be given for no longer than 5 minutes and will be noted in the score sheet. If the player requires another break that day for the same medical issue then that player would be disqualified from competition.[3]

EQUIPMENT

Equipment styles and necessity can vary among the three weapons. Each fencer will be wearing a *mask* that has a metal mesh on the front and a bib that protects the neck. The *jacket* is form fitting and has a strap passed between the legs. Underneath the jacket, a *plastron* is worn to provide added protection. *Chest protectors* can also be used (mostly female fencers). A *glove* is worn on the sword hand with a protection barrier to prevent the blade from going up the sleeve. *Breeches* end below the knee and need to overlap the jacket by 10 cm. *Fencing socks* are worn to cover up to the knee, and can be higher as well. *Fencing shoes* have flat soles and are specifically reinforced in the front and back. Scoring for modern fencing is through electrical equipment and all three weapons utilize them. Specifically for foil and sabre, a *lamé,* which is made of electrically conductive material, is worn over the fencing jacket for scoring. Hits are registered through a body cord which is attached to the weapon and comes out of the back through the inside of the sleeve jacket.[3,4]

> ### >>> Adaptive Sport Key Points: Fencing/Parafencing
>
> Just as in able-bodied competition, athletes can compete in any of the three weapons, but are categorized from "A" to "C" based on the level of disability. For the Paralympic games, players are in category "A" or "B" only, "A" representing those with good trunk control and "B" for those with impairments in the trunk and fencing arm. The target for foil and saber is the same for able-bodied competition. In epee, the target is anything above the waist and a conductive apron is worn below the waist to cancel those touches. The wheelchair must be at 110 degrees angle to the central bar and the player must be seated for the play. There must be a fixed distance between the players; the measurement is to the outer elbow for epee and saber and to the inner forearm for foil.[5]

MEDICAL COVERAGE LOGISTICS

On the day of the event, report to the medical tent at least 1 hour prior to start time to meet the support personnel and other medical providers. It is important to establish an emergency action plan (EAP) and identify communication lines, usually with walkie-talkies. Most competitions are held in large arenas with multiple bouts occurring simultaneously and therefore you will be stationed in the medical tent. To note, depending on the size of the competition, there may be multiple medical tents. If a player needs to be assessed, the referee will communicate the location through the designated communication line and you will attend to the patient on the piste. Injuries records are kept for each fencer.

MEDICAL EMERGENCIES AND MEDICAL BAG ESSENTIALS

Medical emergencies are infrequent in fencing, but can occur. Long competitions require high endurance levels and can be stressful for the body. The protective equipment over the body and prolonged use of the mask can cause the player to faint due to heat-related illness. Although uncommon, penetrating wounds to the chest can lead to pneumothorax and require immediate needle decompression.[6]

EPIDEMIOLOGY

Fencing is a limited-contact sport with a higher incidence of nontraumatic injuries in comparison to traumatic injuries.[4,6-8] Due to protective equipment, serious weapon injuries rarely occur; however, players can get small lacerations and bruising.[6]

Medical Bag Essentials in Fencing	
Medical Emergencies:	**Fractures and Dislocations:**
Automated External Defibrillator (AED)	Immobilizers and Slings
Cricothyrotomy kit	Crutches
14- and 16-gauge needles	**Wound Care:**
Nitroglycerin (sublingual)	Normal saline
Aspirin	Betadine swabs
Epi 1:1,000	Neosporin, mupirocin ointment
Diphenhydramine or another antihistamine	Moleskin
Albuterol inhaler	Elastic bandage
Head and Spine:	Tube stretch gauze
Concussion evaluation form	Sterile gauzes
Stretcher & Spine board	Vaseline
Cervical orthosis	Steri-strips
	Suture tray
	Lidocaine 1%
	Petroleum Jelly

Nontraumatic injuries are due to overload and make up the majority of all injuries in fencing with lower limb injuries more common than upper limbs.[7]

COMMON INJURIES

Spine Injuries

Low back pain is commonly seen in fencers due to the stress placed on the back due to the hyperlordotic stance during practice and competition. Weak core muscles as well as poor biomechanics can lead to intervertebral stress and injury and therefore core strengthening is an integral part of the training and postinjury rehabilitation program. Acute low back pain should undergo a neurologic evaluation to confirm there is no serious injury and then can be treated with rest, heat, and nonsteroidal anti-inflammatory drugs (NSAIDs). If the pain persists, imaging should be considered.[8]

Upper Limb Injuries

Upper limb injuries are due mostly to overuse. **Lateral epicondylopathy** is seen in fencers with tight grips and more commonly in foil fencers as they constantly use the extensor mechanism of the wrist in comparison to epee where the arm moves as a unit. Players will report pain over the lateral elbow and pain when moving the wrist. Hand and wrist injuries can be seen more commonly on the dominant side either through direct contact and/or overuse. **Supinator syndrome** also presents with lateral elbow pain, but the athlete will endorse radiating symptoms down the radial nerve distribution. Treatment will be similar to tennis elbow, but sono-guided hydrodissection with normal saline, local anesthetic, or corticosteroids can be considered for symptom relief. **De Quervain's tenosynovitis** can be assessed with the Finkelstein's maneuver (ulnar wrist deviation) which stresses the abductor pollicis longus and the extensor pollicis brevis. Inflammation of the tendons will cause pain at the base of the thumb and a splint can be used. **Impingement syndrome** in the shoulder can be seen in certain fencers as well, mostly epee, due to the repetitive controlled motion. Treatment for all these conditions includes a thorough examination to rule out neurovascular compromise and then conservative treatment with rest and NSAIDs.[4,6–8]

Lower Limb Injuries

Lower limb injuries are more common and due to overuse as well. Poor biomechanics in combination with the sudden movements of the sport can lead to knee injuries. Frequently seen conditions include **patellofemoral syndrome, patellar tendinopathy, iliotibial band syndrome** and **medial collateral ligament sprain.** Acute knee pain during competition should be assessed for serious injury followed by rest, ice, and bracing/taping if needed. **Quadriceps strains** are common due to the eccentric load on the legs when the knee is in motion. Injury is likely to occur at the myotendinous junction and it is important to evaluate for tears. The player may report pain and weakness with visible hematoma. Imaging can be helpful to assess the extent of injury. Rest and ice are helpful in the acute setting. **Achilles tendinopathy** and **ankle sprains** can result from change in footwear or activity intensity and are seen more often in the back of the foot. Players will report pain and tenderness over the associated tendons and may have limited range of motion. It is important to evaluate for evidence of tendon rupture. Rest, ice, and bracing should be considered. Other injuries to consider are **medial tibial stress syndrome** and **plantar fasciopathy.**[4,6-8]

▓ SUMMARY

Fencing is a limited-contact sport with historic origins as one of the first Olympic sports. Fencers can choose to compete in one of three weapons: foil, sabre, and epee. A thorough understanding of the different weapons, associated rules, and injuries is essential for effectively treating fencers. As medical providers, the care should not only be limited to the acute setting, but also include education on proper training to prevent overuse injuries.

▓ References

1. FIE history. International Fencing Federation website. https://fie.org/fie/history.

2. A comparison of the age profile of participation in major U.S. sports & fencing 2017. National Fencing Club Rankings website. http://nationalfencingclubrankings.com/comparison-age-profile-participation-major-u-s-sports-fencing-2017. Published October 9, 2017.

3. USA fencing rules. https://www.usafencing.org/usa-fencing-rule book. Published August 2019.

4. Roi GS, Bianchedi D. The science of fencing: implications for performance and injury prevention. *Sports Med.* 2008;38(6):465-481. doi:10.2165/00007256-200838060-00003.

5. Parafencing 101. USA Fencing website. https://www.usafencing.org/parafencing-101.

6. Caine DJ, Harmer PA, Schiff MA. *Epidemiology of Injury in Olympic Sports.* Oxford, UK: Wiley-Blackwell; 2009.

7. Harmer PA. Getting to the point: injury patterns and medical care in competitive fencing. *Curr Sports Med Rep.* 2008;7(5):303-307. doi:10.1249/JSR.0b013e318187083b.

8. Murgu A-I, Buschbacher R. Fencing. *Phys Med Rehabil Clin N Am.* 2006;17(3):725-736. doi:10.1016/j.pmr.2006.05.008.

29. FIGURE SKATING

Wilmar G. Pantoja

■ HISTORY

The earliest record of figure skating could be dated back to the 13th century as a means of communication between Dutch villages.[1] Since then the sport has evolved with its official debut in the 1908 London Summer Olympics, becoming the oldest winter sport in the Olympics program.[1]

■ GOVERNING ORGANIZATION

- International: International Skating Union (ISU)
- National: U.S. Figure Skating

■ PARTICIPANTS

As of 2017, U.S. figure skating has had an approximate total of 192,000 registered participants including high school clubs, intercollegiate teams, adult clubs, and U.S. competitors.[2]

■ RULES AND REGULATIONS

Figure skating encompasses a unique combination of strength, endurance, and artistry. It can be divided into four major disciplines which include: single skating, pair skating, ice dance, and synchronized skating. Each discipline has a different focus. Single skating consists of a short program with emphasis on performing jumps and spins. Pair skating performs a short program with moves that include lifts, spirals, throws, and synchronized jumps. Ice dance infuses music and vocals for a performance more focused on intricate footwork and expression of rhythm and how the skating adheres to the music. Synchronized skating is performed by a team of skaters and how they move simultaneously as a group. A standard skating rink is 30 by 60 m in size, with plastic or sliding boards. Figure skaters need ice of the highest quality which is achieved using ice resurfacing machines. The thickness of the ice over its entire surface should not vary by more than 0.5 cm.

■ EQUIPMENT

The **skate** is molded for each skater and proper fitting is integral for the sport. The **boot** is made of thick, stiff leather with extra laces and wide tongues which provide the ankle with both flexibility and support. **Steel blades** are made of high carbon material with concave grooves along their entire length and teeth in the toe of the blade to allow for pushing off when executing certain types of jumps. The skater's **outfit** is made of stretchable, flexible material as the skater needs to perform high-quality moves, yet also encompass a theme and style.

> ### ≫ Adaptive Sport Key Points: Figure Skating
>
> Though not an official sport within the Paralympics, U.S. figure skating offers an adaptive skating program for those with physical disabilities. Depending on the disability level, the skater will have modifications to the skates and may require assistive devices. Consider the use of a helmet and protective padding to avoid serious injury from a fall on the ice.[3]

■ MEDICAL COVERAGE LOGISTICS

Prior to the event, all team members should be aware of available support personnel, especially the physician and paramedic(s). It is important to understand the access route in case of emergency and the entry and exit route should be unobstructed. Also, obtain a copy of the event program and a schematic outline of the venue if available. The ISU recommends that there be medical providers at the diagonal corners of the rink as well as in a separate exam room to treat players in-between competition. If a player needs to be examined on the ice, the ISU has established a protocol for on-ice emergencies that are used during most skating competitions.[4] It is important to use nonslip shoe covers prior to entering the rink. Supplies should be kept close to the entry onto the ice for easy access. Documentation of medical encounters for record keeping and future event planning is important.

■ MEDICAL EMERGENCIES AND MEDICAL BAG ESSENTIALS

Even though most injuries in figure skating are musculoskeletal in origin; it is important for the rink-side physician to be aware of possible medical emergencies. Those that are potentially life-threatening include head, neck, and spine injuries. Regarding on-ice cervical spine emergencies, it is important to understand proper techniques to get the patient onto the spine board and off the ice. It may be beneficial to review with the team on the ice prior to the event. When approaching a fallen athlete with suspected head injuries, the physician should rapidly assess airway, breathing, and circulation and determine the level of consciousness. If ABCs (airway, breathing, circulation) are stable, further neurological examination should be performed. Physical examination should observe for obvious sign of skull fracture, as well for indicators of intracranial bleeding such as asymmetric pupils (anisocoria), periorbital or postauricular ecchymosis, clear otorrhea, rhinorrhea, or hemotympanum. Frequent examination is highly suggested as initial presentation could be normal and then deteriorate. Although rarely reported, nontraumatic emergencies can include cardiac

Medical Bag Essential in Ice Skating	
Medical Emergencies:	**Wound Care:**
Automated External Defibrillator (AED)	Normal saline
Bag valve mask	Betadine swabs
Epi 1:1,000	Neosporin, mupirocin ointment
Diphenhydramine or another antihistamine	Elastic bandage
Albuterol inhaler	Sterile gauzes
	Steri-strips
Head and Spine	Suture tray
Stretcher and spine board	**Musculoskeletal:**
Cervical orthosis	Immobilizers and Slings
Concussion evaluation form	Compression bandages
	Crutches

conditions like arrhythmias and hypertrophic cardiomyopathy (HCM), anaphylaxis, and asthma.

■ EPIDEMIOLOGY

Athletes continue to push the limits of the sport as moves such as the triple axels and quadruple jump are now expected in routines of high-level competitors. Common problems in figure skating include acute musculoskeletal injuries, acute trauma, and chronic overuse injuries. Studies have shown that about 50% of the injuries are traumatic and 50% are due to an overuse mechanism.[5] Events that perform lifts and throws are more prone to acute injuries in comparison to single skaters who are more prone to overuse injuries.[5]

■ COMMON INJURIES

Head and Spine Injuries

Either through direct trauma with the ice or another skater, *cervical spine injuries* and *concussions* are rare, but possible. Given the variability of the clinical presentation associated with concussion, it is important that team physicians and other clinicians responsible for the care of athletes perform a systematic and comprehensive sideline evaluation of each athlete with a suspected concussion.

Upper Limb Injuries

The upper body is essential for an ice skater as a solid strength foundation is needed for jumping, spinning, and both elements in pairs. Male pair skaters and synchronized skaters are at a higher risk of rotator cuff dysfunction. *Rotator cuff tendinopathy* is multifactorial and has been attributed to both extrinsic and intrinsic mechanisms. Extrinsic factors can be seen in subacromial impingement which could be secondary to anatomical variants of the acromion, alteration in scapular or humeral kinetics, postural abnormalities. Other factors are those encroaching the space against posterosuperior rim of the glenoid leading to *internal impingement*; as can be seen with rotator cuff and scapula muscle performance deficits and decreased extensibility of the pectoral muscle. Intrinsic factors are those mechanisms that contribute to rotator cuff degeneration; including tensile/shear overload which ultimately leads to change in tendon biology, morphology, vascularity, and mechanical properties. Clinical feature on examination could present with pain over greater tuberosity (insertion of supraspinatus and infraspinatus) and active range of motion (AROM) abduction and flexion, reproduced with impingement tests and in the apprehension position. Use of ultrasound is useful in ruling out full thickness tear or defining a partial thickness tear. Treatment should first focus on decreasing the acute pain by avoiding aggravating activity, applying ice, and using medication and modalities in combination or solo. If a small or partial thickness tear is present, treatment may be nonsurgical, focused on rehabilitation. Full thickness tears in young athletes require surgical repair and should be discussed with advanced age individuals depending on goals and expectations. Acute injuries also occur in figure skating with the most common being fractures. *Distal radial fractures* occur by the fall on an outstretched hand. One of the most common distal radius fractures is a *Colles fracture*, in which the broken fragment of the radius tilts upward. These injuries tend to result in immediate pain over the site area with possible deformity. Management at rink-side should include a neurovascular evaluation followed by splinting. Patients should be sent to the emergency department as further management is dependent on radiographic imaging to further classify the fracture (intra-articular, extra-articular, or comminuted). **Radial head/neck fractures** are other fractures that occur yet are less common than distal radius fractures. Mechanism is the same as before from falling on an outstretched hand. Patient presents with acute pain located over forearm or elbow. Deformity in radial neck/ head fracture may be more difficult to observe yet acute swelling and limited range of motion is usually present. Management is the same as distal fracture with patients needing to be transported to the emergency department for further imaging, classification, and management.

Lower Limb Injuries

Most common injuries in the lower limbs involve the ankle and foot. **Ankle sprain** is the most common injury in figure skating due to increased risk of foot inversion in multirotation jumps. Skaters would report swelling and tenderness over the lateral aspect of the ankle, which is composed of the anterior talofibular, calcaneofibular, and posterior talofibular ligaments. It is important to determine if further imaging (x-rays) is indicated with reference to the Ottawa Ankle Rules. The skater may not be able to return to play and treatment includes rest, elevation, ice, and/or bracing. **Achilles tendinopathy** involves tendon structure injury secondary to repetitive stress that could lead to a continuum of tendinopathy that ranges from reactive tendinopathy, tendon disrepair, and degenerative tendinopathy. Given the relative lack of dorsiflexion in the skating boot, it is important to address lower leg and ankle flexibility and intrinsic foot and ankle strength in addition to the usual physical therapy prescription for rehabilitating figure skaters with this injury.[6] Due to repetitive stress, inflammation of the bursa between the skin and the medial malleolus can lead to **malleolar bursopathy (bursitis)**. Conservative treatment is recommended and once the pain and inflammation are reduced and motion and strength are restored, the patient gradually returns back to full activities. **Retrocalcaneal bursopathy** is inflammation of the bursa located between the Achilles tendon and calcaneus and may form due to increased ankle dorsiflexion and compression of the retrocalcaneal bursa of the landing leg.[6] Acute treatment should include ice therapy, nonsteroidal anti-inflammatory drugs (NSAIDs), and gradual progressive stretching. **Superficial calcaneal bursopathy** is the second most common lower limb injury due to overuse.[7] Skaters can get inflammation of the superficial bursa located at the back of the heel due to various risk factors including greater boot-foot length difference, less ankle dorsiflexion, and lower jump height.[6] Treatment should include rest, NSAIDs, ice, footwear modifications, therapy, and may consider steroid injections if pain persists. Skaters develop **"lace bite"** or **tenosynovitis of the extensor digitorum and tibialis anterior tendon** due to persistent contact against the skater's boot. Treatment includes modifications of the boots including changing the tongue padding and preventing friction against the tendons as well as NSAIDs, ice, and rest. **Haglund deformity** is a callus or blister formation located over the posterior calcaneus and occurs when the boot is loose, and the heel has constant friction from the upward and downward motion while skating. It is usually resolved by adequate boot fitting, and additional padding. Due to the kinetic chain, repetitive stress on the ankle and foot can translate upward and lead to injury in the knee and hip. **Hamstring strain** most likely occurs while the musculotendinous junction undergoes maximum strain during eccentric contraction. Hamstring strength and flexibility are necessary to perform spiral elements in which the free leg is extended maximally from the hip into an arabesque position.[6] High-impact landings and constant knee extensor activation during routines expose the skater to anterior knee pain. These include injuries such as *Osgood-Schlatter syndrome, patellofemoral syndrome, and patellar tendinopathy*. Quadriceps, hamstrings, and iliotibial band stretching may minimize development of extensor mechanism knee pain.[7]

■ SUMMARY

Figure skating is continually evolving as athletes define the sport each year. Medical providers should have an understanding of the sport to anticipate the most common injuries. Predominance of overuse injuries will be noted more in single skating which reflects the longer training hours and increasing technical difficulties, whereas pair skating has a higher risk of acute injuries with difficult lifts and throws.

■ References

1. Figure skating equipment and history. International Olympic Committee website. http://www.olympic.org/figure-skating-equipment-and-history.

2. 2019-2020 US figure skating factsheet. https://www.usfigureskating.org/sites/default/files/media-files/FactSheet.pdf

3. Adaptive skating. US Figure Skating website. http://www.usfigureskating.org/skate/skating-opportunities/adaptive-skating.

4. International Skating Union. Communication no. 2049-on ice medical emergencies protocol. https://www.isu.org/inside-isu/isu-communications/communications/520-2049-on-ice-medical-emergencies-protocol/file. Published 2018.

5. Porter EB, Young CC, Niedfeldt MW, Gottschlich LM. Sport-specific injuries and medical problems of figure skaters. *WMJ*. 2007;106(6):330-334.

6. Han JS, Geminiani ET, Micheli LJ. Epidemiology of figure skating injuries: a review of the literature. *Sports Health*. 2018;10(6):532-537. doi:10.1177/1941738118774769.

7. Campanelli V, Piscitelli F, Verardi L, et al. Lower extremity overuse conditions affecting figure skaters during daily training. *Orthop J Sports Med*. 2015;3:2325967115596517. doi:10.1177/2325967115596517.

30. GYMNASTICS

Fairen Walker-McCarter

■ HISTORY

Gymnastics has its roots in warfare preparation as it was invented for that purpose by the ancient Greeks. The Romans then continued it after their conquest. However, after the fall of the Roman Empire, gymnastics lost popularity. The modern-day form was originated by Dr. Friedrich Ludwig Jahn of Germany, who is considered the father of gymnastics. It was adopted by the Olympics for the first time in 1896. Disciplines now recognized by the International Gymnastics Federation (FIG) include men's artistic gymnastics, women's artistic gymnastics, rhythmic gymnastics, trampoline gymnastics (including tumbling), acrobatic gymnastics, aerobic gymnastics, parkour, and gymnastics for all.[1] This chapter will focus on the divisions of men's and women's artistic gymnastics.

■ GOVERNING ORGANIZATIONS

- International: International Gymnastics Federation (FIG)
- National: USA Gymnastics (USAG)
- College: National Collegiate Athletic Association (NCAA)
- High School: National Federation of State High School Associations

■ PARTICIPANTS

An estimated 4.81 million male and female athletes over the age of 6 participated in gymnastics in the United States in 2017. A 2007 diversity study survey by USA Gymnastics estimated female to male participation in the sport to be 79.45% to 20.24%, respectively.[2]

■ RULES AND REGULATIONS

Men's Events

Men's artistic events include floor, vault, pommel horse, still rings, parallel bars, and horizontal bar. *Floor:* The athlete performs a routine between 60 to 70 seconds consisting of tumbling passes and strength skills on a 12 m by 12 m spring floor. *Vault*: The athlete uses a 25 m runway and springboard to launch onto a vault (also called "vaulting horse," "vaulting table," or "tongue"). He then performs a twist and somersault combination and lands on a mat. *Pommel Horse*: The athlete performs a routine of leg movements while supporting himself on a pommel horse consisting of a metal body with foam rubber and leather coverings and plastic handles. *Still Rings*: The athlete performs a routine of dynamic movements and at least one static movement on two rings suspended 5.75 m above the ground. *Parallel Bars*: The athlete performs a routine of swings, balances, and releases on two parallel horizontal bars that are typically 2 m above the ground. *Horizontal Bar*: The athlete performs a routine of swings, twists, and releases on a 2.8 cm fiberglass bar with wood laminate that is 2.5 m above the ground.

Women's Events

Women's artistic events include floor, vault, uneven bars, and balance beam. *Floor*: The athlete performs a choreographed routine of up to 90 seconds consisting of tumbling passes, leaps, turns, dance, and acrobatics on a 12 by 12 m spring floor. *Vault*: The athlete uses a 25 m runway and springboard to launch onto a vault (also called "vaulting horse," "vaulting table," or "tongue"). She then performs a twist and somersault combination and lands on a mat. *Uneven Bars*: The athlete performs a timed routine of swings, circles, and release moves on two parallel horizontal fiberglass bars with wood laminate. *Balance Beam*: The athlete performs a choreographed routine of up to 90 seconds consisting of tumbling passes, leaps, turns, dance, and acrobatics on a 5 by 10 cm padded beam.

Each event is scored based on a 10.0 points scale. In nonelite level competition, the score starts at 10.0. At elite levels, including NCAA, the score starts below 10.0 and requires the athletes to acquire bonus points by increasing difficulty levels of skills performed. Judges use preset guidelines to deduct points from the starting score for mistakes either in execution or artistry.

■ EQUIPMENT

See specific equipment used in each event just mentioned. Additionally, gymnasts may use *chalk* ($MgCO_3$) to decrease the moisture in the athletes' hands to decrease friction and help prevent skin tears. *Leather wrist straps* or *grips* are used by female gymnasts for uneven bar routine and by male gymnasts for still rings, parallel bars, and horizontal bar.

>>> **Adaptive Sport Key Points: Special Needs Gymnastics**

Gymnasts with special needs can participate in competitive gymnastics through the Special Olympics and also through HUGS (Hope Unites Gymnastics with Special Athletes), a track within the Gymnastic for All (GFA) discipline. Disciplines through the Special Olympics include Men's Artistic, Women's Artistic and Rhythmic and through HUGS includes Women's Artistic, Men's Artistic, Rhythmic, Trampoline and TeamGym. Modifications for gymnasts with visual and hearing impairments include assistance by coaches, audible and visual cues and further modifications for athletes that require use of a cane or walker.[3,4]

■ MEDICAL COVERAGE LOGISTICS

The role of the on-site physician leader is to organize and coordinate the medical staff, develop an emergency action plan (EAP), and interact with the coaches and officials to help ensure the safety of the athletes and spectators. Prior to the event, it is important to identify available medical staff, support personnel, venue map, and the available medical equipment. Establishing an EAP is the most important task. Protocols and guidelines should include role definition of the medical staff, emergency transportation including personnel, routes, and adequate facilities with the capacity to evaluate and manage possible injuries, and an outline of the chain-of-command and communication standards. During the event the medical team and equipment should be accessible to all apparatus as well as a main medical area. Communication between individual members of the medical staff, coaches, referees, emergency medical staff, and local medical facilities is essential via two or more systems (e.g., hand-held radios and cell phones). Lastly, documentation is essential for review after the game/season to evaluate utilization and plan for future coverage.

■ MEDICAL EMERGENCIES AND MEDICAL BAG ESSENTIALS

The collapsed or unconscious athlete is considered a medical emergency that requires activation of the proper channels of communication and protocols including basic life

Medical Bag Essentials in Gymnastics	
Medical Emergencies:	**Fractures and Dislocations:**
Automated External Defibrillator (AED)	Immobilizers and Slings
Tourniquet	Crutches
Cricothyrotomy kit	**Wound Care:**
14- and 16-gauge needles	Normal saline
Epi 1:1,000	Betadine swabs
Diphenhydramine or another antihistamine	Neosporin, mupirocin ointment
Albuterol inhaler	Moleskin
Head and Spine:	Elastic bandage
Concussion evaluation form	Tube stretch gauze
Stretcher & Spine board	Sterile gauzes
Cervical orthosis	Vaseline
Save a tooth kit	Steri-strips
Protective equipment removal tools	Suture tray
	Lidocaine 1%

support (BLS)/advanced cardiac life support (ACLS). Although rarely reported, non-traumatic emergencies can include cardiac conditions like arrhythmias and hypertrophic cardiomyopathy (HCM), anaphylaxis, and asthma. Musculoskeletal injuries that may become medical emergencies include upper and lower limb fractures or dislocations with neurovascular compromise, traumatic brain injuries with or without spinal cord involvement, and blunt thoracoabdominal trauma with possible internal bleeding.

EPIDEMIOLOGY

Gymnastics has one of the highest injury rates in sports as it combines highly skilled performances with limited safety equipment. The rate of injury in college-level gymnasts is estimated to be 8.78 per 1,000 exposures for male athletes and 9.37 per 1,000 exposures for female athletes. Male gymnasts are at most risk for upper limb injuries, with female athletes being at most risk for lower limb injuries. Both male and female gymnasts are at most risk for injury when performing a floor routine. The most frequent injuries in gymnasts are due to repetitive stress.[5,6]

COMMON INJURIES

Head and Spine Injuries

Head and spine injuries can be serious. **Concussion** can be sustained with falls during a routine or an error that leads to the head striking either the bar, beam, or vault. Symptoms include confusion, dizziness, headaches, nausea, and loss of consciousness. Remove the athlete from the meet and conduct a neurological exam and a Sport Concussion Assessment Tool (SCAT) test. If loss of consciousness along with severe headache, vomiting, seizure, neurological deficit, evidence of head or neck trauma, or a Glasgow Coma Scale (GCS) less than 15 is present, then the athlete should undergo immediate advanced imaging. The athlete should be transferred to an emergency facility for further evaluation. An athlete without the above symptoms should follow up with a sports medicine provider within 24 to 48 hours. **Spinal cord injury** can be sustained with falls during a routine or an error that leads to the head or spine striking either the bar, beam, or vault. Symptoms include motor and/or sensory loss. Spinal cord injuries can be complete or incomplete of which syndromes include central cord, anterior cord, posterior cord, or Brown-Sequard. With any suspected spinal cord injury, remove the athlete from the meet and perform a neurological exam if he or she is stable. In the unstable athlete, start with an evaluation of airway, breathing, and circulation (ABCs) and stabilize the head and neck. The recommended technique to transfer an injured athlete with a suspected cervical spine injury is the lift-and-slide technique. This requires eight individuals: one at the head, three on each side and one controlling the spinal board. The other technique is the log roll. This requires at least four providers: one controlling the head, two the body, and one the spinal board. The athlete should be transferred to an emergency facility for further evaluation.[7] *Spondylolysis* is a defect of the pars interarticularis of the spinal column. *Spondylolisthesis* occurs when there are bilateral pars interarticularis fractures that result in slippage of the vertebral bodies in relation to each other, more commonly at the L5/S1 level followed by the L4/L5 level. Gymnasts are at high risk due to the high stress to the lumbar spine secondary to repetitive hyperextension, presenting with low back pain worse with one-legged hyperextension. Motor or sensory deficits may be present. If deficits are present, then further work-up is warranted. In the absence of neurological deficits, conservative treatment, such as bracing and physical therapy including flexion exercises, can be recommended.[8]

Upper Limb Injuries

Upper limb injuries occur secondary to extensive overhead activity and upper limb weight-bearing associated with most events. Male gymnasts most commonly injure the shoulder followed by the wrist. Female gymnasts' upper limb injuries are most likely to involve the wrist followed by the elbow. *Labrum tears* are more often *superior labrum anterior posterior (SLAP) tears*. Symptoms include pain and weakness of the shoulder. If suspected, the athlete should be removed from the meet. The decision for surgical versus conservative treatment will depend on the type of tear and response to physiotherapy and bracing. *Rotator cuff tendinopathy* symptoms include pain and weakness of the shoulder. Conservative treatment with nonsteroidal anti-inflammatory drugs (NSAIDs), ice, and physical therapy is typically successful. Interventional treatment with sono-guided injections versus surgical intervention can be considered if conservative care is unsuccessful. *Osteochondritis dissecans of the capitellum* is a separation of the articular cartilage from the capitellar subcondral bone. It presents as lateral elbow pain and can have associated swelling, loss of elbow extension, and clicking. Radiographic imaging is required to assess the extent of injury and to determine method of treatment. Conservative treatment includes NSAIDs and activity modification and occasionally bracing or a cast. For unstable lesions, surgical intervention is required. *Distal radial stress injury* is the most common cause for wrist pain in gymnasts. It typically presents as chronic dorsal wrist pain and can be associated with swelling and grip strength weakness. Radiographic imaging should be performed to confirm diagnosis and rule out other pathology, such as scaphoid or ulnar impaction syndrome, dorsal impingement syndrome, and carpal fractures or avascular necrosis which can present similarly. Conservative treatment includes NSAIDs, ice, activity modification, physical therapy, and bracing for immobilization in severe cases.[9] *Blisters* are commonly seen in gymnasts, especially when performing horizontal bar, parallel bar, or uneven bar events. If painful and fluid-filled, then the blister can be drained by inserting a sterile needle at the base. The overlying skin should remain in place. After cleaning, the blister can be covered with antibiotic ointment and a bandage. Chalk and hand grips can be used for blister prevention.

Lower Limb Injuries

Female gymnasts are most likely to sustain a lower limb injury. *Anterior cruciate ligament (ACL) injury* occurs most commonly with the landing during events. Symptoms include a "pop" followed by immediate pain and swelling. Lachman test and pivot-shift test can be performed sideline at the meet. The gymnast should have an MRI performed and be referred to orthopedics for surgical evaluation. *Achilles injury* is common in gymnasts secondary to jumping and landing injuries. *Achilles tendinopathy* typically presents with pain on the posterior heel. There can be associated swelling and/or bone enlargement. Conservative treatment includes NSAIDs, ice, activity modification, physical therapy, and possible bracing for immobilization in more severe cases. Steroid injections should be avoided given the high risk of tendon rupture. Regenerative techniques can be used for chronic recalcitrant cases. *Achilles tendon rupture* typically occurs secondary to a sudden forced dorsiflexion mechanism, typically during a landing. Gymnast will likely report a "pop." Physical examination can reveal weakness of plantarflexion, a defect of the Achilles tendon, and a positive Thompson test. Surgical intervention is recommended. *Ankle sprain* most commonly occurs in the anterior talofibular ligament (ATFL) followed by the calcaneofibular ligament (CFL) and typically occurs secondary to an inversion injury. Symptoms include lateral ankle pain and swelling. Ottawa ankle rules should be used to determine the need for radiographic imaging to rule out ankle fracture. Conservative treatment consists of NSAIDs, ice, bracing, activity modification, and physical therapy. *Sever's disease* is inflammation of the calcaneal apophysis of a young gymnast. It typically presents as pain over the heel area. Achilles tendon tightness along with swelling, erythema, and warmth over the calcaneal apophysis may be found on physical exam. Conservative treatment includes NSAIDs, ice, activity modification, physical therapy, heel cups, and possible immobilization for severe cases. *Plantar fasciopathy* presents as sharp pain along the plantar fascia that is typically worse at the beginning of activity and at the end of the day. On physical exam, dorsiflexion of the foot while palpating the plantar fascia can increase the tenderness to palpation. Conservative treatment includes NSAIDs, ice, activity modification, physical therapy focusing on fascia and Achilles tendon stretches, shoe inserts, and splinting for immobilization in severe cases. Also, regenerative techniques can be considered in recalcitrant cases.

SUMMARY

Gymnastics is a popular high-skill-level sport performed at multiple levels in the United States and around the world. Understanding the events performed and most common injuries is essential for sideline coverage.

References

1. Strauss M. A history of gymnastics: from ancient Greece to modern times. http://www.scholastic.com/teachers/articles/teaching-content/history-gymnastics-ancient-greece-modern-times.html.

2. About USA gymnastics. https://usagym.org/pages/aboutus/pages/about_usag.html.

3. USA gymnastics: hugs program. https://usagym.org/pages/group/pages/hugs.html.

4. Gymnastics. https://resources.specialolympics.org/sports-essentials/sports-and-coaching/gymnastics.

5. Campbell RA, Bradshaw EJ, Ball NB, et al. Injury epidemiology and risk factors in competitive artistic gymnasts: a systemic review. *Br J Sports Med*. 2019;53:1056-1069. doi:10.1136/bjsports-2018-099547.

6. Westermann R, Giblin M, Vaske A, et al. Evaluation of men's and women's gymnastics injuries: a 10-year observational study. *Sport Health*. 2015;7(2):161-165. doi:10.1177/1941738114559705.

7. National Athletic Trainers' Association. Appropriate care of the spine injured athlete. Updated from 1998 document. Prof Rep. 2015.

8. Syrmou E, Tsitsopoulos PP, Marinopoulos D, et al. Spondylolysis: a review and reappraisal. *Hippokratia*. 2010;14(1):17-21.

9. Webb BG, Rettig LA. Gymnastic wrist injuries. *Curr Sports Med Rep*. 2008;7(5):289-295. doi:10.1249/ JSR .0b013e3181870471.

31. SKATEBOARDING

Kevin Frison

■ HISTORY

Skateboarding emerged in the United States sometime in the early 1950s in California. Originally deemed "sidewalk surfing" or "asphalt surfing," the idea of skateboarding was borne out of surfers' desire to emulate surfing during low-tide seasons. Thought of as a fad, it faded out of popularity by 1965 and re-emerged in the 1970s with the help of advancements in technology (i.e., polyurethane wheels).[1] Noted for its high degree of risk, the sport is considered an "extreme sport" and attained mainstream popularity in the mid-90s secondary to ESPN's "Extreme games," later colloquialized to "X-games."[2] Skateboarding will be included in the 2020 Olympic games in Tokyo for the first time ever.[3]

■ GOVERNING ORGANIZATIONS

- International: World Skate
- National: USA Skateboarding
- Major professional league: Street League Skateboarding

■ PARTICIPANTS

Today, there are an estimated 6 to 15 million skateboarders in the United States and there is an increasing number of skateboarders internationally.[4]

■ RULES AND REGULATIONS

As competitive skateboarding is still in its infancy, there are no overarching official rules and regulations. The 2020 Olympic games will include two skateboarding events for men and women: *Street* and *Park*.[3] Street competition is held on a "street-like" course featuring stairs, handrails, curbs, benches, walls, and slopes. Each competitor performs individually and utilizes each course feature to demonstrate a range of skills, or "tricks." Judging considers the following: degree of difficulty of the tricks, height, speed, originality, execution, and composition of moves. Park competitions take place on a hollowed-out course featuring a series of complicated curves. From the bottom of the cavity, the curved surfaces rise steeply with the upper part of the incline being vertical. Competitors for park events are judged on difficulty, quality of execution, use of course, and consistency.

■ EQUIPMENT

Before skating, it is recommended the athletes remove all hard and sharp objects from their pockets and don protective gear. Proper gear consists of a properly fitting helmet, wrist guards, knee and elbow pads, closed-toe shoes, goggles, and a mouth guard. A properly fitted helmet is worn flat on the head with the bottom edge parallel to the ground, sits low on the forehead, has side straps that form a "V" shape around each ear, has a buckle that fastens tightly (there should be room to put only two fingers between the strap and the chin), has pads inside that can be installed or removed so the helmet fits snuggly, does not move in any direction when the head is shaken, and does not interfere with movement, vision, or hearing.[4]

> >>> **Adaptive Sport Key Points: Skateboarding**
>
> For athletes who require a wheelchair, a full suspension wheelchair motocross (WCMX) wheelchair is available to help them adjust. For amputees, specialized prostheses are available, but skateboarding with their normal prosthetic device is possible.[5]

▪ MEDICAL COVERAGE LOGISTICS

The role of the on-site physician is to organize and coordinate the medical staff, develop an emergency action plan (EAP), and interact with the event director to help ensure the safety of the competitors and spectators. Prior to a competition, it is important to identify available medical staff, support personnel, venue map, and medical equipment. The number and types of medical providers required for an event is dependent upon the number of participants and spectators and the number and type of expected injuries. Sports medicine physicians and Emergency Medical Services (EMS) personnel, along with sports medicine fellows, residents, medical students, athletic trainers, or physical therapists can attend expected medical needs. Establishing an EAP is the most important concern. Protocols and guidelines should include role definition of the medical staff, emergency transportation including personnel, routes, and adequate facilities with the capacity to evaluate and manage possible injuries, and an outline of the chain-of-command and communication standards. A medical tent or designated medical area needs to be established with access to all areas of competition and exit route. Lastly, prior to the start of the competition, the medical team should confirm that competitors are wearing proper equipment and there are no obstructions or obvious irregularities on the competing surface. Communication between individual members of the medical staff, support personnel and officials, emergency medical staff, and local medical facilities is essential via two or more systems (e.g., hand-held radios and cell phones). Some professional events may also require a separate area for doping control and drug testing. Proper documentation is essential for review after the event to evaluate utilization and plan for future events.

▪ MEDICAL EMERGENCIES AND MEDICAL BAG ESSENTIALS

It is essential to understand potential medical emergencies that may arise. The collapsed or unconscious athlete is considered a medical emergency. Although rarely reported, nontraumatic emergencies can include anaphylaxis and asthma. Musculoskeletal injuries that may become medical emergencies include upper and lower limb fractures or dislocations with neurovascular compromise, traumatic brain injuries with or without spinal cord involvement, and blunt thoracoabdominal trauma with possible internal bleeding.

▪ EPIDEMIOLOGY

The nature of skateboarding is made up of high-speed and extreme maneuvers with injuries occurring most often when the athlete collides with an immovable object, falls from the skateboard, or is involved in a motor vehicle accident. Most injuries occur because the athlete strikes an irregularity or protuberance in the riding surface, thus

Medical Bag Essentials in Skateboarding	
Medical Emergencies:	**Wound/Laceration/Skin Care:**
Automated External Defibrillator (AED)	Normal saline
Nitroglycerin (sublingual)	Betadine swabs
Aspirin	Neosporin, mupirocin ointment
Epi 1:1,000	Moleskin
Diphenhydramine or another antihistamine	Elastic bandage
Albuterol inhaler	Tube stretch gauze
	Sterile gauzes
Head and Spine:	Vaseline
Concussion evaluation form	Steri-strips
Stretcher & Spine board	Suture tray
Cervical orthosis	Lidocaine 1%
Fractures and Dislocations:	**Others:**
Immobilizers and Slings	Acetaminophen
Crutches	Glucose tabs
	Waterproof SPF 50 sunscreen

lunging the athlete in the direction of travel. The American Academy of Pediatrics recommends against skateboarding for children under the age of 5, as these children have a higher center of mass, immature skeletal development, undeveloped neuromuscular system, and poor judgement.[6] In 2018, there were a total of 124,929 reported skateboarding-related injuries in the United States with males accounting for 70% of them and athletes with ages between 5 and 14, 15 and 24, and 25 and 64 accounting for 33%, 35%, and 29% of reported injuries respectively.[7]

■ COMMON INJURIES

Head and Spine Injuries

Head and spine injuries include intracranial injury, cervical spine and/or skull fractures, soft tissue injury, lacerations, and dental injuries accounting for 3.5% to 13.1% of all skateboarding injuries.[4] Although a higher number of cranial injuries were once seen in younger children (<10 years of age) due to lack of psychomotor development, more recent findings suggest a significant rise in concussions and severe intracranial trauma in adolescent (16 years old) and older populations.[8] *Orofacial injuries,* manifested as craniofacial abrasions, lacerations, and dental subluxations, have become more prevalent, associated with open-road skateboarding as well as increased participation in recreational skateboarding.[9]

Upper Limb Injuries

Upper limb injuries include fractures which account for 32.1% of all fractures and occur most frequently in older skateboarders.[4,10] Upper limb trauma can be attributed to impact with surfaces, rails, and stairs. The elbow is noted to receive a significant portion of trauma with acute injuries ranging from *abrasions, sprains, contusions,* and *hyperextension* following falls.[4] *Ulnar nerve injury* can occur after an elbow dislocation or direct blunt trauma leading to compression. Symptoms include neuritis, arthralgia, and tenderness with concomitant edema ("Swellbow"). Landing directly on the elbow can indirectly cause a *glenohumeral joint dislocation* as well as a hyperextension injury of the cervical spine. The combination of speed and extreme forces transferred proximally up an inflexible limb during a fall often result in *radial* or *ulnar* or *carpal bone fractures*.[4,8,10] Those involving the scaphoid are considered more serious as they can lead to avascular necrosis.

Lower Limb Injuries

Lower limb injuries often involve the left side of the body,[11] because most skateboarders ride with their left foot forward, known as the "normal stance" as opposed to having their right foot forward, or "goofy stance." Lower limb trauma accounts for 17% to 26% of all total injuries and approximately 7.9% of all skateboarding injuries.[4] In skateboarders less than 10 years of age, *femoral fractures* are more common compared to older athletes who are more likely to sustain *tibial fractures*.[8] Although rarely reported, knee trauma consisting of *patellofemoral* arthralgia and inflammation, hyperextension, *meniscal and chondral lesions,* and *cruciate ligament injuries* have been reported.

Thoracoabdominal Injuries

Although infrequent, *thoracoabdominal injuries* can occur. The majority of trauma reported include renal injuries and spleen ruptures, but cases of genitourinary injury and peroneal trauma have been reported.[4]

▨ SUMMARY

As skateboarding is increasing in popularity globally, an increase in the number of injuries is expected. Given the high velocities and challenging stunts incorporated in this extreme sport, it would behoove not only the athlete but the covering physician to be familiar with the potential injuries related to this sport as well as the importance of donning protective equipment for prevention.

▨ References

1. Cave S. A brief history of skateboarding: from an obscure California activity to the mainstream. https://www.liveabout.com/brief-history-of-skateboarding-3002042. Published September 30, 2018.

2. X Games Sports & Competition Information. Skateboarding rules (final). https://xgamessportsandcomp.wordpress.com/rules-documents/skateboard-rules-final.

3. Skateboarding. https://tokyo2020.org/en/games/sport/olympic/skateboarding/. Published December 1, 2018.

4. Shuman KM, Meyers MC. Skateboarding injuries: an updated review. *Phys Sportsmed*. 2015;43(3):317-323. doi:10.1080/00913847.2015.1050953.

5. Skateboarding. https://www.disabledsportsusa.org/sport/skateboarding.

6. Bull MJ, Agran P, Garcia VF, et al. Skateboard and scooter injuries. *Pediatrics*. 2002;109(3):542-543. doi:10.1542/peds.109.3.542.

7. Sports and recreational injuries. Injury Facts. https://injuryfacts.nsc.org/home-and-community/safety-topics/sports-and-recreational-injuries.

8. Lustenberger T, Talving P, Barmparas G, et al. Skateboard-related injuries: not to be taken lightly. A National Trauma Databank analysis. *J Trauma*. 2010;69(4):924-927. doi:10.1097/TA.0b013e3181b9a05a.

9. Hunter J. The epidemiology of injury in skateboarding. *Med Sport Sci*. 2012;58:142-157. doi:10.1159/000338722.

10. Keays G, Dumas A. Longboard and skateboard injuries. *Injury*. 2014;45(8):1215-1219. doi:10.1016/j.injury.2014.03.010.

11. Zalavras C, Nikolopoulou G, Essin D, et al. Pediatric fractures during skateboarding, roller skating, and scooter riding. *Am J Sports Med*. 2005;33(4):568-573. doi:10.1177/0363546504269256.

32. SKIING/SNOWBOARDING

Daniel R. Lueders and Jeffrey Smith

■ HISTORY

The first public ski competition occurred in 1843 and the first ski jump competition in 1862, both in Norway. The International Ski Federation (FIS) governs the sport worldwide and was founded in 1924, the year of the first Winter Olympics, which included cross country, Nordic combined, ski jumping, and military patrol (similar to modern biathlon). Alpine skiing downhill and slalom events were added in 1936, giant slalom in 1952, and super giant slalom (super G) in 1988.[1] In 1965, the first freestyle skiing competition was held in New Hampshire and the discipline was recognized by FIS in 1979 before its first Winter Olympics inclusion in 1988. Mogul skiing was first a medal event in 1992, aerials in 1994, ski cross in 2010, and finally half-pipe and slope style in 2014.[2,3]

The first snowboard competition was held in 1981 in Colorado and the first hal-pipe competition in 1983 at Lake Tahoe. The International Snowboard Federation (ISF) was founded in 1990 but was replaced by FIS and snowboarding was first an Olympic medal sport in the 1998 Nagano games.[4]

■ GOVERNING ORGANIZATIONS
- International: International Skiing Federation (FIS)
- National: U.S. Ski & Snowboard
- Major Professional Leagues: FIS World Cup is the primary professional longitudinal competition. Air & Style and Winter X Games are also annual professional competitions.
- College: United States Collegiate Ski & Snowboard Association (USCSA) includes both and the National Collegiate Athletic Association (NCAA) includes only skiing.
- High School: Organized skiing and snowboarding competitions vary state by state and are more likely to exist in states with terrain suitable for these sports.

■ PARTICIPANTS

There were around 7.0 million active skiers and 2.2 million active snowboarders in the United States during the 2017–2018 season. The percentage of skiers 45 years and older is increasing while participation is decreasing among younger age groups. In contrast, snowboarding has seen consistent growth in those under 18.[5]

■ RULES AND REGULATIONS

Alpine skiing has five separate timed disciplines: downhill, Super G, slalom, giant slalom, and alpine combined. *Downhill* is a timed single run down a long course with widely spaced gates and few turns, facilitating the highest speeds of all alpine events. *Super G* is also single timed run format down a long, fast course but it has more gates that are closer together than in downhill. *Slalom* and *giant slalom* are each determined by the sum of two-timed runs down a more compact course with tightly packed gates. Giant slalom, relatively, has more widely spaced gates and higher speeds. *Alpine combined* adds the time of a slalom run and a downhill or super G run.[6] **Freestyle skiing** has six competitions in its discipline: aerials, moguls, cross, half-pipe, slopestyle, and big air. In *aerials*, an individual performs two separate jumps from a man-made jump and each is scored based on criteria that include the takeoff from the jump, the height and distance obtained from the jump, artistic style, movement precision, and landing form. *Moguls* consists of two runs on a steep course covered in hilly, bumpy terrain called "moguls" where a competitor is scored based on turns, speed, and aerial maneuvers and the higher score of those two runs is used. *Ski cross* involves two to four racers starting at the same time and racing down a specially prepared course of turns, jumps, and other terrain features with the first to cross the finish line the winner. *Half-pipe* involves descending and jumping off the lip of a half-pipe to perform aerial tricks that are scored based on air, difficulty, and technical skill in completion. Two runs are performed and the athlete with the highest summative score wins. *Slopestyle* is a competition of scored jumps and tricks performed on a run down a course containing a variety of features that might be found in a terrain park. *Big air* involves competitors launching off a very large man-made jump and performing aerial maneuvers and tricks while midjump that are scored.[7] **Snowboarding** includes big air, half-pipe, parallel giant slalom, parallel slalom, slopestyle, and snowboard cross events that are timed or scored in the same manner as the analogous skiing event.[8] **Cross-country skiing** involves a mass start of athletes racing a predetermined distance around a closed course of undulating hills. The first athlete to cross the finish line is the winner. In *ski jumping*, the athletes descend a specialized ramp and jump from a take-off table at its base. They then descend and traverse a significant distance in the air toward a targeted "K-point" with a goal of traveling as far as possible. Competitors are scored on distance, style, gate factor, and wind conditions.[9] **Nordic combined** joins ski jumping and cross-country skiing. The ski jump occurs first and is scored as previously noted and those scores are used to determine the order and timing of starts for the cross-country portion, so that the highest scorer starts first and the other racers start with their respective time disadvantages. The first racer to cross the line in the cross-country event is the winner.[9]

▥ EQUIPMENT

The most important equipment for all of these events is **skis** or a **snowboard** along with **bindings** and **boots**. Alpine competitions will have minimum lengths and widths which vary by age group and by the individual discipline and well-defined shape parameters to limit speed or improve safety. In contrast, there are few to no ski guidelines for freestyle events. Additional equipment can include **ski poles, helmet, goggles,** and **specialized clothing,** and **ski poles**. In cross-country skiing, ski length and width have minimum parameters based on skier height and specific guideline regarding shape of the ski. Poles play a greater role in cross-country as a mechanism of propulsion for the athlete. Specific bindings and boots allow the heel to lift away from the ski, permitting greater push off propulsion on flat surfaces and climbs. Ski jump utilizes heavier and longer skis and allow skis that are longer than one's height. Specialized jumping bindings permit an athlete to lean forward while in midair to achieve an aerodynamic shape. There are only minimal regulations of snowboard equipment, usually a minimum board width based upon the length of the gliding surface. All events require the use of a **helmet** that meets industry safety standards for different testing speeds. **Goggles** and **gloves** are not required but will have specifications if used. Specific clothing can vary by event to achieve aims of aerodynamics, comfort, and versatility.

>>> **Adaptive Sport Key Points: Para alpine skiing, cross country skiing and snowboarding**

Para alpine skiing includes downhill, Super G, slalom, giant slalom, and alpine combined events. Specific classification considerations for alpine skiing include arm impairments (one or both arms) and leg impairments (one or both legs) for standing skiers. There are three levels of classification for sit-skiers based upon level of trunk control and function and three classifications given for skiers with visual impairments based on visual acuity and visual field testing. Para cross-country skiing shares standing skier and vision classification levels with alpine skiing. Sit-skiers have five classes that differentiate leg and trunk function. One competitive aspect unique to para cross-country skiing is the percentage-system that multiplies a finishers time by a specified percentage based on each individual's race class, resulting in an adjusted time. Para snowboarding has a less structured classification system than alpine and cross-country skiing with only three total sport classes, two based on leg impairments and one based on arm impairments. Unlike alpine skiing there are no classes for those with trunk impairments or vision impairments. Any proposed orthosis, prosthesis, or specially designed equipment to be used in competition must be inspected and approved prior to competition.[10-12]

■ MEDICAL COVERAGE LOGISTICS

Early arrival and consultation with local ski patrol is important to develop an emergency action plan (EAP). Thorough knowledge of the event course is essential to anticipate where injuries are most likely to occur and to determine where best to monitor an event while permitting efficient access to an injured athlete and to emergency transportation (snowmobile, ambulance, helicopter) to evacuate an athlete if needed. Communication lines, via at least 2 channels (phone and radio) should be open between the medical team, event director, and support personnel. Awareness of and contact information for local/regional hospitals is essential as these events often occur in regions remote from high-level trauma hospitals. It is also important to have a thorough understanding of banned medications specific to the individual sport as regulated by World Anti-Doping Agency (WADA), International Olympic Committee (IOC), or FIS.

■ MEDICAL EMERGENCIES AND MEDICAL BAG ESSENTIALS

Life-threatening emergencies that can occur include severe head trauma, spinal cord injury (SCI), blunt trauma resulting in rib fractures, pneumothorax, or splenic rupture,

Medical Bag Essentials in Skiing/Snowboarding	
Medical Emergencies:	**Wound Care:**
Automated External Defibrillator (AED)	Normal saline
14-and 16-gauge needles	Betadine/Alcohol swabs
Epi 1:1,000	Neosporin, mupirocin ointment
Albuterol inhaler	Gauzes
Pulse oximeter	Steri-strips
Supplemental oxygen	Suture tray
EpiPen	Lidocaine 1%
Head and Spine:	Gloves
	Wound irrigation skit
Concussion evaluation form	
Stretcher & Spine board	**Fractures and Dislocations:**
Cervical orthosis	Immobilizers and Slings
Eye kit	Crutches

and joint dislocations. Nontraumatic emergencies include cardiac arrest, anaphylaxis, and frost bite in athletes or spectators. The most common cause of skiing and snowboarding-associated mortality is cardiac arrest in the recreational population.[13]

EPIDEMIOLOGY

In the alpine skiing World Cup, 36.7 injuries occur per 100 athletes per season. Downhill skiing results in 17.2 injuries per 1,000 runs and slalom 4.9 injuries per 1,000 runs. Males are injured more than females, 12.7 vs 6.2 injuries per 1,000 runs. Professional skiers and snowboarders experience more severe injuries, with 30.9% resulting in more than 28 days missed from practice and competition and only 18.8% causing no time loss.[14] Freestyle skiing in general results in 38.5 injuries per 100 athletes per season, with moguls resulting in 32.6 injuries per 100 athletes per season and the disciplines of aerials and half-pipe resulting in much higher injury rates, 52.3 and 52.8 injuries per 100 athletes per season, respectively. Only 14.4% of freestyle skiing injuries are classified as severe.[15,16] Injury rates in snowboarding World Cup competition are 40.1–56.3 injuries per 100 athletes per season. Injury rates in big air are 2.33 per 1,000 runs, in giant slalom 0.34 per 1,000 runs, in snowboard cross 2.11 per 1,000 runs, and in parallel giant slalom 2.8 injuries per 1,000 runs. Again, males encounter more injuries than females, 6.7 vs 5.9 injuries per 1,000 runs, respectively. Severe injuries that result in greater than 28 days out of practice and competition account for 24.9–30.95 of professional snowboard injuries, while 26.3% do not result in time lost.[16,17] Injury rates in cross country skiing and ski jumping are much lower. Ski jumping results in 21.1 injuries per 100 athletes per season, nordic combined results in 19.2 injuries per 100 athletes per season, and cross-country skiing results in only 11.4 injuries per 100 athletes per season.[16]

COMMON INJURIES

Head and Spine Injuries

Head and neck injuries comprise 12%–13% of skiing and snowboarding injuries, the third most common injury locations with 24% classified as severe injuries. A *subdural hematoma* can be a life-threatening event that occurs after head trauma and constitutes 18.1% of severe head injuries in recreational skiers and snowboarders.[17] Warning symptoms and signs include loss of consciousness, headache, vomiting, dizziness, and seizures, but symptoms as minor as a persistent headache with no improvement should raise concern and prompt evaluation. Serial neurologic examinations should be performed and there should be a relatively low threshold for sending a patient to a hospital for advanced imaging and ongoing monitoring. *Concussion* is the most frequent head injury in recreational and professional skiing and snowboarding.[18] The most common mechanisms of head injury relate to a backward pitching fall, rotation, and hitting the posterior head on the slope.[19] When concussion is suspected, FIS guidelines dictate the immediate removal from competition and the medical evaluation of the athlete utilizing a standardized tool such as the Sport Concussion Assessment Tool to assess for signs of slowed reaction, poor balance, poor attention, and memory loss.[20] U.S. Ski & Snowboard prohibits the athlete from further participation until cleared in writing in which the healthcare professional must certify that he or she has successfully completed a continuing education course in the evaluation and management of concussive head injuries within three years of the day on which the written statement is made.[21] *Cervical spine injuries* should be considered in any athlete who is witnessed or believed to have had an impact with a fixed barrier/object or had a rapid deceleration injury. Any patient who is unconscious or is found with neurologic deficit should be treated as if they have a spinal cord injury (SCI) until proven otherwise. The airway should be urgently assessed and secured if tenuous and then neurologic testing should be done. A helmet should remain in place until a cervical spine injury has been ruled out. Stabilization on a spine board for transportation should be performed using the recommended techniques. X-rays might be accessible on site to assess the cervical spine, but in the event of polytrauma and evacuation to a hospital, CT of the cervical spine should be performed.

Upper Limb Injuries

Skier's thumb is the most common and well-known upper limb injury in skiers and prevalent in 6.6% of all alpine skiing injuries. The mechanism involves a fall onto an open hand with ski poles still in hand which results in forced abduction and extension at the metacarpophalangeal joint (MCPJ) imparting a valgus load to the ulnar collateral ligament. Skiers report ulnar-sided thumb MCPJ pain, pain with pinch-grip, and valgus laxity at the MCPJ. Radiographs should be considered to assess for a distal avulsion fracture before performing valgus stress testing as such testing can result in retracting proximally an avulsed distal tendon into a position that takes an injury that has potential for good nonsurgical recovery and then makes it surgical. A **Stener lesion** is a complete rupture of the distal ulnar collateral ligament (UCL) and proximal retraction that results in interposition of the adductor pollicis aponeurosis between the ligament and its proximal phalanx insertion. The thumb can be stabilized on site with a thumb spica splint and advanced imaging with MRI or ultrasound can be obtained to assess integrity of the UCL. Partial-thickness ligament injuries and nonretracted avulsion injuries can heal to regain valgus stability with spica splinting. Surgical repair or reconstruction is indicated for full-thickness tears and Stener lesions. In snowboarders, **wrist injuries** comprise 8% of all injuries at the World Cup level.[16] The mechanism of injury is backward fall and landing on an outstretched arm and wrist. Fractures account for 77.5% of wrist injuries, most involving the distal radius.[22] With such a high rate of fracture, it is prudent to obtain radiographs and/or CT imaging to assess. The AO classification of a **distal radius fracture** will guide determination of operative or nonoperative approaches. **Scaphoid fractures** make up only 4% of wrist fractures but can be occult in up to 16% of radiographs.[22] Clinical findings have limited specificity, but snuffbox tenderness, scaphoid tubercle tenderness, and discomfort with longitudinal compression of the thumb are clinically useful. The diagnostic sensitivity and specificity of ultrasound for scaphoid fracture reach 80% and 77% respectively, almost double those of radiographs.[23] Management of a scaphoid fracture will most often be surgical given its tenuous blood supply. **Shoulder injuries** in skiing and snowboarding result from direct impact with the ground, barriers, or fixed objects such as trees or poles, and most commonly result in **rotator cuff contusions, anterior glenohumeral dislocations, and acromioclavicular (AC) joint sprains**. Anterior glenohumeral dislocations result from a forceful blow to an abducted, extended, and externally rotated arm and present as anterior shoulder pain, visible shoulder deformity, and palpable subacromial step off. These can be manually reduced on site without sedation with adequate patient relaxation and when seen in the first hour after injury. Follow up imaging (x-rays) is recommended to assess proper relocation and rule out secondary injuries. **AC joint sprains** result from a forceful blow to the acromion resulting in caudal displacement of the acromion relative to the more medial clavicle and can result in tenderness at the AC articulation and a lateral step off at the joint. Treatment depends on the type of injury based on the Rockwood classification. Grades 1–2 are treated nonsurgically, grade 3 nonsurgically or surgically, grades 4–6 surgically. **Clavicle fractures** most commonly result from a direct blow to the clavicle, with only 5% resulting from fall on out-stretched hand (FOOSH) mechanisms, and present as anterior shoulder pain, a shortened clavicle, and pain with active shoulder forward flexion and abduction. Dedicated clavicle radiographs are required to assess the full medial-lateral extent of the clavicle. Treatment is often surgical in those involving the distal aspect and mostly nonsurgical in those involving the middle and proximal aspect of the clavicle.

Lower Limb Injuries

The most common significant lower limb injury in alpine and freestyle skiers is **anterior cruciate ligament (ACL) tear**, and **medial collateral ligament (MCL) sprain** in snowboarders. The most reported mechanism causing ACL injury is the "phantom foot" mechanism where the skier loses balance backward, squats back, shifts weight to the back of the ski, hyperflexes the knee, transfers weight to the downhill ski which then internally rotates the knee, catches a ski in the snow, and the body continues downhill over the downhill lower limb resulting valgus force at the knee.[24] A second common mechanism is known as the "slip catch" in which a skier, in the middle of a turn, loses contact with the snow on the downhill ski and reacts with knee extension to regain contact. This results in the inside edge catching the snow and a forceful tibial internal rotation and valgus stress. Most ACL injuries from snowboarding involve coming down from a jump onto a flat landing instead of a sloped landing. The relative internal rotation of the front tibia combined with an extended rear knee produces an anterior tibial shear force relative to the femur and supramaximal ACL loading and rupture.[25] Lachman has the highest sensitivity, and in combination with the anterior drawer, and pivot shift tests have comparably high specificity.[26] Thirty-two percent of ACL injuries in alpine skiing have concomitant ligamentous injuries, with MCL most associated. Knee radiographs can rule out concomitant fractures. Surgical ACL reconstruction is usually advisable in an active, young adult (18–35 years old).[27] **Fracture of the talus lateral process** is an injury unique to snowboarding, although **fractures of the medial and lateral malleoli** are much more common overall, comprising up two-thirds of ankle fractures. Talus lateral process fractures can present as pain and tenderness anterior and inferior to the tip of the distal fibula, which can be mistaken for an anterior talofibular ligament (ATFL) sprain. The mechanism of injury likely results from either forceful ankle dorsiflexion with foot inversion or dorsiflexion, axial impaction, eversion, and external rotation. Radiographs are the first step in diagnosis although there is no agreed upon "best view" for diagnosis. If this injury is suspected but radiographs are normal, a CT should be obtained as disability can occur if the fracture is missed. Nondisplaced and minimally displaced fractures can be conservatively treated with boot immobilization for 6 weeks, but early surgery can facilitate earlier quicker return to sport in many cases.[28]

Thoracoabdominal Injuries

In high-velocity or high-impact traumas, **rib fractures** are common and secondary **pneumothorax** can occur. Oral medication for pain control can be sufficient for an isolated rib fracture, but supplemental oxygen and early needle decompression may be required if a tension pneumothorax is present or suspected, especially with cardiorespiratory compromise. Snowboarders can be at increased risk for **splenic rupture** and this should be considered after a fall onto the left side presenting with abdominal pain.

■ SUMMARY

Skiing and snowboarding are popular winter sports that involves various competitions with different rules and injury patterns. As a sideline physician, it is important to have a thorough understanding of the various competitions and treating the most common injuries.

■ References

1. Fédération Internationale de Ski. History of snowsports. https://www.fis-ski.com/en/inside-fis/about-fis/history/history-of-snowsports. Published September 17, 2018.

2. Lund M, Miller P. *Roots of an Olympic Sport: Freestyle. Skiing Heritage.* Vol 10: Manchester Center, VT: International Skiing History Association; 1998:11-20.

3. Lund M, Miller P. *Roots of an Olympic Sport: Freestyle, Part 2 Freestyle Comes of Age. Skiing Heritage.* Vol 10. Manchester Center, VT: International Skiing History Association; 1998:19-29.

4. Rebagliati R. *Off the Chain: An Insider's History of Snowboarding.* Vancouver, BC, Canada: Greystone Books; 2012.

5. Gough C. Number of skiers and snowboarders in the U.S. 1996-2018. https://www.statista.com/statistics/376710/active-skiers-and-snowboarders-in-the-us/.

6. Cates E, Damon S, Ehlers JJ, et al. *2019 Alpine Competition Guide.* Park City, UT: U.S. Ski & Snowboard; 2018. https://usskiandsnowboard.org/sites/default/files/files-resources/files/2018/2019_ALP_CompGuide.pdf.

7. Fieguth K, Nyberg A. *2019 Freestyle/Freeskiing Competition Guide.* Park City, UT: U.S. Ski & Snowboard; 2018. https://usskiandsnowboard.org/sites/default/files/files-resources/files/2018/2019_FRE_CompGuide.pdf.

8. Nyberg A. *2019 Snowboarding Competition Guide.* Park City, UT: U.S. Ski & Snowboard; 2018. https://usskiandsnowboard.org/sites/default/files/files-resources/files/2018/2019_BRD_CompGuide.pdf.

9. Lazzaroni R. *2019 Nordic Competition Guide.* Park City, UT: U.S. Ski & Snowboard; 2018. https://usskiandsnowboard.org/sites/default/files/files-resources/files/2018/2019_NOR_CompGuide.pdf.

10. World Para Alpine Skiing. World Para Alpine Skiing classification rules and regulations. https://www.paralympic.org/sites/default/files/document/170803125229547_World+Para+Alpine+Skiing+Classification+Rules+Band+Regulations_Final.pdf. Published 2017.

11. World Para Nordic Skiing. World Para Nordic Skiing classification rules and regulations. https://www.paralympic.org/sites/default/files/document/170803114654801_World+Para+Nordic+Skiing+Classification+Rules+and+Regulations_0.pdf. Published 2017.

12. World Para Snowboard. World Para Snowboard classification rules and regulations. https://www.paralympic.org/sites/default/files/document/170803114835853_World+Para+Snowboard+Classification+Rules+and+Regulations_1.pdf. Published 2017.

13. Ruedl G, Bilek H, Ebner H, et al. Fatalities on Austrian ski slopes during a 5-year period. *Wilderness Environ Med.* 2011;22(4):326-328. doi:10.1016/j.wem.2011.06.008.

14. Flørenes TW, Bere T, Nordsletten L, et al. Injuries among male and female World Cup alpine skiers. *Br J Sports Med.* 2009;43(13):973-978. doi:10.1136/bjsm.2009.068759.

15. Flørenes TW, Heir S, Nordsletten L, Bahr R. Injuries among World Cup freestyle skiers. *Br J Sports Med.* 2010;44(11):803-808. doi:10.1136/bjsm.2009.071159.

16. Flørenes TW, Nordsletten L, Heir S, Bahr R. Injuries among World Cup ski and snowboard athletes. *Scand J Med Sci Sports.* 2012;22(1):58-66. doi:10.1111/j.1600-0838.2010.01147.x.

17. Major DH, Steenstrup SE, Bere T, et al. Injury rate and injury pattern among elite World Cup snowboarders: a 6-year cohort study. *Br J Sports Med.* 2014;48(1):18-22. doi:10.1136/bjsports-2013-092573.

18. de Roulet A, Inaba K, Strumwasser A, et al. Severe injuries associated with skiing and snowboarding: a National Trauma Databank study. *J Trauma Acute Care Surg.* 2017;82(4):781-786. doi:10.1097/TA.0000000000001358.

19. Steenstrup SE, Bakken A, Bere T, et al. Head injury mechanisms in FIS World Cup alpine and freestyle skiers and snowboarders. *Br J Sports Med.* 2018;52(1):61-69. doi:10.1136/bjsports-2017-098240.

20. Harmon KG, Drezner JA, Gammons M, et al. American Medical Society for Sports Medicine position statement: concussion in sport. *Br J Sports Med.* 2013;47(1):15-26. doi:10.1136/bjsports-2012-091941.

21. U.S. Ski & Snowboard. Concussion policy. https://usskiandsnowboard.org/governance/policies/concussion-policy.

22. Idzikowski JR, Janes PC, Abbott PJ. Upper extremity snowboarding injuries. Ten-year results from the Colorado Snowboard Injury Survey. *Am J Sports Med*. 2000;28(6):825-832. doi:10.1177/03635465000280061001.

23. Jain R, Jain N, Sheikh T, Yaday C. Early scaphoid fractures are better diagnosed with ultrasonography than X-rays: a prospective study over 114 patients. *Chin J Traumatol*. 2018;21(4):206-210. doi:10.1016/j.cjtee.2017.09.004.

24. Shea KG, Archibald-Seiffer N, Murdock E, et al. Knee injuries in downhill skiers: a 6-year survey study. *Orthop J Sports Med*. 2014;2(1):2325967113519741. doi:10.1177/2325967113519741.

25. Davies H, Tietjens B, Van Sterkenburg M, Mehgan A. Anterior cruciate ligament injuries in snowboarders: a quadriceps-induced injury. *Knee Surg Sports Traumatol Arthrosc*. 2009;17(9):1048-1051. doi:10.1007/s00167-008-0695-7.

26. Kaeding CC, Léger-St-Jean B, Magnussen RA. Epidemiology and diagnosis of anterior cruciate ligament injuries. *Clin Sports Med*. 2017;36(1):1-8. doi:10.1016/j.csm.2016.08.001.

27. Shea KG, Carey JL. Management of anterior cruciate ligament injuries: evidence-based guideline. *J AAOS*. 2015;23(5):e1-e5. doi:10.5435/JAAOS-D-15-00094.

28. Kirkpatrick DP, Hunter RE, Janes PC, et al. The snowboarder's foot and ankle. *Am J Sports Med*. 1998;26(2):271-277. doi:10.1177/03635465980260021901.

33. SOCCER

Julio Vazquez-Galliano

HISTORY

In virtually every country in the world, it is usual to refer to this game simply as "football" or by the translation of that English word into the native tongue. The term "soccer" is used in North America where its use is made necessary by the fact that Americans and Canadians use "football" to refer to their native, "gridiron" games.[1] The Football Association was established in England in 1863, where it amassed considerable interest and spread to other parts of the globe. It is considered to be the most popular sport in the world and, according to Fédération Internationale de Football Association (FIFA), in 2000 there were 265 million male and female soccer players worldwide.[2]

GOVERNING ORGANIZATIONS

- International: Fédération Internationale de Football Association (FIFA)
- National: United States Soccer Federation
- Major professional leagues: Major League Soccer (MLS), National Women's Soccer League
- College: National Collegiate Athletic Association (NCAA)
- High School: National Federation of State High School Associations

PARTICIPANTS

Classified as a low-static, high-dynamic sport, soccer is one of the fastest growing sports in the United States. Between 2000 and 2006, there was a 54% and 21% increase worldwide in the number of female and male participants registered.[3] In the United States, its participation at the high school level has increased four-fold among boys and 35-fold among girls within the last four decades.[4]

RULES AND REGULATIONS

A match lasts for two equal halves of 45 minutes. Players are entitled to an interval at half-time, not exceeding 15 minutes.[5,6] A match is played by two teams, each with a maximum of 11 players; one must be the goalkeeper. All the surfaces of the body can be used to play the ball, with the exception of the arms and hands, although these are used during throw-ins as well as by the goalkeeper (only within the goal box). A goal is scored when the whole of the ball passes over the goal line, between the goalposts, and under the crossbar. The team scoring the greater number of goals is the winner. If both teams score no goals or an equal number of goals the match is drawn. When competition rules require a winning team after a drawn match, two equal periods of extra time not exceeding 15 minutes each and/or kicks from the penalty mark may be used. Medical stoppages are permitted by competition rules. Medical evaluations are requested by the main referee. If a player suffers a concussion, he or she may not return to play.

If another injury is caused by another player who is penalized, then the player may return to play after cleared by the medical personnel. However, if the injury occurred without violation, then, if the player is substituted, he or she cannot return to play.[6]

■ EQUIPMENT

The *field* is made of natural or synthetic grass. The touchline must be longer than the goal line. Length (touchline): Minimum 90 m (100 yds) and maximum 120 m (130 yds). Length (goal line): Minimum 45 m (50 yds) and maximum 90 m (100 yds).[5]

Minimal equipment is required. The ball must have a circumference of 58 to 61 cm and be of a circular shape. The compulsory equipment of a player includes *shirt with sleeves, shorts, athletic cups for males and chest protectors for women, socks, shin guards* made of a suitable material to provide reasonable protection and covered by the socks and footwear. Goalkeepers may wear tracksuit bottoms and *padded gloves*. For safety reasons, all items of jewelry (necklaces, rings, bracelets, earrings, leather bands, rubber bands, etc.) are forbidden and must be removed. Using tape to cover jewelry is not permitted.

⟩⟩⟩ Adaptive Sport Key Points: Football Five-a-Side

Football five-a-side ("blind football") is an adaptation of soccer for athletes with a vision impairment. Each team is made up of one goalkeeper and four outfield players. Outfield players must be classified as completely blind (i.e., very low visual acuity and/or no light perception), and the goalkeeper must be sighted or partially sighted. To ensure fair competition, all outfield players are required to wear eye shades and all teams may have off-field guides available for assistance, and the ball makes noise, helping players to orient themselves. The duration of a five-a-side match is shorter—50 minutes with two halves of 25 minutes each—than a regulation soccer match (90 minutes).[7]

■ MEDICAL COVERAGE LOGISTICS

Prior to the game, it is important to determine the available medical and support personnel, as well as the medical equipment. Arrive early, at least 30 minutes prior to the game, to assess the medical equipment and support staff. The roles among the personnel need to be established before the game as well, and the Emergency Action Plan (EAP) should be reviewed. Keep note of the nearest hospital, preferably with a trauma center. The provider will introduce him or herself to both coaches, referees, and other staff. The role of the provider along with the support staff needs to be determined prior to the start of the game as well. The equipment should be set up on the home team sideline, but the medical staff can switch sidelines as needed. The referee will notify the head medical provider if an injured player needs to be evaluated on the field.

■ MEDICAL EMERGENCIES AND MEDICAL BAG ESSENTIALS

It is important to understand possible medical emergencies that you may encounter. The collapsed or unconscious athlete is considered a medical emergency and the proper channels should be activated. Nontraumatic deaths can be due to hypertrophic cardiomyopathy, cardiac arrhythmias, heat stroke, and asthma. You should take into account the type of participants, either elite or recreational. The latter are most susceptible to heat illness and dehydration.

Medical Bag Essentials in Soccer	
Medical Emergencies:	**Fractures and Dislocations:**
Automated External Defibrillator (AED)	Immobilizers and Slings
Cricothyrotomy kit	Crutches
Epi 1:1000	**Wound Care:**
Albuterol inhaler	Normal saline
Rectal thermometer	Betadine swabs
Ice bath	Neosporin, mupirocin ointment
Head and Spine:	Moleskin
Concussion evaluation form	Elastic bandage
Stretcher & Spine board	Tube stretch gauze
Cervical orthosis	Sterile gauzes

■ EPIDEMIOLOGY

Soccer, like any sport, places physical demands on its participants and poses a risk for injury. From 2005/2006 to 2013/2014, the overall injury rate in high school soccer players was found to be 2.06 per 1,000 athlete exposure (AE). Typically, more injuries occur during competition than practice. The lower limbs and the head/face were the most commonly injured body areas, specifically the ankle, knee, and thigh. The majority of competition injuries result from player–player contact while the majority of practice injuries result from noncontact mechanisms. Female youth have more soccer injuries than male youth.[4] The rate of head injuries in soccer, which include lacerations, abrasions, concussions, contusions, and facial fractures decreased substantially after 2006, when the direct and deliberate "elbows to head" were punished with a red card.[8] The overall rate of concussion in high school soccer in the United States from 2005/2006 to 2013/2014 was estimated to be 4.5 per 10,000 AE and 2.78 per 10,000 AE, with player–player contact being the most common mechanism of injury.[9]

■ COMMON INJURIES

Head and Spine Injuries

The most common type of **head injury** are **concussions.** This is a type of traumatic brain injury induced by biomechanical forces that may be caused either by a direct blow to the head, face, neck or elsewhere on the body with an impulsive force transmitted to the head.[10] The majority of concussions in soccer occur from direct contact during an aerial challenge, not from purposely heading of the ball. These include head-to-head, elbow-to-head, knee-to-head, foot-to-head, and head-to-ground contact. Concussion results in a range of clinical signs and symptoms that may or may not involve loss of consciousness. Accurate and timely identification of a possible concussion is key, and the evaluation should begin by assessing for cervical spine injury, intracranial bleeding, and other injuries that can present in a similar fashion or in addition to concussion. The sideline concussion evaluation should consist of a symptom assessment and a neurologic examination that addresses cognition (briefly), cranial nerve function, and balance. The Sport Concussion Assessment Tool 5 (SCAT 5) can be used as a screening tool. The player must be taken out of the game and cannot return to play on the same day. If no red flags are observed, then the player may remain on the sideline without his or her equipment. Follow up with a sports physician is recommended in 24 to 48 hours for reassessment and plan for graduated return to sport protocol.

Upper Limb Injuries

Upper limb injuries are not common. **Jersey finger** is an avulsion injury of the flexor digitorum profundus tendon, commonly seen in the ring finger. Mechanism of injury is due to extension of a flexed finger; the typical scenario is when a player tries to grab an opponent's clothing resulting in the distal phalanx being forcibly extended while the athlete is actively flexing. Symptoms include inability to actively flex the distal interphalangeal (DIP) joint. Plain films should be performed to exclude an associated avulsion fracture of the distal phalanx. Management includes surgical repair.

Lower Limb Injuries

Lower limb injuries are common due to the running, kicking, and cutting nature of the sport. **Hamstring strains** typically presents with a sudden, sharp pain localized to the posterior thigh which may be related to an eccentric contraction or an excessive stretch. During the examination, the area should be inspected for visible asymmetry, swelling, or ecchymosis. Palpation of the entire posterior thigh is important to localize the injury, with particular attention to the origin at the ischial tuberosity. In the acute setting, the management involves rest, ice, compression, elevation, and nonsteroidal anti-inflammatory drugs (NSAIDs) followed by rehabilitation with eccentric lengthening exercises. **Quadriceps strains** typically affect the rectus femoris since it is the only one of the four heads of the quadriceps femoris muscle that crosses two joints, the hip and the knee. The most common site of strain is the distal musculotendinous junction. Athletes present with a sudden pain in the anterior thigh during an activity requiring a forceful eccentric contraction of the quadriceps. During examination, the clinician may see ecchymosis and limited range of motion of the knee due to discomfort. Pain is usually elicited with resisted knee extension. Initial treatment includes rest, ice, compression, and elevation. Acetaminophen and/or NSAIDs may be used during the acute phase. For return to play, symmetric pain-free range of motion should be observed, and athletes should be able to demonstrate near normal strength compared to the contralateral side and perform well on functional tests. A **Quadriceps contusion** known colloquially as a "charley horse," is the result of direct blow or trauma to the thigh with resultant focal pain that increases with knee flexion. More significant contusions can result in hematoma formation. Severity of the contusion can be divided into mild, moderate, and severe based on the degree of passive knee flexion after 24 hours. Initial treatment includes rest, ice, compression, and elevation, particularly during the first 24 to 48 hours, to limit the extent of localized bleeding, swelling, and pain. The knee of the contused thigh should be immobilized immediately in 120 degrees of flexion with an elastic wrap. This position of flexion should be maintained for the first 24 hours. Acetaminophen and/or NSAIDs may be used during the acute period. The return-to-play recommendations are similar to the ones for quadriceps strain. **Adductor strains** account for roughly 10% of all injuries in soccer players.[11] Typically, these injuries occur as a result of a rapid acceleration and deceleration, sudden changes in direction and kicking, the adductor longus being the most commonly injured adductor muscle. Usually athletes present with the chief complaint of acute groin pain, located in the medial upper thigh. A complete inspection and palpation of the medial thigh should be performed to look for tenderness, swelling, or defects. Symptoms are commonly accentuated with adduction of the legs against resistance. In many cases, the diagnosis is based solely on the history and physical examination. Adductor strains are managed similar to quadriceps and hamstring injuries. **Anterior cruciate ligament (ACL) injuries** generally occur during a rotational movement or deceleration but can occur with direct contact which may lead to a more complex injury involving the medial meniscus and medial collateral ligament (MCL). Patients often describe an audible "pop" or feeling of "something going out and then going back." Most complete tears of the ACL are extremely painful and associated with a large tense effusion. Physical examination may reveal swelling, restricted movement, and widespread mild tenderness. A combined ligamentous examination (with the anterior drawer, pivot shift, and Lachman testing) has a high sensitivity and specificity for the diagnosis of ACL injuries. Imaging studies including radiographs and magnetic resonance imaging (MRI) can help confirm the diagnosis. Patients may undergo nonoperative or operative management depending on the tear and symptoms. *MCL injury* usually occurs as a result of a valgus stress to the partially flexed knee. This injury can occur in a noncontact mechanism from cutting, pivoting, or twisting, or in contact sports with a blow to the lateral aspect of the leg or lower thigh. Symptoms vary by grades of injury (Grades I–III), with Grade II as a partial tear and Grade III as a complete tear. Focal tenderness without swelling often accompanies a Grade I. A Grade II MCL sprain usually shows marked tenderness and localized swelling, and there is some laxity with valgus stress at 30° of knee flexion. Patients with a Grade III tear of the MCL often complain of a feeling of instability, and on examination the valgus stress applied at 30° of flexion reveals gross laxity without a distinct end point. Most MCL injuries heal reliably with conservative management and a hinged knee brace for 4 to 6 weeks. *Gastrocnemius muscle strains* occur typically when the athlete attempts to accelerate by extending the knee from a stationary position. The medial head of the gastrocnemius is the most common site of injury. This results in immediate pain and tenderness, and in complete muscle tears, there may be a palpable defect. The initial management involves rest, ice, compression, and elevation. Heel lifts may reduce pain by decreasing the stretch of the calf muscles. Rehabilitation consists of a progressive program starting with optimizing the flexibility and range of motion of the ankle and knee, once the pain and swelling have settled. Then, the progression is from active range of motion to strengthening exercises to sport-specific drills. *Ankle sprains* typically involve the anterior talofibular ligament (ATFL) which is the weakest of the lateral ankle ligaments. The most common injury motion is inversion of the plantar-flexed foot. Symptoms include pain, swelling, tenderness along the affected ligaments, and discomfort with weight-bearing. The Ottawa ankle rules can be used to assist the clinician in the decision-making for obtaining plain films. Initial management involves ice, compression, and elevation. Analgesics and/or NSAIDs may be required in the acute phase. Crutches are used in patients with severe sprains who are unable to bear weight. Functional rehabilitation begins with exercises for mobility and strength, and proceeds to exercises for proprioception and activity-specific training. Return-to-sport is advised when functional exercises can be performed without pain. Both external prophylactic measures (bracing or taping) as well as neuromuscular training are equally effective in reducing the risk for ankle-sprain recurrences after an index ankle sprain.[12]

■ SUMMARY

Soccer is among the most popular sports in the world. It is a fast-paced, high-endurance sport, and as a sideline physician it is important to understand the biomechanics of injuries, specifically lower limb injuries.

■ References

1. Crocombe M. The origin, history, and invention of soccer. https://www.liveabout.com/who-invented -soccer-3556873. Published July 22, 2019.

2. Big count survey. https://resources.fifa.com/image/upload/big-count-stats-package-520046.pdf?cloudid =mzid0qmguixkcmruvema

3. Putukian M, Echemendia RJ, Chiampas G, et al. Head injury in soccer: from science to the field; summary of the head injury summit held in April 2017 in New York City, New York. *Br J Sports Med.* 2019;53(21):1332. doi:10.1136/bjsports-2018-100232.

4. Khodaee M, Currie DW, Asif IM, Comstock RD. Nine-year study of US high school soccer injuries: data from a national sports injury surveillance programme. *Br J Sports Med.* 2017;51(3):185-193. doi:10.1136/bjsports-2015-095946.

5. Football (Soccer) rules. https://www.rulesofsport.com/sports/football.html.

6. NCAA soccer 2018 and 2019 rules. http://www.region19.org/d/Soccer_2018-19_Rules.pdf. Published June 2018.

7. History of football 5-a-side. https://www.paralympic.org/football-5-a-side/about.

8. Beaudouin F, aus der Fünten K, Tross T, et al. Head injuries in professional male football (soccer) over 13 years: 29% lower incidence rates after a rule change (red card). *Br J Sports Med.* 2019;53(15):948-952. doi:10.1136/bjsports-2016-097217.

9. Comstock RD, Currie DW, Pierpoint LA, et al. An evidence-based discussion of heading the ball and concussions in high school soccer. *JAMA Pediatr.* 2015;169(9):830-837. doi:10.1001/jamapediatrics.2015.1062.

10. McCrory P, Meeuwisse W, Dvorak J, et al. Consensus statement on concussion in sport—the 5th International Conference on Concussion in Sport held in Berlin, October 2016. *Br J Sports Med.* 2017;51(11):838-847. doi:10.1136/bjsports-2017-097699.

11. Tammareddi K, Morelli V, Reyes M, Jr. The athlete's hip and groin. *Prim Care.* 2013;40(2):313-333. doi:10.1016/j.pop.2013.02.005.

12. Verhagen EA, Bay K. Optimising ankle sprain prevention: a critical review and practical appraisal of the literature. *Br J Sports Med.* 2010;44(15):1082-1088. doi:10.1136/bjsm.2010.076406.

34. SOFTBALL

Alexandra M. Rivera-Vega

■ HISTORY

Softball was invented in 1887 by Chicago reporter George Hancock as a form of indoor baseball that could be played in the winter. The sport was originally called "kitten ball," "diamond ball," "mush ball," and "pumpkin ball" until 1926 when the term "softball" was used. In 1933, the first-ever national amateur softball tournament took place in conjunction with the Chicago World Fair. Soon afterward, the American Softball Association (ASA) was established and softball's popularity spread throughout the world.[1] In 1952, the International Softball Federation (ISF) held its first meeting and would eventually govern the sport around the globe. The first Softball World Championship took place in 1965 when women's teams from five countries competed in Australia. One year later, the first Men's World Championship would be played in Mexico. In 1992, women's fast pitch softball was selected to debut as a medal sport at the 1996 Olympic Summer Games in Atlanta.[1]

■ GOVERNING ORGANIZATIONS
- International: World Baseball Softball Confederation (WBSC) since 2014 when the International Baseball Federation (IBAF) and the International Softball Federation (ISF) merged
- National: USA Softball (formerly the Amateur Softball Association [ASA] and ASA/USA Softball)
- Major Professional League: National Pro Fast pitch (NPF), formerly the Women's Pro Softball League, is a professional women's softball league in the United States.
- College: National Collegiate Athletic Association (NCAA)
- High School: The National Federation of State High School Associations (NFHS)

■ PARTICIPANTS

Men and women play softball both recreationally and competitively in over 100 countries around the world. The WBSC has 113 member countries (excluding dependent territories). The former ASA, now USA Softball, has overseen more than 80,000 teams annually within their youth programs and encompass more than 170,000 teams with 2.5 million adult participants annually.[2] Approximately 1.3 million athletes belong to fast pitch and slow pitch teams. As per the NFSHSA report, during the 2010 to 2011 school year, 1,548 boys and 389,455 girls competed in either fast or slow pitch teams. At the NCAA level, 950 women's fast pitch teams with a total of 17,154 participants were competing in 2007-2008.

■ RULES AND REGULATIONS

Two nine-player teams play for seven innings on a field that has as a focal point a diamond-shaped dirt infield with a home plate and three other bases, 60 ft (18.29 m) apart.

This forms a circuit that must be completed by a base runner in order to score. The central offensive action entails hitting a pitched ball with a wooden or metal bat and running the bases. The winner is the team scoring the most runs. The ball used in this game is a sphere approximately 12 in. (30.5 cm) in circumference with a twine-covered center of cork or polyurethane mixture covered by stitched horsehide and is typically optic yellow in color. Specifically to softball, there are fewer innings and a smaller field than baseball. Bases are 60 ft apart (vs. 90 ft in baseball). The pitcher throws from a flat pitching circle (vs. a raised mound in baseball). Either an 11-in or 12-in circumference ball is used. Regulation softball weight ranges between 6.25 and 7 oz (vs. 5 oz of baseball). The underhand pitching technique (windmill pitch) is one of the most important differences with baseball.[2]

EQUIPMENT

A *helmet, chest protector,* and *shin guards* are the main equipment required for safety. To play softball, a *ball, a bat, gloves,* and *uniforms* are required.

>>> Adaptive Sport Key Points: Softball

Wheelchair softball was started in 1975 by a few individuals with spinal cord injuries and lower limb impairments in the Midwest. The game is played under the official rules of the 16-in. slow pitch softball as approved by the ASA of America with 15 exceptions that are geared toward the wheelchair user. Among those are: players compete on hard surfaces, such as a parking lot, instead of a normal baseball field, and use a 16-in. softball, which allows wheelchair players to keep one hand on the wheelchair while catching the softball without a glove. Similar to wheelchair basketball, teams are balanced by using a scoring system. Quad (any) = 1 point; Class I = 1 point; Class II = 2 points; Class III = 3 points. At no time in a game shall a team have players participating with a total value of points greater than 22.[3]

MEDICAL COVERAGE LOGISTICS

Arrive as early as possible (30–45 minutes prior to the game) to determine the available personnel (medical and support) as well as the medical equipment beforehand. Some games will have on-site EMT personnel while others will have them on call in case of emergencies. Establish the roles of the personnel and review the Emergency Action Plan before the game starts. Keep notes of the emergency medical technician (EMT) contact numbers and nearest hospital (preferably a trauma center). The provider will introduce him- or herself to coaches, umpires, and other event support staff. The umpire will notify the medical staff if a player needs evaluation.

MEDICAL EMERGENCIES AND MEDICAL BAG ESSENTIALS

Possible medical emergencies that one might encounter in a softball game include: a collapsed or unconscious athlete if hit by a thrown or batted ball to the head; chest injury and/or cardiac injury secondary to possible commotio cordis; acute joint injury resulting in fracture, instability, or dislocation. Heat-related injuries are less common in softball, but one should be prepared, particularly with catchers, to treat athletes for potential heat illness.

EPIDEMIOLOGY

The National High School Sports Related Injury Surveillance system collected longitudinal data from 2005 to 2008 school years. It found a higher injury rate for competitive

Medical Bag Essentials in Softball	
Medical Emergencies:	**Fractures and Dislocations:**
Automated External Defibrillator (AED)	Immobilizers and Slings
Epi 1:1,000	Crutches
Diphenhydramine	**Wound Care:**
Albuterol inhaler	Normal saline
Ice bath	Betadine/Alcohol swabs
Thermometer	Neosporin, mupirocin ointment
Head and Spine:	Gauzes
Concussion evaluation form	Vaseline
Stretcher & Spine board	Steri-strips
Cervical orthosis	Suture tray

games (1.74 per 1,000 athlete exposures [AE]) compared with practices (0.742 per 1,000 AE). Severe injury rate (loss of sport participation of more than 21 days) was 0.3 per 1,000 AE for games and 0.12 per 1,000 AE for practices. The knee (30.7%) and the ankle (19.2%) were the most common severely injured body areas. Fractures (41.3%) and ligament sprains/tears (33.3%) were the most common etiology of severe injuries. Collision with bases (21.3%) was the most common form of trauma. Catastrophic injuries in softball are rare.[2] Most softball injuries are due to contact with the ground, the ball, or an object such as a wall or the base. Sliding lesions can make up to 23% of all game injuries. Lesions unique to softball are associated mainly with the windmill pitching technique. These include biceps tendinopathy, forearm stress fractures, and ulnar neuritis.[4]

■ COMMON INJURIES

Head and Spine Injuries

The majority of **head trauma** include direct cranial blows, ocular, mouth, and dental injury.[4] For **concussions** in any sport, and regardless of level of play, providers must be up-to-date on the appropriate treatment. This includes immediate removal from play and a full neurological assessment including the administration of a Sport Concussion Assessment Tool (SCAT) test. For minors, periodic assessment throughout the game or practice should be performed until cleared to leave with a parent if under age. Further evaluation with a sports medicine provider and/or concussion specialist will be required for further assessment in the next 1 to 2 days.

Upper Limb Injuries

Hand and wrist trauma include various **finger** and **thumb sprains**, primarily attributable to batting mishaps and from falling on outstretched arms during sliding. **Wrist tendinopathies, metacarpal stress fractures** and diminished neurological sensation are especially prevalent among pitchers.[4] Injuries include **interphalangeal joint sprain/dislocation, mallet finger** and **thumb ulnar collateral ligament sprain**. Management includes immobilizing; rest, ice, compression, elevation (RICE); and obtaining x-rays for assessment of a fracture/irreducible dislocation that requires surgical evaluation. The majority of emergency cases involve **spiral and oblique fractures of the humerus**. **Radial nerve damage** associated with denervation and palsy distal to the elbow can happen following abrupt cubital extension and hyperextension.[4] A common injury is **ulnar collateral ligament sprain/tear at the elbow** which may require surgical repair if a complete tear.

Lower Limb Injuries

Anterior cruciate ligament (ACL) tear, medial collateral ligament (MCL) sprain, meniscal tear, patellar subluxation/dislocation are common injuries. Obtaining a detailed history (including the mechanism of injury) and a thorough exam for diagnosis purposes is extremely important. Initial x-Ray imaging is required for assessing fractures, dislocations, and avulsion fractures needing surgical evaluation. *Ankle sprains* (lateral, medial, or high ankle sprain), *tibial fracture (acute or stress), fibula fracture, ankle dislocation* can also occur. On-site treatment usually requires RICE. The Ottawa ankle rules may help to indicate when x-Rays are needed. They should include anteroposterior (AP) and lateral views of the ankle, tibia and fibula, as well as mortise view. Nonoperative treatment with RICE, immobilization, and a functional rehabilitation program are the first line of treatment for ankle sprains without diastasis instability or concomitant fracture. *Hip contusions and hip/adductor strains* may also be seen. Symptoms include local pain and swelling. RICE is recommended as initial treatment. The player can return to play once strength is equal to the contralateral side.

Dermatologic Injuries

Since softball is played outdoors, there is risk of *sunburn* and *heat -elated illness*. Players can also get *abrasions, blisters,* and *contusions*. Treatment includes local care with normal saline and triple antibiotic.

■ SUMMARY

Softball is a unique sport played by female and male athletes from young age until adulthood. Knowing the sport and the most common injuries are key elements for sideline coverage.

■ References

1. History. Softball New Zealand. https://www.softball.org.nz/Softball+NZ/History.html.

2. Briskin SM. Injuries and medical issues in softball. *Curr Sports Med Rep.* 2012;1(5):265-271. doi:10.1249/JSR.0b013e3182699489.

3. Meyers MC, Brown BR, Bloom JA. Fast pitch softball injuries. *Sports Med.* 2001;31(1):61-73. doi:10.2165/00007256-200131010-00005.

4. Softball. https://www.wheelchairsportsfederation.org/adaptive-sports/softball. Updated December 11, 2009.

35. SURFING

Claudia Jimenez-Garcia, Jose R. Vives-Alvarado,
and Luis Baerga-Varela

HISTORY

The exact origin of surfing is not known. Research suggests it developed in Western Polynesia over 3,000 years ago, where it was used to assert dominance by community chiefs. Surfing was first described by Lieutenant James King of the British Navy in the 18th century when he wrote about surfboard riding by the locals of Kealakekua Bay on the Kona coast of Hawaii. In the early 20th century it spread from Hawaii to California and Australia and has continued to evolve and spread worldwide ever since.[1]

GOVERNING ORGANIZATIONS

- International: International Surfing Association
- Major professional league: World Surf League

PARTICIPANTS

Surfing is a popular recreational and competitive sport, which has grown dramatically since the 1960s. There are an estimated 37 million surfers worldwide, 2.1 million in the United States alone.[2,3]

RULES AND REGULATIONS

In the first circuit, the World Qualifying Series (WQS), pro surfers compete to reach the elite circuit called the World Championship Tour (WCT) where 34 males and 17 females compete at the highest level. In contests by the International Surfing Association (ISA), each country sends a team of three males and three females to compete for medals. For the Tokyo 2020 Summer Olympics, 20 men and 20 women will compete in shortboard.[4,5] In Olympic competition, the format will progress through initial and main rounds which eventually lead to gold medal and bronze medal matches. The initial rounds will have four- and five-person heats, and the main rounds will have two-person heats where the winner advances to the next round and the loser is eliminated. The length of a heat is normally 30 minutes and is decided by the Technical Director depending on the conditions of the day. In this time, athletes will be allowed to ride a maximum of 25 waves, and their two highest scoring waves will count toward their heat total which creates their heat result. The following five criteria are used to score waves: commitment and degree of difficulty, innovative and progressive maneuvers, combination of major maneuvers, variety of maneuvers, and speed, power, and flow.[5]

EQUIPMENT

There are four main board categories: *longboards, shortboards, SUP boards, and tow-in boards*. In terms of recreational surfing, surf equipment may vary by where the sport is

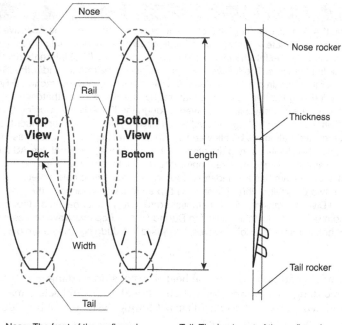

Nose: The front of the surfboard
Rocker: The curve applied to the
nose and tail

Tail: The back part of the surfboard
Rail: The shape of the sides of the
surfboard

Figure 35.1 Surfboard anatomy.
Source: Adapted from Parts of a surfboard. https://calimasurf.com/news/parts-of-a-surfboard.
Courtesy of Calima Surf School, Lanzarote.

practiced geographically due to changing water and weather temperatures and conditions. The anatomy of surfboards is seen in Figure 35.1. Protective equipment has been developed such as temperature-appropriate **wetsuits** protecting against hypothermia, as well as protected, rounded, and shock-absorbing surfboard noses and fin-trailing edges. A **board leash** should be used to keep the board close at hand, and the board can be used as a flotation device should a surfer become exhausted or injured. Regulatory bodies also restrict the use of any equipment other than a surfboard (inflatable boats, SUPs, paddles, surf skis, water patrols' board or jet skis, photographers' craft, or previous or current heat Surfers' or other Caddies surfboards), unless the surfer is in a life-threatening situation as deemed by water patrol. Water caddies are permitted only under extreme conditions by ISA.

■ MEDICAL COVERAGE LOGISTICS

Prior to an event it is important to determine logistical information for deployment of emergency services teams including: personnel, deployment of personnel, dress standards and appearance, access to arenas, equipment, communications, vehicle access, and alternative venues. An ambulance dedicated to the event should be present at all times during the competition. A local hospital with trauma level-1 capabilities and emergency room should also be designated to receive any medical emergencies from the competition. The medical personnel and organizing committee should also evaluate weather and surf conditions prior and during competition to determine whether it is necessary to postpone, cancel, or relocate all or parts of a competition. Adverse

>>> **Adaptive Sport Key Points: Surfing**

Under the ISA Adaptive Surfing Guidelines, in order to compete in the Adaptive Surfing competitions, an athlete must have an eligible impairment under the list of Eligible Impairments presented in the International Paralympic Committee (IPC) International Standard for Eligible Impairments. The following are the eligible impairments under the ISA for adaptive surfing: impaired muscle power, impaired passive range of motion (PROM), limb deficiency, leg length difference, short stature, hypertonia, ataxia, athetosis, vision impairment. Athletes are assessed and reviewed through the ISA Adaptive Surfing Classification Review Committee (ASCRC) and classified as Eligible, Not Eligible, or Under Review. Each national federation will be allowed to field a team of up to eight athletes in the following six classifications: two athletes-AS 1 (stand/kneel), two athletes-AS 2 (stand/kneel), one athlete-visually impaired, one athlete-upright, one athlete-prone, one athlete-assist. Each team has a mandatory spot for at least one female athlete. All athletes will surf in two Qualifying Round heats and top surfers will advance to the Final Round(s). An Overall Division Ranking will be established for every surfer based on the top two wave score points from either Qualifying Rounds 1 or 2 (top two wave scores can be from same round). In terms of judging waves, Standard ISA Judging Criteria are used.[6]

weather includes conditions of extreme heat or cold, storms, dangerous surf or swell, and associated dangers to competitors. Occupational health and safety matters should also be considered. Tools such as Surf Hazard Rating System have been developed to aid in the assessment of risk management.[7]

■ MEDICAL EMERGENCIES AND MEDICAL BAG ESSENTIALS

Most surfing-related injuries presenting to U.S. emergency departments appear to be consistent with acute traumatic injuries as opposed to chronic overuse injuries. Some of the most severe injuries in surfing have occurred in shallow beaches with hard bottoms when surfers hit the bottom head first.[8] Very little has been reported on the topics of submersion injuries, drowning or death during surfing. However, although infrequent, these are often fatal. Most *submersion injuries* are usually related to head injury. Many surfers have described near-death experiences, especially in big wave surfing, after getting caught under water by multiple subsequent waves. However, in the absence of trauma, drowning is rare among experienced surfers. Among inexperienced surfers, risk factors for drowning are poor swimming skills, lack of aerobic capacity, and inebriation, especially in the setting of rip currents.[9] Nontraumatic deaths can be due to hypertrophic cardiomyopathy, cardiac arrhythmias, anaphylaxis, and asthma. *Fin-related injuries* are mostly superficial, however, fatal and near fatal fin lacerations of the aorta and femoral arteries have been described as well as evisceration and rectal injuries.[9] Cases of splenic rupture and pneumothorax have been reported secondary to blunt trauma to the abdomen and chest respectively and liver lacerations have also been reported. Severe *surfboard*-related ocular injuries have been reported, occasionally resulting in global ruptures and permanent monocular vision loss. Ocular injuries often occur due to the recoil of the leash causing the pointed nose of the board to strike the surfer's eye. A surfer's *leash* can also contribute to drowning if it gets caught on the ocean floor. Finger amputations caused by getting caught in a loop within the leash during a wipe out have been reported. Tympanic membrane injuries sometimes occur when surfers are hit by the lip of a large forceful wave or by hitting the water with a high-speed wipeout. Tympanic membrane injuries can cause immediate conductive hearing loss, ear pain, and bloody discharge. *Spinal cord injuries* due to surfing have been reported to be similar to injuries seen in shallow water diving accidents.

The usual mechanism has been reported to occur when the surfer wipes out and strikes the bottom head first leading to excessive axial loading, hyperextension, hyperflexion, or rotational injury to the cervical spine Headfirst injury at sand bottom beaches has also resulted in a number of cases of quadriplegia in young surfers. Any surfer found floating on the surface or with complaints of severe neck pain after a wipeout should be presumed to have suffered an unstable cervical spine fracture until proven otherwise. An improvised backboard can be made by using the surfboard as a backboard and immobilizing the patient's spine by using towels on either side of the surfer's neck and head and around the neck. The board's leash may be used to immobilize the surfer's waist around the board while the patient is transported to a medical facility.[9]

Medical Bag Essentials in Surfing	
Medical Emergencies:	**Fractures and Dislocations:**
Automated External Defibrillator (AED)	Immobilizers and Slings
Tourniquet	Crutches
Cricothyrotomy kit	**Wound Care:**
14- and 16-gauge needles	Normal saline
Epi 1:1,000	Betadine swabs
Diphenhydramine or another antihistamine	Neosporin, mupirocin ointment
Albuterol inhaler	Moleskin
Rectal thermometer	Elastic bandage
Ice bath	Tube stretch gauze
Head and Spine:	Sterile gauzes
Concussion evaluation form	Vaseline
Stretcher & Spine board	Steri-strips
Cervical orthosis	Suture tray
	Lidocaine 1%

EPIDEMIOLOGY

The rates of surfing injuries are highly variable depending on the style of surfing and the competitive level at which it is practiced. There are 5.7 injuries per 1,000 athlete exposures in competitive surfing.[3] Acute injury rate in both competitive and recreational surfers was found to be 1.79 major injuries per 1,000 hours of surfing. A total of 131,494 injuries were seen in ED in 2012–2013.[8] Injuries were classified by anatomical region, injury type, and level of care. The anatomical region most commonly affected was lower limbs (25.9%), followed by face (23.1%), and head and neck (22.7%). Upper limbs and trunk accounted for 16.7% and 8.6% of injuries respectively. The most common injury type was found to be lacerations (40.7%), followed by sprains and strains (14.4%), contusions (12.9%), and fractures (11.9%). Approximately 96% of surfing injuries that arrived to the ED were treated and released. However, in patients older than 60 years, trunk injuries, fractures, and internal organs were admitted at increased frequency.[8] The most common mechanism overall was direct contact with the surfer's board or ocean floor.[3,8]

COMMON INJURIES

Head and Spine Injuries

Head and neck injuries include traumatic spinal cord injuries (SCI) as discussed in Medical Emergencies. **Lacerations** are the most common type of head, face, and neck injury accounting for 62.7% of laceration injuries.[8] These tend to result from direct trauma with either a surfer's board or contact with the ocean floor. Treatment depends on the severity of the laceration. **Cervical sprains** and **strains** account for 28.8% of all sprains and strains in surfing. **Concussions** are infrequent in surfing and account for only 2.7% of all injuries,[2,8] but they may be under-reported. The use of helmets or protective headgear has been proposed to reduce the risk of head injuries, but most surfers are not willing to wear a helmet due to underestimation of risk of injury and surf culture fashion.[10] A complete assessment should be performed with a concussion assessment tool like the Sport Concussion Assessment Tool 5 (SCAT 5). Rest and symptomatic management are the mainstay of treatment followed by a graduated return-to-sport progression.

Although **trunk injuries** account for only 8.6% of injuries, the trunk is one of the most common anatomic regions requiring hospitalization (10.3%).[8] Surfer's myelopathy is a form of nontraumatic SCI that typically affects young, thin males learning how to surf, especially first-time surfers. It presents with nontraumatic back pain, progressing to paraparesis with sensory and urinary symptoms. MRI may show increased signal involving the lower thoracic cord in long TR sequences. There is usually complete or near complete recovery of symptoms with rare cases of residual paraplegia.[11] Thoracic spinal cord changes are thought to be caused by ischemia secondary to kinking or vasospasm of spinal arteries secondary to prone hyperextension during paddling. Treatment depends on neurologic deficits. **Paraspinal muscle strains** in the lumbar and cervical spine are common due to the sustained isometric contraction required while lying prone on the board while paddling. Neck soreness may result with neck hyperextension as a compensatory mechanism for inadequate back extension due to fatigued muscles or lack of lumbar or thoracic flexibility. Dynamic warm-up and routine stretching of low back muscles, hamstrings, and hip flexors, together with a good core-strengthening program are important factors in helping prevent these injuries. However, as low back extension is repetitive, spondylolysis involving the pars interarticularis should be kept in mind when focal low back pain is observed in young surfers.

Upper Limb Injuries

Sprains and strains are the most common upper limb injuries. **Shoulder injuries** commonly result from paddling as a surfer spends 50% of the time paddling, 45% still, and only 3% to 5% wave riding. Muscle strength imbalance between the internal rotators and the external rotators of the shoulder together with scapular instability have been proposed as cause for these types of injuries. Overdevelopment and shortening of pectoralis and anterior deltoid relative to weaker scapular stabilizers lead to scapular protraction resulting in **impingement syndrome** and secondary **rotator cuff tendinopathy** and/or **tears**.[9] Core and back extensor weakness or fatigue may also result in reduced lumbar extension leading to a more unstable shoulder position while paddling, also contributing to impingement syndrome and rotator cuff tendinopathy. Rehabilitation should involve a period of relative rest and physical therapy modalities. If a bursopathy is present without significant evidence of tendinopathy or tendon tears on sonography, an ultrasound-guided low dose corticosteroid bursa injection may be considered for short-term symptom relief. A rehabilitation program should include pectoralis and posterior capsule stretching, strengthening of scapular stabilizers and rotator cuff, along with core-strengthening exercises. Once the athlete achieves painless range of motion (ROM) and is able to paddle without pain, gradual return to surfing may be started. **Lateral epicondylopathy** and **triceps tendinopathy** are also seen from the forces exerted while duck diving and popping up. These may be treated with physical therapy and rehabilitation exercises. Regenerative techniques including prolotherapy, platelet-rich plasma, and extracorporeal shockwave may be considered.[9] **Fractures** are more common in the upper limbs (31.7%).[8] These will require immobilization in the field and transfer to the hospital for x-rays and definitive treatment. It is important to rule out neurovascular compromise before and after immobilization. **Dislocations** which account for only 4.5% of all injuries are more common in the upper limbs (84.9%), mainly the shoulder.[8] If possible, reduction of the shoulder dislocation should be done immediately. Neurovascular evaluation must be performed before and after reduction. X-rays should be obtained following a reduction to ensure proper relocation and to evaluate for possible concomitant fractures. A proper shoulder rehabilitation protocol should follow.

Lower Limb Injuries

Lower limb injuries account for approximately 25.9% of all injuries.[8] **Lacerations** are the most common lower limb injuries. Treatment will vary depending on the severity and location of the laceration. **Ankle sprain** is the second most common type of injury.[8] These result from direct trauma, wave riding, and aerial maneuvers. Landing awkwardly or abruptly on the board during an aerial maneuver is a common mechanism for ankle and knee injuries including *ankle sprains, fractures, anterior cruciate ligament (ACL),* and *medial meniscus injuries.*[9]

▓ SUMMARY

Surfing is a rapidly evolving and popular wave-riding sport considered relatively safe when compared to more traditional sports in terms of injury rates. However, it is important to remember that these rates are highly variable and dependent on the style of surfing that is practiced. It is important to keep up with trends and innovations in both the sport and its equipment as surfing evolves in order to understand injury mechanisms, become familiar with common injuries, and be able to provide optimal safety and sideline coverage at future surfing events.

▓ References

1. Warshaw M. *The History of Surfing.* San Francisco, CA: Chronicle; 2010.

2. Furness J, Hing W, Walsh J, et al. Acute injuries in recreational and competitive surfers. *Am J Sports Med.* 2015;43(5):1246-1254. doi:10.1177/0363546514567062.

3. Nathanson A, Bird S, Dao L, Tam-Sing K. Competitive surfing injuries: a prospective study of surfing-related injuries among contest surfers. *Am J Sports Med.* 2007;35(1):113-117. doi:10.1177/0363546506293702.

4. World Surf League. *WSL Rule Book 2019.* Santa Monica, CA: Association of Surfing Professionals; 2019.

5. Surfing. https://tokyo2020.org/en/games/sport/olympic/surfing/.

6. International Surfing Association. ISA para surfing sport rules and regulations. https://www.isasurf.org/wp-content/uploads/downloads/2019/06/ISA-Rulebook_-13-June-2019.pdf. Published January 2020.

7. McCoy GK, de Mestre NJ. Surf hazard rating: a decision-making system for application to competition through the surf zone. *J Coastal Res.* 2014;72:122-126. doi:10.2112/SI72-023.1.

8. Klick C, Jones CM, Adler D. Surfing USA: an epidemiological study of surfing injuries presenting to US EDs 2002 to 2013. *Am J Emerg Med.* 2016;34(8):1491-1496. doi:10.1016/j.ajem.2016.05.008.

9. Mei-Dan O. *Adventure and Extreme Sports Injuries: Epidemiology, Treatment, Rehabilitation and Prevention.* London, UK: Springer; 2013.

10. Taylor DM, Bennett D, Carter M, et al. Perceptions of surfboard riders regarding the need for protective headgear. *Wilderness Environ Med.* 2005;16(2):75-80. doi:10.1580/1080-6032(2005)16[75:POSRRT]2.0.CO;2.

11. Thompson TP, Pearce J, Chang G, Madamba J. Surfer's myelopathy. *Spine.* 2004;29(16):e353-e356. doi:10.1097/01.brs.0000134689.84162.e7.

36. TRACK AND FIELD (HIGH JUMP, POLE VAULT)

Jasmine H. Harris

■ HISTORY

The origins of pole-vaulting can be traced to the Netherlands in the 13th century in the form of a practical way of traversing natural obstacles, such as marshy terrains, canals, and brooks. By the mid-19th century, modern pole-vaulting would be adopted in German gymnastics. Initially composed of bamboo, the poles would later become steel, followed by flexible fiberglass, and lastly carbon fiber by mid-20th century.[1,2] Meanwhile, the high jump appeared first in Scotland in the 1800s with its first recorded contest utilizing a feet-first approach. Today's modern form of the running high jump has used the Frosbury flop technique since the 1960s.[3] The pole vault and high jump were both incorporated as Olympic events in 1896 as part of the first modern games,[2,3] and introduced as a collegiate event in the 1920s.[4]

■ GOVERNING ORGANIZATIONS

- International: International Association of Athletics Federation (IAAF)
- National: USA Track & Field (USATF)
- Major professional leagues (organization): none
- College: National Collegiate Athletic Association (NCAA)
- High School: National Federation of State High School Associations (NFHS)

■ PARTICIPANTS

Track and field (T&F) has the most participants of all high school sports with nearly 1.1 million athletes participating each year. It has the highest number of high school participants among girls' sports and the second highest among boys' sports after American football.[5] The NFHS does not provide a breakdown for the specific number of high school pole vaulters and high jumpers, but the estimated total number of high school pole vaulters from 2008 to 2010 was 80,000.[2]

■ RULES AND REGULATIONS

The high jump is an unassisted jump from a running approach. The only requirement in the high jump is the athlete must takeoff on one foot, instead of two. The pole vaulter also attempts to clear a bar with a running approach, however in this case with the aid of a pole. Competitors may use their own poles. The pole must have a smooth surface, otherwise there are no restrictions on the composition, length, or diameter of the pole. Pole vaulters are allowed to use gloves or gripping substance on their hands or on the pole for improved grip during the competition.[6]

Jumpers and vaulters may request bar placement at any height above the required minimum height. The competitor is given three attempts to clear a crossbar at a specified height. On the other side of the bar is a landing pit composed of well-padded material to break the fall. The crossbar, supported by two upright poles, is designed to fall easily if touched. With each successive height clearance, the bar is raised. Three unsuccessful attempts at a given height eliminates the competitor and the last height cleared is recorded. If competitors are tied on the same height, the winner will have had the fewest failures at that height. If competitors are still tied, the winner will have had the fewest failures across the entire competition. Thereafter, a jump-off will decide the winner.[2,3]

■ EQUIPMENT

A competitor may compete bare feet or with *footwear*. The sole of the shoe is allowed any number up to 11 spikes. High jumper's shoes can have a maximum thickness of 13 mm in the sole and 19 mm in the heel.[6] A *pole* is used by the vaulter to pass over the bar. The pole may be composed of any material, but typically carbon fiber is used due to its high flexibility. Pole is designed with one side stiffer than the other to facilitate the bending after the plant.[6] The use of *helmets* on pole vaulters is optional but may be required in some states. If the athlete chooses to use a helmet, a lacrosse type helmet without face gear or visor is recommended.[7]

Adaptive Sport Key Points: High Jump
High Jump Is a Paralympic sport. Para athletes compete in groups with similar classifications based on functional limitation. Visually impaired athletes may have up to two guides, depending on their classification. For athletes with amputations, if a prosthesis is used and lost during the run-up, the athlete is able to adjust the prosthesis within the allowed time or continue without the prosthesis with no penalty. If the athlete is wearing the prosthesis at take-off, both the athlete and the prosthesis must clear the bar.[8]

■ MEDICAL COVERAGE LOGISTICS

The role of the medical director and/or on-site physician leader is to organize and coordinate the medical staff, develop an emergency action plan (EAP), and interact with the meet director to help ensure the safety of the competitors and spectators. Prior to a competition, it is important to identify available medical staff, support personnel, venue map, and the available medical equipment. It is important to ensure that medical services have clear access for the pole vault and high jump events. Protocols and guidelines should include role definition of the medical staff, emergency transportation including personnel, routes, and adequate facilities with the capacity to evaluate and manage possible injuries, and an outline of the chain-of-command and communication standards. T&F competitions pose challenges as track events generally take place at the same time as field events. On-site medical care should be located in a well-marked medical tent or room with convenient access to both track and field events. If the event is taking place outdoors, ensure there is appropriate coverage of the treatment area from the environment and ambient weather. Communication between individual members of the medical staff and meet officials, emergency medical staff, and local medical facilities is essential via two or more systems (e.g., hand-held radios and cell phones). Lastly, documentation is essential for review after the event to evaluate utilization and plan for future events.

▦ MEDICAL EMERGENCIES AND MEDICAL BAG ESSENTIALS

The nature of jumping and falling from elevated heights as seen in high jump and pole vault make athletes vulnerable to severe or even fatal injuries. In fact, the most catastrophic sports injuries seen in track and field have occurred with pole vaulting. These athletes are at high risk for severe head trauma and spinal cord injury as a result of landing on or outside of the landing pit.[9] The collapsed or unconscious athlete is considered a medical emergency that requires activation of the proper channels of communication and protocols including basic life support (BLS)/advanced cardiac life support (ACLS). Although rarely reported, nontraumatic emergencies can include anaphylaxis, asthma, and heat-related illness, specifically heat stroke.

Medical Bag Essentials in Track and Field: High Jump and Pole Vault	
Medical Emergencies:	**Wound/Laceration/Skin Care:**
Automated External Defibrillator (AED)	Normal saline
Nitroglycerin (sublingual)	Betadine swabs
Aspirin	Neosporin, mupirocin ointment
Epi 1:1,000	Moleskin
Diphenhydramine or another antihistamine	Elastic bandage
Albuterol inhaler	Tube stretch gauze
Rectal thermometer	Sterile gauzes
Ice bucket	Vaseline
Head and Spine:	Steri-strips
Concussion evaluation form	Suture tray
Stretcher & Spine board	Lidocaine 1%
Cervical orthosis	**Others:**
Cricothyrotomy kit	Acetaminophen
Fractures and Dislocations:	Glucose tabs
Immobilizers, Splints, and Slings	Waterproof SPF 50 sunscreen
Crutches	

▦ EPIDEMIOLOGY

Pole-vaulting has the highest risk for contact-related catastrophic injuries in T&F. To prevent severe or fatal injuries in the pole vault, competition regulations and field official education have been modified and adapted.[5] Most jumping injuries involve the lower limbs with ankle sprains as the most common injury. Lumbar spine and hamstring muscle injuries are the most common injuries seen in vaulters.[10]

▦ COMMON INJURIES

Head and Spine Injuries

Head and cervical spine trauma is a potential high risk for pole vaulters and high jumpers. Athletes can travel from heights as high as 20 ft in pole vaulting. Mechanism for catastrophic head injury typically occurs on landing.[11] The vaulter either completely misses or lands partially on the landing pad resulting in a head strike on a surrounding hard surface. Another mechanism of injury is seen when the vaulter does not gain enough momentum during pole-planting phase, releases the pole prematurely, and strikes the head by landing in the vault box. **Lumbar muscle strains, spondylosis** and **spondylolysis** can be seen in pole vaulters. Most lower back injuries are typically muscle strains due to overuse and the repetitive forced lumbar hyperextension that occurs during planting and takeoff to drive upward momentum off the ground. Spondylosis and spondylolysis, which is a stress-related fracture of the pars interarticularis, should be suspected in an athlete complaining of frequent or persistent low back pain. High suspicion should prompt imaging including plain radiographs and MRI to further evaluate and rule out a fracture. If spondylolysis is diagnosed, the athlete should be cautioned for potential severity and progression as this may result in a season-ending injury. Athletes and trainers should ensure proper form especially during pole planting and take off to reduce injury occurrence and reinjuries.[10]

Upper Limb Injuries

Upper limb injuries involve mostly the shoulder. **Rotator cuff tendinopathy** can occur in pole vaulters with repetitive poor pole placement in the vault box. Acute injuries like **shoulder dislocation** or **proximal humerus fracture** can be seen with vaulters and jumpers when falling on an outstretched arm during landing.

Lower Limb Injuries

Lower limb injuries are more common. **Hamstring muscle strains** occur primarily during the sprinting approach phase of the vault. Also pole vaulters incorporate sprint training both preseason and throughout the season. Athletes and trainers should place proper attention to hamstring strength and conditioning to prevent injury occurrence.[10] **Patellar tendinopathy,** also known as "jumper's knee," is a chronic injury commonly seen in explosive-jumping athletes. If an athlete develops sudden acute pain in the patellar tendon, he or she should be evaluated for a possible **rupture**. Exam findings typically include painful palpation over the patella tendon. Tape may be tried to return the athlete back to competition with patellar tendinosis, but the athlete should be warned about the risk of rupture before returning to competition. **Ankle sprains** are the most common injuries in jumping events usually as a result of inadvertently landing the foot in a plantar-flexed and inverted position. Evaluation should be performed to rule out fracture. Acute management of mild ankle sprains includes icing and applying supportive tape. The athlete may return to competition but should have follow-up with a therapist and/or trainer to ensure proper rehabilitation. **Achilles tendinopathy** or **tendon rupture** may occur when there is an eccentric load placed on the tendon as when a jumper takes off. The athlete usually feels as if struck from behind in the calf but sometimes only feels a pop. The athlete will not be able to continue and should be splinted in equines, iced, and sent for further evaluation. **Heel bruise, plantar fasciopathy, plantar fascia rupture,** or **fat pad atrophy** may also occur with jumpers and vaulters. The heel pad consists of a fatty layer of multiple arcades and septae to cushion heel strike. The heel can be injured acutely on one particular landing or through repetitive trauma. Chronic injury such as fat pad atrophy with plantar heel pain can be caused and aggravated by walking, jumping, and running on hard surfaces. Physical examination reveals a heel that appears atrophic, feels soft, and has a persistent imprint from the knuckle when pressure is applied. Acute care involves applying a cushion to the heel.

■ SUMMARY

High jumpers and pole vaulters have a high risk of catastrophic head trauma and cervical spine injury regardless of skill level. These injuries, along with the more common overuse injuries, are a result of poor technique and form. Medical personnel should be assigned to provide sideline coverage during these events to ensure quick access and evaluation of serious injuries.

■ References

1. Tomlinson A. Pole vault. A dictionary of sports studies. New York, NY: Oxford University Press; 2010. https://www.oxfordreference.com/view/10.1093/acref/9780199213818.001.0001/acref-9780199213818-e-888.

2. World Athletics. Pole vault. https://www.iaaf.org/disciplines/jumps/pole-vault.

3. World Athletics. High jump. https://www.iaaf.org/disciplines/jumps/high-jump.

4. Pole vault. Encyclopædia Britannica. https://www.britannica.com/sports/pole-vault. Published 2019.

5. National Federation of State High School Associations. Participation statistics. http://www.nfhs.org/ParticipationStatics/ParticipationStatics.aspx.

6. USA Track & Field 2020 competition rules. http://www.usatf.org/About/Competition-Rules.aspx.

7. Boden BP, Pasquina P, Johnson J, Mueller FO. Catastrophic injuries in pole-vaulters. *Am J Sports Med.* 2001;29(1):50-54. doi:10.1177/03635465010290011301.

8. Adaptive Track & Field USA. Rules. http://atfusa.org/RULES/2020/2020%20ATFUSA%20Rulebook_V1_FINAL%20_2_19_20%20.pdf. Published 2020.

9. Pendergraph B, Ko B, Zamora J, Bass E. Medical coverage for track and field events. *Curr Sports Med Rep.* 2005;4(3):150-153. doi:10.1097/01.CSMR.0000306198.59617.3d.

10. Rebella G, Edwards J. A prospective study of injury patterns in collegiate pole vaulters. *Med Sci Sports Ex.* 2014;46:761.

11. Krauss MD. Equipment innovations and rules changes in sports. *Curr Sports Med Rep.* 2004;3(5):272-276. doi:10.1249/00149619-200410000-00007.

COVERAGE ESSENTIALS FOR NONCONTACT SPORTS

Yusik Cho, Lawrence G. Chang,
and Gerardo Miranda-Comas

HISTORY

Archery was an important military and hunting skill, featured prominently in the mythologies of many cultures for at least 10,000 years. The first-known archery competition relatable to modern times was held in Finsbury, England in 1583. As a sport, archery was first included in the Olympic Games in 1900 and has remained on the Olympic Program since 1972. Para-archery has been featured in the Paralympic Games since 1960.

GOVERNING ORGANIZATIONS

- International: World Archery Federation (WAF), International Field Archery Association (IFAA)
- National: USA Archery, National Field Archery Association (NFAA)

PARTICIPANTS

In the United States in 2017 there were about 7.77 million archery participants. There are two common forms of archery competition: Target and Field archery. Target archery involves standing at a shooting line and firing at a target at a known distance. This modality is included in the Olympic Games in both individual and team competition for men and women. Field archery involves shooting at targets of varying and unmarked distances, typically in woodland and rough terrains.

RULES AND REGULATIONS

Archery is a sport with a high safety record because of the constant attention to safety in planning an archery shooting range. The range should be free of obstructions and provide a safety buffer behind the target of at least 50 m. Allow at least 15 m of clear and restricted space on either side of the target (Figure 37.1).

Target archery is divided into outdoor and indoor and includes two bow-styles: recurve and compound (Table 37.1). For outdoor target archery, recurve athletes shoot at targets set 70 m away and compound athletes shoot targets at 50 m away. The recurve target is 122 cm in diameter with a 10 ring 12.2 cm in diameter (Table 37.1). For Indoor target archery, both recurve and compound athletes shoot at targets set 18 m away. Outdoor and indoor target archery includes individual, team and mixed team competitions at international events.

Field archery is a form of modern archery that takes place on a multitarget course on all kinds of terrain. Athletes shoot at black- and yellow-colored target faces set at distances of up to 60 m. The targets have six concentric rings, four black and two gold. The inner gold ring scores six points, outer gold ring five points, and black rings four to one point.

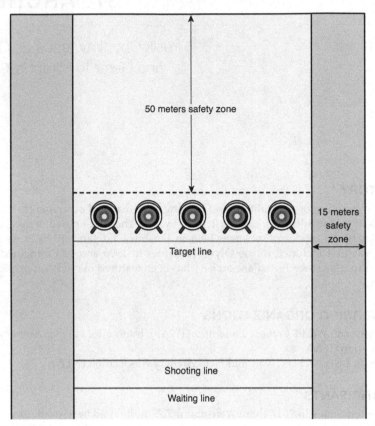

Figure 37.1 Outdoor range.

■ EQUIPMENT

Equipment includes bows (recurve and compound, Table 37.1), bowstring, wax, stabilizers, plunger, clicker, sight, arrow rest, arrows (arrowhead, shaft, and fletchings), and
other accessories like arm guard, chest protector, gloves, bow sling, finger sling, finger
tab, quiver.

> **》》 Adaptive Sport Key Points: Archery**
>
> Para archery is open to athletes with physical impairments, who can use competi-
> tion-classified assistive devices allowed for shooting. Para archery competition clas-
> sifications currently consist of open, W1, and visually impaired categories. The official
> shooting lane width is expanded to 1.25 m to accommodate archers using wheelchairs. If
> approved, athletes may shoot using a wheelchair, a stool, a foot block or wedge, a mouth
> tab, or a bow arm. Adaptations for athletes with hearing impairments could include a flag
> system, or the light system. Some electronic timing systems have buzzer settings which
> can be useful for athletes with visual impairments.

■ MEDICAL COVERAGE LOGISTICS

Pre-event preparation is imperative to improve safety measures, reduce risks to
athletes and spectators during the event, and provide appropriate medical care.

Table 37.1 Bow Styles and Targets

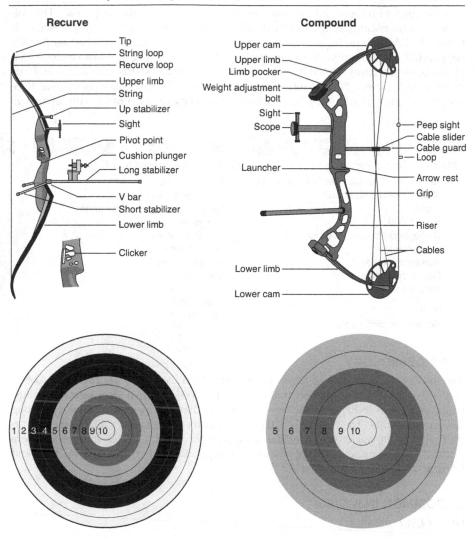

Medical providers should ensure that all equipment needs are met, and know what supplies are available on-site and what is available at local medical facilities, in addition to the proper channels of communication via at least two methods like cell phones and radios. The medical staff should arrive at least an hour early before the start of the event to inspect the venue. It is critical to ensure that team members know the role they play in an emergency and review the Emergency Action Plan (EAP). The medical staff should assess and manage the illnesses and injuries, determine if the patient requires treatment on site or urgent/emergency transportation, and if the athlete may return to play. After the event, it is also important to review injuries that occurred and follow up injured athletes along with proper documentation.

■ MEDICAL EMERGENCIES AND MEDICAL BAG ESSENTIALS

It is essential to understand potential medical emergencies that may arise. The collapsed or unconscious athlete is considered a medical emergency that requires activation of the EAP and protocols including basic life support (BLS)/advanced cardiac life support (ACLS). Although rarely reported, nontraumatic emergencies can include anaphylaxis, asthma, heat-related illness, especially heat stroke, status epilepticus, and cardiopulmonary arrest. Participants with uncontrolled epilepsy cannot participate. Rare severe traumatic injuries include puncture wounds by direct contact with an arrow.[1]

Medical Bag Essentials in Archery	
Medical Emergencies:	Wound/Laceration/Skin Care:
Automated External Defibrillator (AED)	Normal saline
Nitroglycerin (sublingual)	Betadine swabs
Aspirin	Neosporin, mupirocin ointment
Epi 1:1,000	Moleskin
Diphenhydramine or another	Elastic bandage
antihistamine	Tube stretch gauze
Albuterol inhaler	Sterile gauzes
Rectal thermometer	Vaseline
Ice bucket	Steri-strips
Others	Suture tray
Waterproof SPF 50 sunscreen	Lidocaine 1%

■ EPIDEMIOLOGY

Archery is safe. Archery had lower injury rates than basketball, soccer, and baseball and one of the lowest youth sports injuries. In the 2004 National Electronic Injury Surveillance System (NEISS) study, archery has less than 1% incidence of injury among 1,000 participants. The Sports and Fitness Industry Association (SFIA) reported archery had no change in injury incidence from 2007 to 2014. Overuse injuries are more common due to muscle weakness, excessive repetitions when drawing the bow and firing arrows, and poor technique.[1-5]

■ COMMON INJURIES

Upper Limb Injuries

Most injuries occur in the upper limbs. Shoulder injuries accounted for half of total injuries archers reported by the 1996 FITA medical committee. The second most common archery injury is at the elbow. *Rotator cuff tears/impingement* and/or *bicipital tendinosis* are common on the bowstring limb. These occur with drawing the bow due to repetitive use of deltoid and shoulder girdle muscles. Archers who have posterior shoulder injuries while firing an arrow present poor static stabilization of the scapula and glenohumeral joint. Dislocations are rare. Treatment should focus on strengthening scapular and the rotator cuff muscles to decrease the upper/lower trapezius strength ratio.

The *elbow* of the bow arm is the second most common overuse injury anatomic area due to asymmetric use of forearm muscles. Both bow arm and bowstring elbow are subject to much stress. As one brings the bow to full draw, the bow elbow is held in extension and bow string elbow is flexing. Repetitive stress from this can lead to *medial/lateral epicondylopathy* and/or *elbow median nerve compression* with traumatic synovitis. Preventative measures include the use of protective gear, a lightweight bow, forearm flexor muscles conditioning, and modifications in drawing the bowstring. Stretching, massage, heat/ice, muscle strengthening, and injections are effective treatments. Acute *wrist* and *hand injuries* occur after mishandling of bows and arrows. These include *laceration of digital nerve* or *artery, puncture wounds, contusions, introduction of foreign bodies,* and *compression neuropathy of digital nerves* from the bowstring. Hematomas usually occur in the arm due to cuts from a fractured bow. For cuts, irrigate wound and apply dry dressing. Bacitracin can be for infection prophylaxis. For hematomas, the protocol to use is rest, ice, compression, elevation (RICE) therapy. Overuse injuries around the wrist include *De Quervain's tenosynovitis, extensor tendon tenosynovitis,* and *median nerve compression at the wrist.* Spica splinting and injections are usually successful treatments.

Back pain results from acute and/or repetitive microtrauma. In a single day of archery, a person can pull about 3,000 lbs on average. Acute injuries affect the intervertebral disks, end plates, or ring apophyses and contribute to early degenerative process seen in archers. Early prevention is key with core strengthening and proper training.

■ SUMMARY

Archery has a much lower incidence of injuries compared to other sports. Archers nevertheless can develop acute and overuse injuries in various body regions. In order to prevent these injuries, safety measures are necessary through a team-based approach involving doctors, coaches, trainers, and rehabilitation therapists.

■ References

1. Palsbo SE. Epidemiology of recreational archery injuries: implications for archery ranges and injury prevention. *J Sports Med Phys Fitness.* 2012;52(3):293-299. https://www.minervamedica.it/en/journals/sports-med-physical-fitness/article.php?cod=R40Y2012N03A0293

2. Rayan GM. Archery-related injuries of the hand, forearm, and elbow. *South Med J.* 1992;85(10):961-964. doi:10.1097/00007611-199210000-00007.

3. Niestroj CK, Schöffl V, Küpper T. Acute and overuse injuries in elite archers. *J Sports Med Phys Fitness.* 2018;58(7-8):1063-1070. doi:10.23736/S0022-4707.17.07828-8.

4. Lin J-J, Hung C-J, Yang C-C, et al. Activation and tremor of the shoulder muscles to the demands of an archery task. *J Sports Sci.* 2010;28(4):415-421. doi:10.1080/02640410903536434.

5. National Archery in the Schools Program. Archery safety brochure 2016. https://www.naspschools.org/wp-content/uploads/2017/11/2016ArcheryTradeSafetyBrochure.pdf. Published July 5, 2016. Accessed July 10, 2020.

38. BADMINTON

Michael Chiou

HISTORY

Badminton emerged in the United Kingdom in the mid-19th century as a variant of the earlier game of battledore and shuttlecock. Despite originating in Europe, international competition has as of late been dominated by Asian nations.

GOVERNING ORGANIZATIONS

- International: Badminton World Federation (BWF)
- National: USA Badminton (USAB)
- College: National Collegiate Athletic Association (NCAA)

PARTICIPANTS

Badminton is widely considered to be the second most popular participatory sport in the world with over 6.43 million estimated participants.[1]

RULES AND REGULATIONS

The aim of badminton is to hit the shuttlecock with your racquet so that it passes over the net and lands inside your opponent's half of the court. Each game is played to 21 points, with players scoring a point whenever they win a rally regardless of whether they served. A match is the best of three games. Competitive badminton is always played indoors.

EQUIPMENT

Badminton *racquets* are lightweight and composed of many different materials ranging from carbon fiber to solid steel. Rules limit racquet size and weight. A *shuttlecock* (often abbreviated to shuttle and sometimes called a "birdie") is a high-drag projectile, with an open conical shape. There are rules for testing the shuttlecock for the correct speed. Badminton *shoes* are lightweight with soles of rubber or similar high-grip, non-marking materials. They have little lateral support as badminton requires powerful lateral movements.

>>> **Adaptive Sport Key Points: Para Badminton**

This sport is governed by the Badminton World Federation (BWF) and will make its first Paralympic appearance at Tokyo 2020. Athletes are divided into six classes (two wheelchair classes and four standing classes including lower limb amputees) with the rules of Badminton followed except for minor modifications.

■ MEDICAL COVERAGE LOGISTICS

The role of the medical director is to establish an Emergency Action Plan (EAP), co-ordinate with event personnel and referees, to ensure the safety of all players and spectators. Protocols and guidelines should include role definition of the medical staff, emergency transportation including personnel, routes, and adequate facilities, and an outline of the chain-of-command and communication standards. An accessible and centrally located area for medical evaluation, medical equipment, and personnel must be established prior to play time. Communication between medical personnel, referees, and event organizers is essential for proper medical coverage and can be facilitated by two-way radios, cell phones or walkie-talkies. Each medical encounter must be documented properly for continuity of care and planning for future events.

■ MEDICAL EMERGENCIES AND MEDICAL BAG ESSENTIALS

The collapsed or unconscious athlete is considered a medical emergency that requires activation of the proper channels of communication and protocols including basic life support (BLS)/advanced cardiac life support (ACLS). Nontraumatic emergencies include asthma, anaphylaxis, cardiac arrhythmias, or hypertrophic cardiomyopathy.

Medical Bag Essentials in Badminton	
Medical Emergencies:	**Fractures and Dislocations:**
Automated External Defibrillator (AED)	Immobilizers, Crutches.
Nitroglycerin (sublingual)	Slings
Aspirin	
Epi 1:1,000	
Diphenhydramine or another antihistamine	
Albuterol inhaler	

■ EPIDEMIOLOGY

Badminton is a noncontact racquet sport with repetitive arm motions and agile foot-work. Strains/sprains are the most common type of injury followed by soft tissue injuries, then skin-level injuries and fractures. The lower limbs are the most commonly injured body area, specifically the ankle.[2,3]

■ COMMON INJURIES

Spine Injuries

Lumbar spine muscle strains/sprains are caused by damage to the muscles and ligaments of the back when performing strenuous activity, twisting, or falling. Symptoms include dull, achy back pain that is exacerbated by activity without neurologic symptoms. Treatment includes rest, ice, and pain relievers.

Upper Limb Injuries

Badminton has the most overhead strokes out of all the racquet sports; therefore, overuse **upper limb injury** is common. **Shoulder impingement syndrome** involves **rotator cuff tendinopathy or tendonitis** through the subacromial space, most commonly the supraspinatus tendon, that occurs with repetitive overhead movements. Symptoms include pain, weakness, and decreased range of motion ("painful arc") in the affected shoulder. Treatment should start conservatively with rest, cessation of painful activity, and initiation of physical therapy to maintain range of motion and improve posture and strength. In severe cases, arthorscopic or open surgery may be necessary. **Lateral epicondylopathy,** also known as **tennis elbow,** is the most common overuse syndrome in the elbow. It is a forearm extensor muscle tendinopathy and can be caused by poor backhand technique where the player has a soft or bent wrist. Symptoms include pain, most commonly on the outside of the elbow. Treatment should start conservatively with rest, ice, pain relievers, and physical therapy. An elbow brace may help. **Medial epicondylopathy,** also known as **golfer's elbow,** is caused by excess or repetitive stress of the common flexor tendon. Symptoms include pain, most commonly on the inside of the elbow, and may be associated with elbow stiffness and hand/wrist weakness. Treatment includes rest, ice, pain relievers, and physical therapy. An elbow brace may help. **Wrist injuries** include **extensor** or **flexor tenosynovitis/tendinopathy** ranging from acute or overuse injury. Symptoms include pain in the wrist that may be sharp, dull, or throbbing. Treatment includes rest, ice, pain relievers, and physical therapy.

Lower Limb Injuries

Lower limb injuries include **muscle strains affecting the hamstrings, quadriceps,** or **adductors.** Symptoms include pain, swelling, bruising, and in severe cases, a loss of function in the affected muscle. Muscle strains can be associated with muscle cramps, which are painful, involuntary contractions also caused by overuse of a muscle or de-hydration. Treatment should start with protection, rest, ice, compression, and elevation. **Patellofemoral pain syndrome** is a condition in which the cartilage under the kneecap is damaged due to excessive overload, overuse, or direct trauma to the kneecap (falling on the knee). Symptoms include diffuse pain in and around the kneecap. **Patellar tend-inopathy,** also known as **jumper's knee,** is an overuse injury that occurs gradually over time, most commonly seen in athletes who jump the highest and most frequently or who have recently increased training volume. Symptoms include knee pain, swelling, and stiffness. Treatment involves improving body biomechanics to eliminate inciting factors through a structured training program to improve strength, mobility, and mus-cle control. Work load should be assessed and monitored. **Meniscal tears** can be caused by sudden twisting movements of the knee during footwork. Symptoms include knee pain, swelling, stiffness, and classically locking, clicking, and buckling. Collateral or cruciate ligament injuries can be associated with meniscus tear. Treatment should start with rest, ice, pain relievers, and physical therapy, but if not responding to conserva-tive treatment, then surgical intervention should be considered. **Medial tibial stress syn-drome,** also known as **shin splints,** is an overuse injury of the bone tissue overlying the tibia. The main symptom is lower leg pain after exercise or vague pain along the shin bone. Treatment includes rest, ice, pain relievers. The most important thing to do is to find the underlying cause of the problem, such as addressing risk factors or adjusting the training routine. **Ankle sprains** occur most frequently when stopping, turning, jump-ing, or landing. The foot inverts or everts, which may cause injury of one or more of the ligaments in the ankle. Symptoms include swelling, tenderness, and pain on the inside or outside of the ankle. Treatment should start with protection, rest, ice, compression, and elevation. Physical therapy should start as soon as possible. Consider supporting tape or a brace. Plantar fasciopathy is an overuse injury of the plantar fascia, a band of tissue that supports the arch of the foot. Pain develops gradually underneath the heel and along the foot arch. At first, it can be painful in the morning, but better with activity. Without treatment, pain increases during and after exercise and can persist for a long time. Treatment includes rest, ice, pain relievers, and physical therapy focusing on strengthening exercises for the foot and calf muscles. Orthotics may help. Severe cases may benefit from regenerative medicine interventions. **Achilles tendinopathy or rupture** is a partial or complete disruption of the tendon just above the heel caused by forceful jumping or pivoting, or sudden accelerations, that can overstretch the tendon and cause a tear. Symptoms include sudden pain, a popping or snapping sensation, swelling on the back of the lower leg, and difficulty walking. Treatment should start with rest, ice, compression, and elevation. The decision of whether to proceed with surgery or nonsurgical treatment is based on the severity of the rupture and the patient's health status and activity level.

■ SUMMARY

Badminton is a very popular noncontact sport that can be played at all levels. Understanding the game, positions, and most common injuries is essential for sideline coverage.

■ References

1. Statistica. Number of participants in badminton in the United States from 2006 to 2017 (in millions). https://www.statista.com/statistics/191754/participants-in-badminton-in-the-us-since-2006. Published July 2018.

2. Nhan DT, Klyce W, Lee RJ. Epidemiological patterns of alternative racquet-sport injuries in the United States, 1997-2016. *Orthop J Sports Med*. 2018;6(7):2325967118786237. doi:10.1177/2325967118786237.

3. Krøner K, Schmidt SA, Nielsen AB, et al. Badminton injuries. *Br J Sports Med*. 1990;24(3):169-172. doi:10.1136/bjsm.24.3.169.

■ Further Reading

Lam W-K, Lee K-K, Park S-K, et al. Understanding the impact loading characteristics of a badminton lunge among badminton players. *PLoS One*. 2018;13(10):e0205800. doi:10.1371/journal.pone.0205800.

Vuurberg G, Hoorntje A, Wink LM, et al. Diagnosis, treatment and prevention of ankle sprains: update of an evidence-based clinical guideline. *Br J Sports Med*. 2018;52(15):956. doi:10.1136/bjsports-2017-098106.

39. BOBSLED, LUGE, AND SKELETON

Rachel Santiago

■ HISTORY

Bobsledding and the luge were started in the alpine regions of Europe in the 1800s. Bobsledding became an Olympic sport in 1924 and skeleton was first introduced to the Olympics in 1924, becoming a permanent sport in 2002.[1] Luge became an official Olympic sport in 1964 with events in men's singles, women's singles, and doubles teams.

■ GOVERNING ORGANIZATIONS

- International: International Bobsleigh and Skeleton Federation (IBSF), International Luge Federation (ILF)
- National: United States Bobsled and Skeleton Federation (USBSF)

■ PARTICIPANTS

The majority of participants in the bobsled, luge, and skeleton are experienced athletes. Modified recreational bobsled, luge, and skeleton experiences are available at various ice tracks.

■ RULES AND REGULATIONS

Bobsled athletes are allowed a 15-m running start for initiation of movement. The bobsled is steered using a pulley system. Athletes speed down the ice track at speeds over 150 km/hour in the seated position and stop using a braking system.[2] Skeleton athletes propel themselves down the ice track with a 30-m running start. Steering is achieved by minimal shifts in body weight. Speeds over 100 km/hour are achieved and stopping the sled is achieved by friction of feet on the ice. Luge athletes use gloved hands to propel themselves forward by pushing off of the ice track. They race down in the supine position with the neck flexed to visualize the track. There are single- and double-rider events for this sport. Athletes use handles, body weight shifts, and leg muscle pressure to steer down the track at speeds over 100 km/hour. The luge is stopped using leg muscles by friction of feet on the ice. To compete in an IBSF event, athletes must be at least 15 years old. To compete in youth Monobob events, athletes must be at least 13 years old.

■ EQUIPMENT

All athletes must wear a racing **helmet** with a face shield protecting the forehead and chin.[3] The helmet is usually made of fiberglass. **Brush spiked shoes** have a maximum diameter of spikes 1.5 mm, maximum length of 5 mm. A skintight **racing speed suit** promotes aerodynamics and speed. **Elbow and shoulder pads** are optional and worn under the racing suit. **Gloves** used in the luge are spiked to assist with push off from the ice.

The **bobsleigh** must be a minimum weight of 170 kg for two-man/woman bobsleigh and 210 kg for a four-man/woman bobsleigh, and a maximum weight of 330 kg for a two-woman bobsleigh, 390 kg for a two-man bobsleigh, and 630 kg for a four-man bobsleigh.[1] **Skeleton** sled frames are made from steel. They are not permitted to have any steering or brake system. Handles and bumpers are along the sides to secure athletes during the race. **Luge** sleds are made of fiberglass and steel, custom built for each athlete. Luge sleds weigh between 22 and 27 kg. There is a built-in flexible runner to which athletes apply pressure in order to steer the sled.

> **⟫ Adaptive Sport Key Points: Bobsled**
>
> Para-Bobsled began in the early 2000s with its first World Cup event in 2014–2015. The current category is a seated category for athletes who have spinal cord injuries, above-the-knee amputations, and other injuries which medically fit that classification.

▦ MEDICAL COVERAGE LOGISTICS

As per IBSF regulations, a medical specialist, known as a "race doctor," must be available during race heats, official training days, and race days. The role of the race doctor is to organize and coordinate the medical staff, develop an emergency action plan (EAP), and interact with the race or event director to help ensure the safety of the competitors and spectators. Protocols and guidelines should include role definition of the medical staff, emergency transportation including personnel, routes, and adequate facilities with the capacity to evaluate and manage possible injuries, and an outline of the chain-of-command and communication standards. An ambulance stocked with resuscitation equipment must be present. A medical tent or room for fast evaluation and treatment clearly marked must be present. During World Cup Championship races there must be two ambulances present and, if both are utilized concurrently, the race will be stopped. The race doctor must examine athletes after every crash and give clearance to participate in further training or racing. If a concussion is suspected, then the athlete must be removed from training and competition, and the Jury President of the IBSF must be notified.[2]

▦ MEDICAL EMERGENCIES AND MEDICAL BAG ESSENTIALS

Medical emergencies must be recognized and assessed immediately. The collapsed or unconscious athlete is considered a medical emergency that requires activation of the EAP and protocols including basic life support (BLS)/advanced cardiac life support (ACLS). Musculoskeletal injuries that may become medical emergencies include upper and lower limb fractures or dislocations with neurovascular compromise, traumatic brain injuries with or without spinal cord involvement, and blunt thoracoabdominal trauma with possible internal bleeding. Partial or full ejection of the sled from the track has occurred and resulted in fatalities.

▦ EPIDEMIOLOGY

Bobsled, skeleton, and luge are high-velocity sports. The majority of injuries are contusions and sprains that occur during the initial sprint or during impact when stopping the sled at the end of the track. Injuries to the head and neck are common and occur secondary to the high forces experienced by athletes during turns on the track. Severe injuries occur when athletes lose control of the sled resulting in collision with the ice or ejection from the racetrack. There have been few fatalities secondary to ejection from the track or overturning of the sled.[3–5]

Medical Bag Essentials in Bobsled, Skeleton, and Luge	
Medical Emergencies:	**Wound/Laceration/Skin Care:**
Automated External Defibrillator (AED)	Normal saline
Nitroglycerin (sublingual)	Betadine swabs
Aspirin	Neosporin, mupirocin ointment
Epi 1:1,000	Moleskin
Diphenhydramine or another antihistamine	Elastic bandage
Albuterol inhaler	Tube stretch gauze
Rectal thermometer	Sterile gauzes
	Vaseline
Head and Spine:	Steri-strips
Concussion evaluation form	Suture tray
Stretcher & Spine board	Lidocaine 1%
Cervical orthosis	
Fractures and Dislocations:	
Immobilizers and Slings	
Crutches	
Splints	

■ COMMON INJURIES

Head and Spine Injuries

Head and spine injuries can be severe. ***Concussion*** is most common when athletes lose control of the sled, hitting the track and flipping the sled over.[3] Direct head trauma occurs when the athlete's head is hit against the ice or the sled. Symptoms include headache, photosensitivity, vomiting, and loss of consciousness. A complete neurologic exam and concussion assessment must be performed. Sledding athletes also report "sled head" after performing multiple runs down the track without a specific trauma.[4] Symptoms include headaches, dizziness, and lightheadedness. Players in bobsled, skeleton, and luge experience forces up to five times the force of gravity when turning down the track. Additionally, athletes in the luge must keep the neck-unsupported in flexion and, in the skeleton, the neck is unsupported in extension making it vulnerable to injury. It is unclear if the symptoms of sled head are related to neck strain or a type of concussion. Some Olympic teams have limited the number of runs during practice to three a day due to the symptoms.[3,4] ***Cervical spine instability*** occurs when athletes lose control of the sled and crash. Cervical spine stabilization and precautions should be initiated immediately and the athlete transported to a suitable medical facility for further evaluation and possible surgical stabilization. ***Trapezius muscle strain*** is a common injury in the bobsled, skeleton, and luge event. This presents with tenderness over the trapezius muscle and may be associated with tension, headache, and pain when lifting arms over the head. ***Deep cervical muscle strain*** secondary to contusions and repetitive use injury is also common. Treatment is conservative with physiotherapy. ***Thoracic spine injuries*** have been documented in older athletes participating in recreational bobsledding. This occurrence is not as common since the majority of participants in sledding events are elite and experienced athletes. The mechanism of this injury is thought to be secondary to the high forces experienced during sledding. Those with underlying osteoporosis are at higher risk of compression fracture.[5] ***Rib fracture*** has been reported and is related to the collision/landing from sprint onto the skeleton. This also occurs when the sled is derailed from the track. Associated intraabdominal injury can occur.

Treatment is supportive with ice, nonsteroidal anti-inflammatory drugs (NSAIDs), and taping.

Upper Limb Injuries

Upper limb injuries include acute injuries to the shoulder, forearm, and hand. **Acromio-clavicular (AC) joint sprain/separation** can occur as a result of direct impact and collision occurring during the landing from the sprint onto the skeleton. Partial sprains can be treated with conservative measures of ice and NSAIDs and may be placed in a sling for comfort for 1 to 2 weeks. More severe tears may require follow-up and possible surgical intervention. Those in the luge and skeleton are at risk of **hand contusions** and **hand fractures**, the most common being the **triquetral bone, the third metacarpal**, and **fifth metacarpal bones.** Injuries occur after a collision of the hand with the ice track. Players will present with tenderness and swelling at the base of the digit. Initial treatment includes ice and splinting. These injuries rarely require surgical intervention. Overuse injuries include **ulnar stress fractures.** These occur due to the positioning of the hands during repetitive strain on the arms when pushing the sled or landing onto the skeleton or luge. The force on the ulna increases with wrist flexion, ulnar deviation, and forearm pronation. Stress fractures may be managed conservatively, although a referral should be made to assess for surgical intervention.

Lower Limb Injuries

Acute and overuse lower limb injuries can involve muscle, tendon, or bone. **Hamstring strain** or **tear** is one of the most common injuries in bobsled and skeleton events. This occurs secondary to the sprints at the beginning of the race. A hamstring strain will present as pain over the muscle belly or insertion point of hamstring with pain in the ischial region during knee flexion. If severe, consider radiographs to assess for avulsion fracture over the ischial tuberosity, but further imaging with MRI or ultrasound may be needed to better assess location and severity. Initial treatment is with ice and compression. Injury to the **medial collateral ligament of the knee** may present as acute pain at the medial knee with stiffness over the course of several hours. Athlete will endorse tenderness along the medial joint line with medial instability when applying valgus stress. Initial treatment with bracing and physiotherapy can be recommended. Acute **ankle sprains** are common in the luge event, likely related to the athletes using their feet to stop the sled at the end of the track, involving the anterior talofibular ligament. Depending on the severity, they may be treated with conservative management and early mobilization. Acute and overuse fractures in the foot can occur. **Jones's fracture** is a fracture through the fifth metatarsal. Injury may occur when stopping the luge with the feet. X-ray and possibly MRI/CT are recommended. Athlete should be nonweight-bearing for 6 weeks and may need surgical intervention. **March fracture** is a metatarsal stress fracture that should be managed with rest and immobilization, but may require surgical fixation as there is risk of fracture displacement. A **metatarsal pha-langeal sprain** occurs during the sprint and take off in the skeleton, luge, and bobsled events. Radiographs should be obtained to rule out a fracture and treatment is conservative. **Achilles tendinopathy** can present due to the high velocity eccentric muscle contraction that occurs during the sprint. Short-term bracing or splinting may be utilized along with stretching and eccentric strengthening of the gastroc-soleus muscle complex.

■ SUMMARY

The majority of sledding sport participants are experienced and elite athletes. EAP is essential to avoid complications from traumatic injuries. When assessing novel recreational participants, consider higher risk injuries. Understanding mechanisms of injuries in these sports is necessary for appropriate medical coverage.

■ References

1. International Bobsleigh and Skeleton Federation. International bobsleigh rules 2018. http://www.ibsf.org/images/documents/downloads/Rules/2018_2019/2018_International_Rules_BOBSLEIGH.PDF. Published September 2018.

2. International Bobsleigh and Skeleton Federation. International skeleton rules 2018. http://www.ibsf.org/images/documents/downloads/Rules/2018_2019/2018_International_Rules_SKELETON.PDF. Published September 2018.

3. McCradden MD, Cusimano MD. Concussions in sledding sports and the unrecognized "sled head": a systematic review. *Front Neurol.* 2018;18(9):772. doi:10.3389/fneur.2018.00772.

4. Stuart CA, Richards D, Cripton PA. Injuries at the Whistler Sliding Center: A 4-year retrospective study. *Br J Sports Med.* 2015;50(1):62-70. doi:10.1136/bjsports-2015-095006.

5. Severson E, Sofianos D, Powell A, et al. Spinal fractures in recreational bobsledders: an unexpected mechanism of injury. *Evid Based Spine Care J.* 2012;3(02):43-48. doi:10.1055/s-0031-1298617.

40. CURLING

Jasmin Harounian

HISTORY

Curling originated in 16th century Scotland. It was introduced to the United States in 1832, and curling clubs began to form across the country by 1855. Although curling initially debuted as a medal sport in the 1924 Olympic Winter Games, it was not recognized as a permanent medal sport again until the 1998 Olympic Winter Games in Nagano, Japan. Curling is occasionally called "The Roaring Game," which originates from the rumbling sound made by the heavy stones as they travel across the ice.[1]

GOVERNING ORGANIZATIONS

- International: World Curling Federation (WCF)
- National: United States Curling Association (USCA)
- Regional: 11 USA Curling Member Clubs
- College: College Curling USA

PARTICIPANTS

There are up to 1.5 million curlers worldwide, including participants at the collegiate and youth levels.[2] There are approximately 20,000 individual member curlers in the USCA. Canadians make up about 80% of the worldwide curling population, with up to 870,000 curlers.[3]

RULES AND REGULATIONS

Curling is played indoors on refrigerated ice, and the playing surface is also known as the "sheet of ice" (Figure 40.1). There are two four-person teams that are in play. Each team comprises the lead, the second, the third (or vice), and the skip (strategist). All four players on each team throw two stones per end (eight stones per team), alternating with the corresponding player on the opposite team. An end is over once all 16 stones have been thrown. When throwing or delivering a stone, each curler starts at the hack line, which is similar to a runner's starting block, and pushes off in a lunge position, gripping the stone handle in one hand and a broom or stabilizer in the other hand. The stone must be released before it reaches the hog line closest to their side of the sheet of ice, and it must cross the far hog line in order for it to be considered in play. The two curlers not throwing the stone in play serve to sweep in front of the stone to influence its trajectory. The fourth curler, or the skip, often stands at the house (or target) and is the main strategist who determines the game plan for each stone. Scoring is determined after each end is completed, and only one team can score per end. A stone is in the scoring area if it is in or touching the opponent team's house. In order to win an end, a team must get more stones closer to the middle of the house than their opponent. Each game is made up of eight ends (similar to innings) and typically lasts 2 hours. In the Olympic setting, games are usually made up of 10 ends and can last 2.5 hours.[4]

Playing Surface/Sheet of Ice:
16.5" W x 150" L

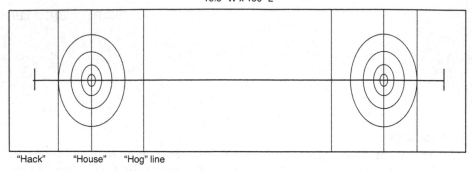

"Hack"   "House"   "Hog" line

Figure 40.1 Curling playing surface.

▉ EQUIPMENT

Curling *shoes* have a specialized surface which aids in sliding or gripping. Slider shoes have a sliding sole made of Teflon, and often come in step-on or strap-on varieties. Gripper shoes have a soft rubber sole that allows the curler to better "grip" the ice. A *broom* is used by curlers to sweep the ice in front of the stone that is being thrown, made either of synthetic materials, hog hair, or horse hair. A *stabilizer* is often used while delivering the stone to help curlers with balance. Curling *stones* are made of granite and are approximately 42 lbs in weight, with smaller stones available for use by youth curlers.

> **≫ Adaptive Sport Key Points: Wheelchair Curling**
>
> Teams consist of four players and must include both male and female players. The stones are thrown from a stationary wheelchair with both feet on foot pads and assistance from a delivery stick. There is no sweeping involved. Games are eight ends in duration with time limits of 68 minutes per team as opposed to 73 minutes. Eligibility is limited to those who use a wheelchair for daily mobility.

▉ MEDICAL COVERAGE LOGISTICS

The role of the on-site doctor is to organize and coordinate the medical staff, develop an emergency action plan (EAP), and interact with the event director to help ensure the safety of the competitors and spectators Protocols and guidelines should include role definition of the medical staff, emergency transportation including personnel, routes, and adequate facilities with the capacity to evaluate and manage possible injuries, and an outline of the chain-of-command and communication standards.

▉ MEDICAL EMERGENCIES AND MEDICAL BAG ESSENTIALS

Although curling is relatively safe compared to other ice sports, it is important to understand possible medical emergencies that you may encounter. Falls can lead to acute fractures or concussions in curlers. Additionally, cardiovascular fitness of curlers comes into play especially when sweeping, as this activity can produce an average heart rate of 170 bpm. Thus, medical providers should be aware of the potential risks of nontraumatic medical emergencies, such as hypertrophic cardiomyopathy and cardiac arrhythmias.

Medical Bag Essentials in Curling	

Medical Emergencies:
   Automated External Defibrillator (AED)
   Nitroglycerin (sublingual)
   Aspirin
   Epi 1:1,000
   Diphenhydramine or another
   antihistamine
	Head and Spine:
	   Concussion evaluation form
	   Stretcher & Spine board
	   Cervical orthosis
	
	 Fractures and Dislocations:
	   Immobilizers and Slings
	   Crutches
	   Splints

EPIDEMIOLOGY

Musculoskeletal injuries occur in 79% of curlers, most commonly involving the knee (54%), back (33%), and shoulder (20%). Sweeping and delivering the stone are the most common mechanisms of injury.[2]

COMMON INJURIES

Head and Spine Injuries

Concussion is not commonly seen in curling, but may account for up to one-third of all acute injuries in less experienced curlers.[3] Mechanism of injury includes falling backward on the ice, often due to improper footwear, thus leading to direct trauma to the head. Symptoms can include confusion, dizziness, headaches, nausea, vomiting, and occasionally, loss of consciousness. The athlete should be removed from play, and a neurological exam, including a concussion specific assessment like the Sport Concussion Assessment Tool (SCAT), should be administered. If no red flags are observed, then the player may remain on the sideline for the duration of the game with sports medicine follow-up in 24 to 48 hours for further assessment.

Lumbar disc herniation occurs when the annulus fibrosus of the vertebral disc is torn, thus enabling the nucleus to herniate or extrude into the spinal canal. The mechanism of injury is typically due to prolonged or repetitive spinal flexion, gradual disc degeneration due to torsional strain, as well as heavy lifting. In curlers, this can occur when throwing the heavy 42-pound stones across the ice or due to the overall kyphotic posture during sweeping. Symptoms can include axial back pain, radicular pain to the buttock or leg with associated weakness. Management is often nonoperative, involving rest, nonsteroidal anti-inflammatory drugs (NSAIDs), with progressive activity and spinal extension exercises as tolerated.

Upper Limb Injuries

Upper limb injuries include shoulder overuse injury and distal limb acute injuries. Shoulder impingement syndrome is caused by extrinsic compression of the rotator cuff between the humeral head and the acromion. Bursitis can also develop if the subacromial bursa becomes inflamed. Mechanism of injury is due to repetitive use of the affected arm, which can be seen in curlers during delivery of the stone and during sweeping. Symptoms include decreased range of motion and pain, especially with overhead activities and lifting objects away from the body. Management involves oral anti-inflammatory medications, physical therapy for rotator cuff strengthening and periscapular stabilization, and subacromial injections. **Distal radius fracture** and associated soft tissue injuries can be seen in curlers who lose their balance on the ice.

Mechanism of injury is usually a fall on out-stretched hand (FOOSH). Symptoms include ecchymosis and edema, diffuse tenderness, and a possible visible deformity if the fracture is displaced. Management involves either closed reduction and splint/cast immobilization or surgical intervention for more unstable, comminuted fractures. *Carpal tunnel syndrome* results from compression of the medial nerve within the carpal tunnel at the wrist. The mechanism of injury is usually overuse with repetitive wrist movements as well as prolonged forceful grip which occurs during sweeping. Symptoms include nighttime hand pain, clumsiness, and numbness or tingling in the median nerve distribution. Management in mild cases includes bracing, grip modification, and NSAIDs. Moderate to severe cases may require sono-guided steroid injections, or carpal tunnel release.

Lower Limb Injuries

Lower limb injuries are the most common. *Chondromalacia patella* or *patellofemoral syndrome* occurs with malalignment of the patella causing subsequent damage to the cartilage on its posterior surface. Mechanism of injury is multifactorial but involves patella maltracking and prolonged knee flexion as seen with the lunge position during stone delivery in curling. Symptoms include diffuse pain in the anterior and peripatellar regions of the knee. Management involves initial rest, ice, and NSAIDs followed by physical therapy with emphasis on strengthening of the leg and pelvic stabilization. *Adductor strain* results from injury to the adductor muscle group, with the adductor longus being the most commonly affected. Mechanism of action is due to forceful external rotation of an abducted leg, which can be seen after a curler pushes off the hack in the lunge position during delivery of the stone. Symptoms include tenderness at the site of injury with radiation to the groin and pain with resisted leg adduction. Management includes rest, ice, and return to play when patient is asymptomatic. Immobilization should be avoided as it promotes further muscle tightness.

▓ SUMMARY

Curling is a noncontact sport that can be played at all levels. Understanding the game, positions, and most common injuries is essential for sideline coverage.

▓ References

1. Curling Equipment and History - Olympic Sport History. International Olympic Committee. https://www.olympic.org/curling-equipment-and-history.

2. Reeser JC, Berg RL. Self reported injury patterns among competitive curlers in the United States: a preliminary investigation into the epidemiology of curling injuries. *Br J Sports Med*. 2004;38(5):e29. doi:10.1136/bjsm.2003.010298.

3. Ting DK, Brison RJ. Injuries in recreational curling include head injuries and may be prevented by using proper footwear. *Health Promot Chronic Dis Prev Can*. 2015;35(2):29-34. doi:10.24095/hpcdp.35.2.01.

4. USA Curling. Team USA. https://www.teamusa.org/USA-Curling/About-Us/About-USA-Curling/Curling-101.

▓ Further Reading

Bradley JL. The sports science of curling: a practical review. *J Sports Sci Med*. 2009;8(4):495-500. https://www.ncbi.nlm.nih.gov/pmc/articles/PMC3761524

Juan C. Perez-Santiago and Robert Pagan-Rosado

HISTORY

Cycling emerged in the early 19th century following the invention of the bicycle primarily as a mode of transportation. It was initially devised and refined in Europe. The first race officially recorded dates back to 31 May 1868 at the "Parc de Saint-Cloud," in Paris. Road cycling has been part of the Olympic Games program since its first edition in 1896.[1]

GOVERNING ORGANIZATIONS

- International: International Cycling Union (UCI- Union Cycliste Internationale)
- National: USA Cycling
- Major professional leagues: American Bicycle Association (ABA)
- College: National Collegiate Cycling Association (NCCA)
- High School: National Federation of State High School Associations

PARTICIPANTS

There are approximately 2 billion bicycle users worldwide, among which several million are active in competition.[1] Cycling disciplines include road and track, mountain bike, extreme biking (BMX), triathlon, and cyclocross across all age groups in both men and women.

RULES AND REGULATIONS

There are multiple disciplines within competitive cycling. The rules and regulations vary according to the discipline and event type (Table 41.1). These events may be individual or team competitions. Especially in road cycling, events vary by distance, 40 to 50 km to longer than 200 km, and single day to multiple day events.[2]

EQUIPMENT

Equipment can slightly vary depending on the discipline, but overall consists of a properly fitted cycling *helmet, cleats or shoes, padded shorts* to protect the skin from shear forces, and the *bicycle* itself (Figure 41.1).[3] Aerobars and solid disk rear is prohibited in road events.[2]

MEDICAL COVERAGE LOGISTICS

The role of the medical director and/or on-site physician leader is to organize and coordinate the medical staff, develop an emergency action plan (EAP), and interact with the race or event director to help ensure the safety of the competitors and spectators.[2] Prior to a competition, it is important to identify available medical staff, support personnel,

Table 41.1 Types of Events

Track	Road	Off Road
• Keirin*	• Individual Time Trial*	• BMX Race*
• Sprint*	• Road Race*	• Mountain Bike- Cross-Country*
• Omnium*	• Hill Climb	
• Team Pursuit*	• Road Stage Race	• Mountain Bike- Downhill
• Team Sprint*	• Road Criterium	• Mountain Bike-4X
• Points Race	• Sportive	• Mountain Bike-Enduro
• Madison	• Triathlon	• Mountain Bike-4X
• Scratch Race	• Duathlon	• Alpine Snow Bike
• Elimination Race		• Cyclo-Cross
		• BMX Freestyle

*Olympic Events for Men and Women
Source: Adapted from Union Cycliste Internationale. https://www.uci.org.

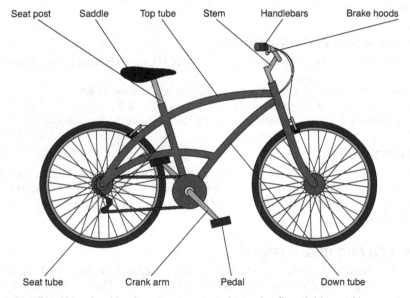

Seat post   Saddle   Top tube   Stem   Handlebars   Brake hoods

Seat tube   Crank arm   Pedal   Down tube

Figure 41.1 Road bicycle with relevant components impacting fit and rider position.
Source: Reproduced with permission from Silberman M, Webner D, Collina S, Shiple BJ. Road bicycle fit. *Clin J Sport Med.* 2005;15(4):271-276. doi:10.1097/01.jsm.0000171255.70156.da.

>>> Adaptive Sport Key Points: Cycling

The sport was developed in the 1980s and was first open to visually impaired athletes who competed in tandem with a sighted pilot. It is divided according to bike including standard, tandem, tricycle, and handbike. The choice of bike used depends on the athlete's disability.

- **Tandem:** used by cyclists who are visually impaired teamed with a sighted pilot.
- **Handbike:** used mainly by paraplegic, quadriplegic, and amputees of one or both lower limbs.
- **Tricycle:** used mainly by cyclists with brain injury to provide more stability.
- **Standard:** can be used with or without adaptations for mild brain injuries, limb amputations, or any other upper or lower limb limitations.

race course or venue map, and the available medical equipment. Sports medicine physicians and Emergency Medical Services (EMS) personnel, along with sports medicine fellows, residents, medical students, athletic trainers, or physical therapists can attend to expected medical needs. Establishing an EAP is the most important concern. Protocols and guidelines should include role definition of the medical staff, emergency transportation including personnel, routes, and adequate facilities with the capacity to evaluate and manage possible injuries, and an outline of the chain-of-command and communication standards. Contingency plans should be made for extreme temperature, humidity, and other weather conditions that may involve race cancellation, modification of start time, or an increase in the number of food and resupply stations. Lastly, prior to the start of the competition, the medical team should confirm that competitors are wearing proper equipment. On a road race, medical stations are established along the course to attend to emergencies and first aid. Larger recreational events may also employ volunteer medical staff carrying basic first aid and medical supplies to ride along with the participants.[2] Communication between individual members of the medical staff and with the race director, race officials, emergency medical staff, and local medical facilities is essential via two or more systems (e.g., hand-held radios and cell phones). In stage or road cycling races, the medical staff travels as part of the caravan of cars behind the main group of cyclists. The physician's car is usually in the forward portion of the caravan behind the head official.[2] A medical station at the finish line should be located within a secured area with access limited to medical staff and athletes. Some professional events may also require a separate area for doping control and drug testing. For larger races with a large number of spectators, a first aid tent for spectators may be established in a convenient location.[2] Lastly, documentation is essential for review after the event to evaluate utilization and plan for future events.

■ MEDICAL EMERGENCIES AND MEDICAL BAG ESSENTIALS

The collapsed or unconscious athlete is considered a medical emergency that requires activation of the proper channels of communication and protocols including basic life support (BLS)/advanced cardiac life support (ACLS). Although rarely reported,

Medical Bag Essentials in Cycling	
Medical Emergencies:	**Wound/Laceration/Skin Care:**
Automated External Defibrillator (AED)	Normal saline
Nitroglycerin (sublingual)	Betadine swabs
Aspirin	Neosporin, mupirocin ointment
Epi 1:1,000	Moleskin
Diphenhydramine or another antihistamine	Elastic bandage
Albuterol inhaler	Tube stretch gauze
Rectal thermometer	Sterile gauzes
Ice bucket	Vaseline
Head and Spine:	Steri-strips
Concussion evaluation form	Suture tray
Stretcher & Spine board	Lidocaine 1%
Cervical orthosis	**Others:**
Cricothyrotomy kit	Acetaminophen
Fractures and Dislocations:	Glucose tabs
Immobilizers and Slings	Waterproof SPF 50 sunscreen
Crutches	

nontraumatic emergencies can include anaphylaxis, asthma, and heat related illness, specifically heat stroke. Musculoskeletal injuries that may become medical emergencies include, upper and lower limb fractures or dislocations with neurovascular compromise, traumatic brain injuries with or without spinal cord involvement, and blunt thoracoabdominal trauma with possible internal bleeding.

■ EPIDEMIOLOGY

Injury prevalence and incidence varies according to each individual discipline.[4–11] Injuries may be classified into traumatic and overuse injuries. Traumatic injuries occurred in 48% and overuse in 52% of elite road cyclists.[4] Two-thirds of traumatic injuries occur in the upper limbs and two-thirds of overuse injuries occur in the lower limbs; however, overall the lower back is the most commonly injured body area.[4]

■ COMMON INJURIES

Head and Spine Injuries

Head and spine injuries can vary from facial and skull fractures to traumatic brain injury with or without spinal cord injury. **Traumatic Brain Injuries (TBIs)** and **cervical spine injuries** may occur secondary to a fall or collision.[10] Cyclists found to be unconscious or with neck pain and neurological symptoms should be removed from the event and have the cervical spine immobilized with a full neurological examination performed. Spinal cord injury and cervical stability are always a concern when evaluating multiple body trauma secondary to falls in mountain biking and BMX sports.[7] Any cyclist diagnosed with a concussion should not be allowed to return to the event on the day of the injury. If medically warranted, the athlete may need to be transferred to the pre-established medical facility with the capacity to attend brain and spine injury. **Cervical myofascial** and **facet mediated pain** occurs secondary to sustained riding position. Symptoms include cervical and upper trapezius pain with cervical extension and tenderness to palpation along the upper trapezius and deep neck extensors. Management includes changing handlebar grip, adjusting stem and handlebar elevation. Postural corrective exercises, strengthening of cervical spine stabilizers, physical modalities, and using a lighter helmet can also aid in managing neck pain.[5,6] **Low back pain** is the most commonly reported injury secondary to overuse in all cyclists.[4] Mechanism of injury may be caused by prolonged lumbar kyphosis or trauma. Symptoms include axial lower lumbar pain while trunk in sustained flexion. Management includes adjusting the handlebar and saddle in order to reach a tolerable degree of lumbar flexion. Mid-ride stretches and varying hand position are helpful throughout the ride. Acute low back pain requires evaluation and imaging for disc disease or herniation followed by therapeutic exercises and physical modalities.

Upper Limb Injuries

Acute/traumatic upper limb injuries commonly occur after a fall. Common injuries include clavicular and radial head fractures. **Clavicular fractures** are caused by a direct blow to the shoulder from falls, often going from the front bar. Symptoms include tenderness over the distal third of the clavicle with possible bony deformity due to clavicle displacement. Management includes immobilization in nonoperative cases to surgical correction depending on clavicle displacement and/or shortening. Displacement can be assessed by x-ray imaging and in the case of a suspected sternoclavicular (SC) joint injury, a CT is indicated to rule out a posterior dislocation. Operative treatment is indicated for posterior dislocation of SC joint. **Radial head fractures** are commonly caused from falls on an outstretched hand. Symptoms include tenderness to palpation near the radial styloid, swelling, and reduced range of motion of the wrist. Management includes immobilization, icing, nonsteroidal anti-inflammatory drugs (NSAIDs), and aspiration of hemarthrosis with anesthesia infiltration in some cases. Most athletes with nondisplaced fractures can return to riding in 7 to 14 days. Surgical correction may be necessary if displacement is noted. Overuse injuries include **compression neuropathies** involving the median or the ulnar nerve at the wrist, carpal tunnel syndrome, and ulnar neuropathy at the wrist (Cyclist's palsy), respectively. Mechanism of injury may occur secondary to overuse or previous history of focal entrapment neuropathy. Symptoms include numbness, tingling or weakness in median or ulnar distribution while riding. Management includes evaluating frequent position change, flexed elbows while riding, adding cushioning to bars or gloves, raising handlebars and shortening their reach, and correcting a nose-down tilted saddle.[3,6]

Lower Limb Injuries

Lower body limb injuries are mostly overuse due to training errors like increase in riding distance or times and improper equipment or technique. Gluteal pain etiology includes **ischial bursitis, proximal hamstring tendinopathy** and **saddle sores**. Symptoms include pain and discomfort to palpation near the ischial tuberosity and proximal hamstring origin. Management includes evaluation of saddle shape, increased saddle padding, and skin lubrication. **Pudendal neuropathy** is caused by vibration, traction, or compression of the blood supply and nerves to the genital region. Symptoms include positional scrotal pain and numbness or urinary incontinence. Management includes switching to a wider saddle, correcting excessive saddle tilt, weight distribution analysis, and padded cycling shorts. Severe cases may require pulsed radiofrequency lesioning and blocking of the pudendal nerve.[6] Hip pain may include underlying **hip osteoarthritis, adductor strain, femoroacetabular impingement (FAI), labral tear, greater trochanteric pain syndrome secondary (GTPS)** including trochanteric bursitis, gluteal tendinopathy, and/or iliotibial band (ITB) syndrome. Mechanism of injury includes weak hip abductors, saddle height, longer riding distances, and direct trauma. Symptoms may include pain during cycling, crepitus and pain with internal or external rotation of hip joint. Evaluation and management include imaging, physical therapy, pain modalities or interventions like injections, and bike adjustments. The differential diagnosis of knee pain includes: **Patellofemoral pain syndrome (PFPS or cyclist's knee), patellar and quadriceps tendinopathy, medial plica syndrome,** and **ITB friction syndrome**. Symptoms include knee pain, swelling, or clicking during cycling. Management includes equipment and technique modification, and pain control modalities and interventions. **Achilles tendinopathy** in cyclists may occur secondary to excessive plantar flexion from a high saddle and excessive dorsiflexion from a low saddle. Mechanism of injury includes use of softer shoes, pes planus, and excessive riding forces due to poor equipment fit. Symptoms include pain with dorsiflexion while cycling and tenderness to palpation over the Achilles tendon, at the insertion or midportion. Management includes diagnostic imaging, physical therapy that may include manual therapy and eccentric strengthening, and bike fit and technique modification. **Morton's neuroma** is due to compression of interdigital nerves from a fixed cleat-pedal interface and narrow rigid cycling shoe. Symptoms include pain, numbness and tingling to palpation between metatarsal bones. Management may include imaging, cleat adjustment, wider toe box, wider pedals, metatarsal pads, or steroid injection. Surgical neurectomy via plantar or dorsal approach may be necessary in some cases.[6]

Dermatologic Injuries

Skin abrasion (road rash) and contusions are common injuries. Mechanism of injury includes shear stress to skin with contact during collision or crash. Management includes rapid scrubbing and debridement with soap and water to prevent infection. Wounds should not be left uncovered using semipermeable films, hydrocolloid dressings or bio-occlusive bandages. The most common site for contusions is the quadriceps from direct contact after a fall. Immediate placement of the knee in 120 degrees of flexion for 24 hours may allow an earlier return to sports. In case of contusion-induced hematomas, ultrasound-guided aspiration may be performed.

Abdominal Injuries

Abdominal contusions from crashes occur most commonly in BMX and mountain biking.[7] The mechanism of injury is most often blunt trauma with the horizontal bar ends. Symptoms include abdominal pain, although symptoms may be nonspecific. Major visceral injuries including spleen, lungs, and kidney lacerations or ruptures need to be evaluated with appropriate imaging studies. Management includes vital signs monitoring, a full abdominal and pulmonary physical examination with transfer to the ED. Most intraabdominal contusions are treated with serial observation. Return to cycling may take from 1 to 2 months.

■ SUMMARY

Cycling sporting events have increased substantially in the last decades. It is important to understand common injuries, anatomical factors, technique errors, and fit/equipment contribution for an adequate sideline and event coverage assessment.

■ References

1. Union Cycliste Internationale. https://www.uci.org.

2. Martinez JM. Medical coverage of cycling events. *Curr Sports Med Rep*. 2006;5(3):125-130. doi:10.1097/01.csmr.0000306301.80201.3d.

3. Silberman MR, Webner D, Collina S, Shiple BJ. Road bicycle fit. *Clin J Sport Med*. 2005;15(4):271-276. doi:10.1097/01.jsm.0000171255.70156.da.

4. De Bernardo N, Barrios C, Vera P, et al. Incidence and risk for traumatic and overuse injuries in top-level road cyclists. *J Sports Sci*. 2012;30(10):1047-1053. doi:10.1080/02640414.2012.687112.

5. Kotler DH, Babu AN, Robidoux G. Prevention, evaluation, and rehabilitation of cycling-related injury. *Curr Sports Med Rep*. 2016;15(3):199-206. doi:10.1249/JSR.0000000000000262.

6. Silberman MR. Bicycling injuries. *Curr Sports Med Rep*. 2013;12(5):337-345. doi:10.1249/JSR.0b013e3182a-4bab7.

7. Ansari M, Nourian R, Khodaee M. Mountain biking injuries. *Curr Sports Med Rep*. 2017;16(6):406-412. doi:10.1249/JSR.0000000000000429.

8. Barrios C, Bernardo ND, Vera P, et al. Changes in sports injuries incidence over time in world-class road cyclists. *Int J Sports Med*. 2014;36(3):241-248. doi:10.1055/s-0034-1389983.

9. Dahlquist M, Leisz MC, Finkelstein M. The club-level road cyclist: injury, pain, and performance. *Clin J Sport Med*. 2015;25(2):88-94. doi:10.1097/JSM.0000000000000111.

10. Broe MP, Kelly JC, Groarke PJ, et al. Cycling and spinal trauma: a worrying trend in referrals to a national spine centre. *Surgeon*. 2018;16(4):202-206. doi:10.1016/j.surge.2017.07.004.

11. Decock M, De Wilde L, Bossche L, et al. Incidence and aetiology of acute injuries during competitive road cycling. *Br J Sports Med*. 2016;50:669-672. doi:10.1136/bjsports-2015-095612.

Raúl A. Rosario-Concepción, Ana Ortiz-Santiago,
and Fernando L. Sepúlveda-Irizarry

HISTORY

Although debated, the modern game of golf is said to have been developed in 15th century Scotland. In 1754, the Royal and Ancient Golf Club of St. Andrews was founded, which still remains the oldest golf organization to date. Golf continued to grow in popularity and eventually the game spread to the British colonies, including the United States of America (USA). Subsequently, the United States Golf Association (USGA) was formed in 1894. As of 2019, there were around 16,752 courses in the United States; approximately 50% of the golf courses worldwide.[1]

GOVERNING ORGANIZATIONS

- International: International Golf Federation (IGF)
- National: United States Golf Association (USGA)
- Professional: Professional Golf Association (PGA), Ladies Professional Golf Association (LPGA)
- College: National Collegiate Athletic Association (NCAA)
- High School: National Federation of State High School Associations (NFHS)

PARTICIPANTS

Golf is played in 206 countries worldwide by around 55 million people. It is practiced by people of all ages. Recently, the world appeal has increased to the point that golf was reintroduced as an Olympic sport at the 2016 Olympic Games in Rio de Janeiro.

RULES AND REGULATIONS

The main goal of golf is to get the ball into the cup in the fewest strokes possible. Each swing of the golf club is considered a stroke with "par" being the amount of strokes that was intended per hole by the course designer. Most golf tournaments are played according to "stroke play," consisting of 18 holes with the winner being the player with the fewest strokes at the end. The majority of the PGA tournaments consist of 4 days of "stroke play." "Match play" is a competition between two golfers, with the player with fewer strokes in a hole winning the hole. The winner is declared when one player has a bigger lead than the number of holes remaining. In amateur-level golf tournaments, there is a handicap system that allows golfers of different skill levels to compete equitably. The handicap system is not used at the professional level. A golfing event starts with the first swing at the first tee and ends when the player completes the 18-hole course. On a tournament, in the case of a tie after 18 holes, extra holes are played until someone wins a hole. Actual game times vary depending on how busy the golf course is, the number of golfers playing each hole, and the skill level.[2]

EQUIPMENT

The golf *club* is used for striking the ball. It comes in different forms depending on the shape of the club head and the intended use: driver, woods, irons, hybrids, wedges, and putters. Overall length is at least 18 in and may not exceed 48 in, with the exception of the putter. *Golf balls* must conform to specific categories, including weight, size, spherical symmetry, initial velocity, and overall distance standard. The dimpled surface reduces aerodynamic drag. The weight of the ball may not be greater than 45.93 g, but may be as light as the manufacturer desires. The diameter may not be less than 1.68 in, yet there is no maximum size. Initial velocity must not exceed the limit specified under the R&A and the USGA rules.[3] The *tee* is a device used to raise the ball off the ground. It may not be longer than 4 in, influence the movement of the ball, or assist the player in making a stroke. *Gloves* are optional, used mainly to aid in a player's grip of the club. It must be made of smooth material that does not provide substantial thickness, adhere to material on the grip, or bind digits together. As part of the golf etiquette, nearly all golf courses require that men wear collared shirts. Women's golf tops vary greatly, but all adhere to a traditional sense of modesty. *Shoes* that aid in a player's stance may be used. Nonetheless, their use to assist in player's alignment or making a stroke is prohibited.

>>> **Adaptive Sport Key Points: Golf**

There are multiple associations around the world that incorporate adaptive golf. One of them is the National Amputee Golf Association (NAGA). In 2001, the PGA TOUR established a 12-person "Golf Disability Review Board" that reviews TOUR professional requests on the use of a cart during competition. The USGA also developed a form for the applicant's physical limitations and requires the submission of medical certification of impairment and disability by a licensed physician. In addition, under the rule 14-3/15, orthotic and prosthetic devices are permitted in the USGA.[4]

MEDICAL COVERAGE LOGISTICS

The level of medical coverage in golf events depend on the number of participants and/or spectators, weather conditions, access to local health care facilities, and tournament resources.[5] The medical director must establish an emergency action plan (EAP), define roles, and establish a communication command chain. Just like marathons and road races, medical coverage of golf tournaments presents with unique challenges due to the large setting of golf courses. They typically cover more than 100 acres for which access to all parts of the course is essential. A designated medical area with appropriate equipment and staff is needed in order to handle minor emergencies. Having dedicated medical communications networks (walkie-talkies or cell phones) in order to communicate with a mobile response team is important so they can travel to the different holes of the golf course. In order to manage emergencies, multiple Automated External Defibrillators (AEDs) and an emergency cooling area with oral and intravenous hydration are needed. Advanced planning with emergency services is necessary in order to transport serious injuries to the emergency department. It is necessary to establish a weather policy in addition to having a lightning detection system in order to prevent any lightning injuries or death.[5]

MEDICAL EMERGENCIES AND MEDICAL BAG ESSENTIALS

Emergencies in golf are rare but may be seen after a fall from a golf cart, getting hit by a club or golf ball, or struck by lightning. Although infrequent, golf events have the highest sports incidence of lightning-strike deaths in the United States.[6] On hot

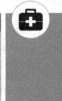

Medical Bag Essentials in Golf	
Medical Emergencies: AED Nitroglycerin (sublingual) Aspirin Epi 1:1,000 Diphenhydramine or another antihistamine	Albuterol inhaler Rectal thermometer Ice bath IV normal saline IV lines

days, heat-related injuries must be evaluated and managed. Rapid identification of emergencies, like the collapsed athlete, is important and the proper channels should be activated.

EPIDEMIOLOGY

There is an overall incidence of 15.8 injuries per 100 golfers, with 46% of all injuries occurring during the swing phase and 23.7% during ball impact.[7] The lower back is currently the most common site of injury, followed by the elbow, shoulder, and ankle.[7]

COMMON INJURIES

Head and Spine Injuries

Head injuries are infrequent in golf, but are the most common golf-related injuries that require evaluation in an emergency department.[6,8] Injuries in children are most frequently secondary to being struck with a club while adults are due to getting hit by a golf ball. Quick neurological examination is essential to determine the seriousness of the injury. If neurological deficit is found, the patient needs to be transferred to the emergency department. Concussion evaluation will be important to determine the adequate management and return to play. *Injuries of the lumbar spine* are the most common complaint in professional golfers. This may be secondary to the high acceleration forces the trunk needs in order to generate power in the golf swing. The elevated loads on the spine experienced with compression, lateral-bending, and rotational movement can predispose golfers to develop *muscle strains, herniated intervertebral discs, stress fractures of the vertebral body and pars interarticularis, spondylolisthesis, and facet arthropathy.*[6] The medical provider should be able to distinguish from mechanical back pain and radicular pain with special emphasis on the identification of red flags like saddle anesthesia, bowel and bladder involvement, significant unintentional weight loss, and night sweats. Conservative management of low back pain (LBP) should include relative rest, ice, nonsteroidal anti-inflammatory drugs (NSAIDs), physical therapy, stabilization exercises with biomechanics, and swing analysis. Advanced imaging is usually needed when neurological deficit is found on physical examination or when back pain has not improved in 6 weeks.

Upper Limb Injuries

Shoulder degenerative joint disease is very prevalent in golf due to high participation from the geriatric population. Patients may develop *acromioclavicular (AC) joint degenerative joint disease* due to the repetitive adduction of the lead shoulder at the top of the takeaway phase, which adds stress loads on the AC joint. Most patients respond to conservative treatment with physical therapy, swing modification, and steroid injections. Surgical treatment with distal clavicle excision is usually not needed. *Labral tears* are common injuries that include superior labral tear from anterior to posterior (SLAP) lesions that can often cause pain in the lead shoulder during the end of the takeaway phase or the beginning of the forward swing. Conservative treatment includes physical therapy, NSAIDs, and glenohumeral joint and biceps sheath cortisone injections. Surgical management is considered in young golfers with acute tears or patients who did not respond to conservative management. *Rotator cuff impingement and tendinopathy* is a common source of pain in golfers. They often experience symptoms at the extremes of the golf swing, such as at the top of the backswing phase or the end of the follow-through.[7] A common problem is subacromial impingement of the rotator cuff which can create tendinopathies or tears. Conservative treatment includes relative rest, physical therapy focusing on strengthening exercises of the rotator cuff and scapular stabilizers muscles, NSAIDs, and subacromial corticosteroid injections. Recent studies have looked at a possible role for regenerative medicine procedures like platelet rich plasma (PRP) in rotator cuff tendinopathies and tears.[9] In rotator cuff tears, surgical management may be indicated including acromioplasty and rotator cuff repair. Acute and overuse *injuries at the elbow* are the most common complaint in amateur golfers due to a poor swing technique.[7] Acute injuries may occur after a sudden deceleration of the golf swing by hitting the ball through heavy rough or grass. *Lateral and medial epicondylopathy* is the most common elbow injury in golfers. Lateral epicondylopathy usually presents in the lead arm with medial epicondylopathy presenting in the trailing arm. Patients present with tenderness on the tendon insertion in the epicondyles. Conservative treatment will include relative rest, NSAIDs, forearm straps, physical therapy, deep friction massage, nitroglycerin patches, and/or extracorporeal shockwave therapy (ESWT). Equipment evaluation and fitting is important, with some patients feeling better when they change from heavy steel to lighter graphite shafts. Also, increasing the grip size can help. Recent evidence supports the avoidance of corticosteroid injections for this problem. However, in refractory cases, there may be an indication for corticosteroid injections, percutaneous ultrasonic tenotomies, or PRP. Surgical debridement is reserved when a patient does not respond to conservative management or procedures. *Wrist injuries* usually affect the lead hand. Acute injuries commonly occur after hitting the firm ground or hitting the shot fat. Overuse injuries can occur secondary to the repetitive nature of the golf swing. Athletes with poor golf swing technique can develop *tendinopathy of the extensor carpi ulnaris (ECU)*. Wrist pain can develop on the early follow-through swing phase of the golf swing. At this stage the wrist undergoes accelerated ulnar deviation causing disruption of the ECU tendon sheath that can result in painful tendon snapping with wrist movement. Conservative treatment includes relative rest, splinting, and hand therapy. Some cases require repair of the tendon sheath. *Triangular fibrocartilage complex (TFCC) injuries* occur due to the repetitive wrist motion during the golf swing. Acutely, a forceful ground hit during ulnar deviation can develop an acute injury to the TFCC. It presents with ulnar-sided pain with possible palpable click on forearm rotation. Initial treatment includes relative rest, immobilization or splinting, NSAIDs, or corticosteroid injection. Surgical management is usually done if conservative treatment is unsuccessful. *Fracture in the hook of the hamate* is very important to identify on the hand holding the end of the club after a forceful hit to the ground. Golfer presents with direct tenderness to palpation on the hook of the hamate. Radiographs are recommended but can be initially normal. If high suspicion, a hand CT scan or MRI is needed in order to confirm the diagnosis. Initial treatment includes relative rest and immobilization. If pain persists, surgical management involves removing the hook of the hamate.[7]

Lower Limb Injuries

Hip injuries include **acetabular labral tears**. In this particular sport, repetitive rotational velocities experienced at the hip during forward swing result in elevated joint stress. Although not as prevalent as lumbar injuries, of the 2.8% hip injury incidence in golf, 78% are attributed to wear and tear. Treatment is aimed at strengthening internal hip rotators in order to further improve hip range of motion (ROM). Surgical intervention has been moving toward arthroscopies, yet it still has limited indications for osteoarthritis. **Knee injuries** account for 18% of all golf injuries.[10] Most knee injuries associated with golf are a result of overuse or mechanical faults. During the swing phase, there is increased internal and external rotation of the femur and the tibia. Most patients may be treated conservatively with NSAIDs and therapy; if needed, corticosteroid injections may also be performed. Platelet-rich plasma injections may provide benefit for golfers with mild to moderate knee osteoarthritis (OA). If a golfer presents with mechanical symptoms, knee arthroscopy may be indicated. Eventually, severe and advanced degenerative changes may lead to a total knee arthroplasty. Orthopedic surgeons commonly recommend golf as a good rehabilitation activity following total knee arthroplasty due to its low impact nature.[10] **Ankle injuries** are usually secondary to accidents, like slipping or tripping over something. This can cause sprains around the ankle. In the absence of fracture, initial management includes relative rest, ice, bracing, NSAIDs, and proprioceptive training.

Most orthopedic surgeons feel comfortable with patients returning to low-impact sporting activities such as golf after shoulder, hip, and knee arthroplasties, with patients reporting good outcomes in performance after surgery.[11]

SUMMARY

Golf is a very popular noncontact sport. Most injuries are caused by overuse disorders. However, when covering an event, it is imperative to be prepared to manage medical emergencies caused by trauma or weather-related events.

References

1. The R&A, United States Golf Association. *Golf Around the World. Edition 3.* St Andrews: The R&A, USGA; 2019

2. The rules of golf. https://www.randa.org/en/rog/2019/pages/the-rules-of-golf.

3. The equipment rules. https://www.randa.org/RulesEquipment/Equipment/EquipmentRules.

4. Parziale J. Golf in the United States: an evolution of accessibility. *PM R.* 2014;6(9):825-827. doi:10.1016/j.pmrj.2014.04.002.

5. Wadsworth L. Sideline and event management in golf. *Curr Sports Med Rep.* 2011;10(3):131-133. doi:10.1249/JSR.0b013e31821d040b.

6. Murray A, Daines L, Archibald D, et al. The relationships between golf and health: a scoping review. *Br J Sports Med.* 2016;51(1):12-19. doi:10.1136/bjsports-2016-096625.

7. Zouzias I, Hendra J, Stodelle J, Limpisvasti O. Golf injuries: epidemiology, pathophysiology, and treatment. *J Am Acad Orthop Surg.* 2018;26(4):116-123. doi:10.5435/JAAOS-D-15-00433.

8. Walsh B, Chounthirath T, Friedenberg L, Smith GA. Golf-related injuries treated in United States emergency departments. *Am J Emerg Med.* 2017;35(11):1666-1671. doi:10.1016/j.ajem.2017.05.035.

9. Le ADK, Enweze L, DeBaun MR, Dragoo JL. Current clinical recommendations for use of platelet-rich plasma. *Curr Rev Musculoskelet Med.* 2018;11(4):624-634. doi:10.1007/s12178-018-9527-7.

10. Baker ML, Epari DR, Lorenzetti S, et al. Risk factors for knee injury in golf: a systematic review. *Sports Med.* 2017;47(12):2621-2639. doi:10.1007/s40279-017-0780-5.

11. Papaliodis D, Photopoulos C, Mehran N, et al. Return to golfing activity after joint arthroplasty. *Am J Sports Med.* 2016;45(1):243-249. doi:10.1177/0363546516641917.

43. LONG DISTANCE RUNNING

Allison C. Bean

HISTORY

According to legend, in 490 BCE, an Athenian *hemerodromos,* or day-long runner named Pheidippides, was sent from Athens to Sparta to request help against the invading Persians. He ran 140 miles in 2 days to deliver this message. Upon arrival, the Spartans told him they would aid in the battle, but could not leave until the next full moon 6 days later, as they were celebrating the festival of Carnea. Pheidippides then ran back to Marathon to convey the bad news. Unexpectedly, the Athenians decided to attack the Persians, and eventually prevailed. Pheidippides is then said to have run the approximate 25 miles from Marathon to Athens to deliver the good news to the Athenian people, collapsing and dying immediately after.[1] At the 1896 Athens Olympics a 40 km (24.85 miles) run was organized to commemorate Pheidippides and his famous run from Marathon to Athens. In 1921, the distance was standardized to 26 miles and 385 yards, the distance run during the 1908 London Olympics.

GOVERNING ORGANIZATIONS
- International Amateur Athletic Federation
- Association of International Marathons and Distance Races

PARTICIPANTS

In 2018, there were approximately 1.1 million marathon participants globally. Marathon participation has more than doubled since the early 2000s. The average age of marathon participants is 40 years old. Over 30% of marathon finishers are women. The average finishing time is 4 hours and 32 minutes.[2] The number of participants in a marathon varies widely, with the largest races having more than 50,000 participants.

RULES AND REGULATIONS

Long distance running events typically involve distances ranging from 5 km, 10 km, 21 km (half-marathon), or 42 km (marathon). Runners attempt to complete the established distance as fast as possible.

EQUIPMENT

Running shoes and **socks** are typically worn. These have different characteristics to match the needs of the individual runner. Running **shorts** and **shirts** are worn. Participants must wear official **numbered bibs** provided to them for identification. These bibs typically have space on the back for the athlete to fill out emergency contact information and any pertinent personal medical information. Depending on the weather conditions, additional gear may be used to protect the runner against an adverse environment.

■ MEDICAL COVERAGE LOGISTICS

An Emergency Action Plan (EAP) must be established and reviewed. For large events, a Mass Casualty Disaster (MCD) plan should be part of the EAP as well. Marathons typically include several medical aid stations/medical tents at different locations throughout the course and at the finish line. The finish line medical tents are often larger and have additional supplies/equipment due to the higher number and medical acuity of participants requiring care at the end of the event. For large events, there may also be medical professionals on bicycles throughout the course who can provide aid to participants who require immediate care in the areas between aid stations. Each aid station should have an experienced physician team leader or "tent captain" who oversees patient care and other medical personnel, and communicates with the medical director during the event as needed. Most medical personnel are volunteers with various types and levels of experience and may include licensed professionals as well as trainees. The medical personnel should arrive at least 1 hour before the time that the first participants are expected to reach their aid station/medical tent. Medical personnel should be assigned roles based on individual qualifications by the team leader. The EAP for evacuating any participants to a higher level of care should be reviewed. Aid stations/medical tents should have an ambulance located next to it or an established plan in place to allow an ambulance access to the area. The team leader should check that all medical equipment and supplies are present and in working order. The type of treatment that can be provided at the aid stations/finish line tents may vary. Some marathons will have the ability to initiate intensive care including IV fluids and monitors, while others will have only basic life support capabilities. It is important for medical personnel to know what supplies are available prior to the event.

■ MEDICAL EMERGENCIES AND MEDICAL BAG ESSENTIALS

The collapsed or unconscious athlete is considered a medical emergency that requires activation of the proper channels of communication and protocols including basic life support (BLS)/advanced cardiac life support (ACLS). Nontraumatic emergencies include asthma, anaphylaxis, heat- or cold-related illness, electrolyte disturbances, cardiac arrhythmias, or hypertrophic cardiomyopathy.

■ EPIDEMIOLOGY

Musculoskeletal and dermatologic complaints are the most common reason for athletes to seek medical aid during marathons. Illness involving other organ systems including cardiovascular, pulmonary, renal, and gastrointestinal systems may also occur, but are rarer. Marathon participants may experience acute or chronic injuries. Chronic injuries are common due to the high training load required for marathon preparation. It has been estimated that 25% of runners are injured at any given time, with individuals who have suffered a previous injury or who train more than 40 miles per week

Medical Bag Essentials in Long Distance Running or Endurance Events	
Medical Emergencies:	**Wound Care/Dermal Injuries:**
Automated External Defibrillator (AED)	Normal saline
Sublingual nitroglycerin	Betadine/Alcohol swabs
Epi 1:1,000	Neosporin, mupirocin ointment
Albuterol inhaler	Gauzes
Pulse oximeter	Mole skin
Supplemental oxygen	Vaseline
Rectal thermometer	Tongue depressors/applicators
Bear huggers	Wound irrigation kit
Blankets	Sterile needle
Ice baths	**Musculoskeletal:**
Sunscreen	Crutches
Water	Topical analgesics
Sports drink	Oral Acetaminophen tabs/caps*
Pretzels	Tourniquets
Salt packets	
I-STAT	
Syringes	
Glucometer	
Glucose testing strips	
Finger lancet	
Glucose tabs	
Oral ondansetron	
IV lines	
IV bags	

*Use of oral analgesics during marathon events warrants specific discussion. Many athletes will seek treatment with oral analgesics during the event for various types of pain. Nonsteroidal anti-inflammatory drugs (NSAIDs) are not recommended due to the increased risk of adverse events including electrolyte abnormalities, gastrointestinal cramping/bleeding, renal dysfunction, and cardiovascular events.[3] Acetaminophen/paracetamol is considered a safer option, and a single dose (500 to 1,000 mg) may be provided for pain relief. Athletes who are given acetaminophen should have their bib clearly marked (e.g., a large red dot) to signal to other medical providers that the athlete has received the medication in order to avoid potential overdose.

(common for many marathon participants) at increased risk.[4] Athletes with chronic injuries who choose to participate in the marathon event may experience acute worsening of their symptoms during the event. The incidence of injury or illness during marathon events can be variable, and may depend on several factors including climate, course difficulty, and participant skill level. A study conducted during the Chicago Marathon from 2012 to 2016 found that 2.92% of participants received medical care at an aid station along the course or a medical tent at the finish line; 3.4% of participants who received medical care required transport to a local hospital.[5]

▪ COMMON INJURIES

Medical Illnesses

Exercise-associated collapse (EAC) most commonly occurs at the marathon finish line after an athlete stops running. This is a benign condition that occurs in the absence of neurologic, electrolyte, or thermal abnormalities. EAC occurs as a result of venous pooling in the lower limbs secondary to decreased peripheral vascular resistance and reduced baroreflex response, leading to postural hypotension.[6] Management of EAC focuses on restoring hemodynamics, by placing the patient's legs above his or her head (Trendelenburg) and providing oral hydration. *Cardiopulmonary arrest* occurs in approximately 1 in 100,000 marathon participants, with men at higher risk than women. Younger athletes are more likely to suffer sudden cardiac death due to hypertrophic cardiomyopathy, while older athletes are more likely to have cardiac arrest due to myocardial infarction in the setting of underlying atherosclerotic disease.[7] Rapid initiation of cardiopulmonary resuscitation by bystanders or medical personnel increases the likelihood of survival,[7] followed by activation of the EAP, implementation of CPR/ACLS by the medical team on site, and transfer to the hospital. *Environmental illnesses* including *hypothermia* and *hyperthermia* occur most frequently with events that take place in extreme temperatures or when weather changes rapidly. Climate acclimatization prior to the event, fitness status, and hydration status influence the risk of developing heat- or cold-related illness. Core temperature should always be measured rectally for improved accuracy. Treatments should focus on restoration of normal core temperature. *Exercise-associated hyponatremia (EAH)* is rarely severe enough to cause symptoms in runners, but is essential to recognize due to risk of severe cerebral edema, which may lead to herniation and death in severe cases. Hyponatremia is defined as a serum Na^+ less than 135 mmol/L, and is often asymptomatic in mild cases. Symptomatic EAH typically occurs if the serum Na^+ drops below 125 mmol/L, or if it rapidly falls to between 125 to 130 mmol/L. Symptoms in mild EAH may include lightheadedness, dizziness, nausea, and weight gain; while athletes with severe EAH may present with headache, vomiting, altered mental status, seizure, or coma as a result of cerebral edema.[8] Symptoms of EAH overlap with other conditions including heat illness, EAC, and hypernatremia. Thus, it is essential to measure serum sodium (typically with point-of-care i-STAT) prior to initiating treatment. Risk factors for development of hyponatremia in runners include overconsumption of hypotonic beverages, slow pace, high or low body mass index, inexperience, and limited training. Athletes with asymptomatic hyponatremia should be treated with oral hypertonic fluids (e.g., concentrated bouillon, 3% NaCl with flavoring) to prevent further reduction in serum Na^+ levels. Oral or IV hypotonic or isotonic fluids should be avoided in asymptomatic hyponatremia until the athlete is freely urinating. Severe hyponatremia resulting in encephalopathy should be considered a medical emergency and rapidly treated with boluses of intravenous 3% NaCl to reduce cerebral edema and risk of herniation.[8]

Exertional rhabdomyolysis occurs as a result of muscle breakdown leading to release of myoglobin into the circulation. Risk factors for development of rhabdomyolysis in runners include recent illness, NSAID use, hyperthermia, and sickle cell anemia. Typical symptoms include muscle pain, low-grade fever, and dark urine. High concentrations of myoglobin may precipitate in the kidney tubules leading to acute renal failure. Rhabdomyolysis may also lead to disseminated intravascular coagulation, hyperkalemia, and cardiac dysrhythmias.[9] Management of rhabdomyolysis is typically supportive, with aggressive IV hydration to prevent kidney injury. *Exercise-associated muscle cramping (EAMC)* often occurs in the gastrocnemius/soleus complex, the hamstrings, and the quadriceps. EAMC may occur at any temperature in the setting of fatigue; however, it is more commonly seen with warmer temperatures. Management may include massage, stretching, and ice. Sports drinks and salt may also provide some benefit, particularly for athletes known as "salty sweaters" who may lose greater amounts of salt during activity; however, the exact contribution of dehydration and salt-loss to the development of cramping remains unclear.[10] Widespread and/or persistent severe cramping should raise concern for potential development of rhabdomyolysis.

Lower Limb Injuries

Tendinopathies and **other soft tissue injuries** are common injuries suffered by runners. Often these injuries are chronic, occurring as a result of repetitive mechanical overloading of the tissues. Many marathon athletes will have experienced symptoms during training prior to the event, with potential exacerbation during the event. The most common areas affected are the Achilles tendon, patellar tendon, iliotibial band, plantar fascia, and proximal hamstring tendon. Acute tendon and ligament injuries are less common in marathon athletes due to limited explosive and cutting movements, but may occur in athletes with previous injury or in the event of a misstep resulting in an abnormal twisting motion, particularly at the knee or ankle. A focused physical exam should be completed for any athlete with acute onset of pain and difficulty with weight-bearing to determine the severity of injury. Supportive treatment including compression, ice, and/or oral or topical analgesia may be provided. **Bone stress injuries (BSIs)** are common in long distance runners due to structural fatigue as a result of repetitive loading. BSIs occur on a spectrum, ranging from inflammation of the periosteum to complete cortical fracture. **Medial tibial stress syndrome (MTSS),** commonly known as "shin splints," is a form of mild BSI that typically presents as pain in the posteromedial aspect of the middle to distal tibia more than 5 cm in distance. Supportive treatment including compression, ice, and/or oral or topical analgesia may be provided during the event. The most common locations for BSIs in marathon athletes are the tibia, fibula, and metatarsals. BSIs may also develop in the tarsals, calcaneus, femur, pelvis, and lumbar spine.[12] BSI should be suspected in marathon athletes who develop focal bony pain and tenderness with percussion over the area. Pain elicited with a single-leg hop test or fulcrum test can also raise suspicion of BSI. If BSI is suspected on the marathon course, the athlete should be advised to stop his or her participation in the event to prevent injury progression. Ice and acetaminophen may be provided for pain relief. If stress fracture is suspected, weight-bearing on the affected area should be avoided and the athlete should follow up with a physician to obtain imaging as soon as possible.

Muscle strains are the result of overstretching of muscle fibers. Muscles crossing two joints including the gastrocnemius, hamstrings, and rectus femoris are at highest risk. Clinical assessment should include palpation, range of motion (ROM), and strength testing. Acute on-course or finish line management of low grade muscle injuries are focused on pain relief and may include topical analgesics, ice, compression, and/or acetaminophen. Long-term management should include a rehabilitation program focused on progressive strengthening and gradual return to activity. High grade injuries with extensive muscle fiber disruption are uncommon in runners. In these cases, the athlete may describe a sudden "popping" sensation followed by severe localized pain and loss of motor function. A palpable defect and/or rapid formation of a hematoma may be noted. Athletes with high-grade muscle injuries should have close physician follow-up; in some cases surgical intervention may be warranted. Large hematomas also have potential to cause neurovascular compromise leading to compartment syndrome or deep vein thrombosis,[11] and athletes should be counseled to seek immediate care if pain and/or swelling significantly worsens in the days following injury.

Dermatologic Injuries

Blisters are common in runners, occurring most frequently on the feet and ankles due to repetitive friction between the skin and sock or running shoes leading to separation between epidermal cells. For all stages of blisters, care should be taken to ensure the surrounding area is clean and dry before further treatment. Early blister formation is typically felt as a "hot spot," with skin appearing erythematous and raw. Hot spots can be managed by covering the area with a bandage, moleskin, athletic tape, or event duct tape. Once a blister becomes fluid-filled, adhesive bandages should not be utilized over the delicate skin of the blister. Painful, unruptured blisters can be treated by creating a small hole at the edge of the blister using a sterile needle or scalpel, allowing the fluid to drain while maintaining the roof of the blister. The blister should then be covered with a nonadhesive bandage. Moleskin can be cut into a doughnut shape with the inner hole approximately the size of the blister and adhered to the surrounding unaffected skin. If the roof of the blister has torn off, antibiotic ointment should be applied followed by a nonadhesive dressing. **Subungual hematomas** typically occur in runners as a result of repetitive trauma of the toe against the front of the shoe. Blood may collect between the nail bed in the toenail, causing pain due to increased pressure. Painful subungual hematomas can be treated by boring a hole into the nail using an 18-gauge needle at a 90-degree angle over the central area of the hematoma. Once the hematoma is drained, there is typically complete relief of pain.

▨ SUMMARY

Long distance running, "Marathon," is a popular sport with participants ranging from elite to recreational athletes. While nonemergent musculoskeletal and dermatologic injuries are the primary reasons for athletes to require medical care, the extended time of exertion required to complete the 26.2-mile distance can result in more serious systemic illnesses, particularly in less experienced individuals, and must be efficiently recognized and managed by medical providers.

▨ References

1. Grogan R. Run, Pheidippides, Run! The story of the Battle of Marathon. *Br J Sports Med.* 1981;15(3):186-189. doi:10.1136/bjsm.15.3.186.

2. Andersen JJ. The state of running 2019. RunRepeat. https://runrepeat.com/state-of-running.

3. Küster M, Renner B, Oppel P, et al. Consumption of analgesics before a marathon and the incidence of cardiovascular, gastrointestinal and renal problems: a cohort study. *BMJ Open.* 2013;3(4). doi:10.11 36/bmjopen-2012-002090.

4. Fields KB, Sykes JC, Walker KM, Jackson JC. Prevention of running injuries. *Curr Sports Med Rep.* 2010;9(3):176-182. doi:10.1249/JSR.0b013e3181de7ec5.

5. Chan JL, Constantinou V, Fokas J, et al. An overview of Chicago (Illinois USA) marathon prehospital care demographics, patient care operations, and injury patterns. *Prehosp Disaster Med.* 2019;34(3):308-316. doi:10.1017/S1049023X19004345.

6. Asplund CA, O'Connor FG, Noakes TD. Exercise-associated collapse: an evidence-based review and primer for clinicians. *Br J Sports Med.* 2011;45(14):1157-1162. doi:10.1136/bjsports-2011-090378.

7. Hart L. Marathon-related cardiac arrest. *Clin J Sport Med.* 2013;23(5):409-410. doi:10.1097/01. jsm.0000433155.97054.c8.

8. Hew-Butler T, Rosner MH, Fowkes-Godek S, et al. Statement of the 3rd International Exercise-Associated Hyponatremia Consensus Development Conference, Carlsbad, California, 2015. *Br J Sports Med.* 2015;49(22):1432-1446. doi:10.1136/bjsports-2015-095004.

9. Clarkson PM. Exertional rhabdomyolysis and acute renal failure in marathon runners. *Sports Med.* 2007;37 (4-5):361-363. doi:10.2165/00007256-200737040-00022.

10. Eichner ER. Muscle cramping in the heat. *Curr Sports Med Rep.* 2018;17(11):356-357. doi:10.1249/JSR.000 0000000000529.

11. Alessandrino F, Balconi G. Complications of muscle injuries. *J Ultrasound.* 2013;16(4):215-222. doi:10.1007/ s40477-013-0010-4.

12. Tenforde AS, Kraus E, Fredericson M. Bone stress injuries in runners. *Phys Med Rehabil Clin N Am.* 2016;27(1):139-149. doi:10.1016/j.pmr.2015.08.008.

44. RACQUETBALL

Michael Harbus and Priya B. Patel

■ HISTORY

Evolving from paddleball and closely related to handball and squash, racquetball is an indoor racquet sport developed in 1950 by Joe Sobek, who wanted a sport that was faster than paddleball, but less demanding than handball. It uses a stringed racquet and a hollow rubber ball within a four-walled 20 ft wide to 40 ft long court. Further, it is relatively easy to learn, provides a great workout, and is a great alternative to tennis in bad weather.[1,2]

■ GOVERNING ORGANIZATIONS

- International: International Racquetball Federation
- National: USA Racquetball
- Major professional tours: International Racquetball Tour, Ladies' Professional Racquetball Tour

■ PARTICIPANTS

Recent estimates of participants in the United States are in the 3 to 4 million range. This is down from the estimated 7 million in the United States, and 8.5 million worldwide, when Mr. Sobek passed away in 1998.[3]

■ RULES AND REGULATIONS

The size of the racquet and type of ball are different in racquetball from squash, but the games are similar in fundamental ways: a stringed racquet is used to hit a ball within four enclosed walls, and you score a point when your opponent fails to hit the ball to the front wall before it bounces twice. Specifically, your opponent must return your shot either in midair before it bounces, or after just one bounce. In contrast to squash, ceiling shots are fair, as are shots at the lower portion of the front wall (squash has a tin at the bottom of the front wall which is out of bounds). Games are played to 15 points, and you can score a point only if you are serving. If you are serving and your opponent wins the rally, he or she gets to serve. Serves are made from inside a service zone, and must hit the front wall first before hitting any other wall. If the first serve is "short" (bounces before the short line) or "long" (hits the back wall on a fly), these are faults. The server gets a second service try, but no more. Once the serve is in play, the players alternate in hitting the ball to the front wall until one fails to return a fair shot. Returns can hit side walls first, or the ceiling, as long as the ball hits the front wall before hitting the floor.

EQUIPMENT

The *court* is 20 ft wide and 40ft long and 20 ft high (front wall, two side walls, back wall, ceiling). Equipment consists of *goggles*, used to protect the eyes, a string *racquet* and a bouncy, hollow rubber *ball, racquetball sneakers* with good traction, an ankle support for side to side movement, and a *glove* for better grip on the racquet handle.

》》 Adaptive Sport Key Points: Wheelchair Racquetball

The standard rules for racquetball are generally used, with the exception that the ball is allowed to bounce twice. There is also a division which allows more than two bounces. The wheelchair is considered part of the body as applies to ball contact. Adapted rules also exist for visually impaired competitors. Visual impaired players are permitted to try to hit the ball until it has stopped bouncing, until it has been touched, or until it has rolled past the short line after hitting the back wall.

MEDICAL COVERAGE LOGISTICS

The role of the medical director is to establish an Emergency Action Plan (EAP), coordinate with event personnel, officials, and referees to ensure the safety of all players and spectators. Protocols and guidelines should include role definition of the medical staff, emergency transportation including personnel, routes, and adequate facilities, and an outline of the chain-of-command and communication standards. An accessible and centrally located area for medical evaluation, medical equipment, and personnel must be established prior to play time. Communication can be facilitated by two-way radios, cell phones, or walkie-talkies. If a player suffers from a treatable medical condition, the player must communicate with the referee who will notify the medical personnel. In cases of acute injury, the player may request to be evaluated and treated immediately. Each medical encounter must be documented properly for continuity of care and planning for future events.

MEDICAL EMERGENCIES AND MEDICAL BAG ESSENTIALS

Life-threatening events are quite rare in racquetball. The collapsed or unconscious athlete is considered a medical emergency that requires activation of the proper channels of communication and protocols including basic life support (BLS)/advanced cardiac life support (ACLS). Other conditions considered to be urgent include facial, dental, or eye injuries with racquets or balls. Other nontraumatic emergencies include asthma, anaphylaxis, cardiac arrhythmias, or hypertrophic cardiomyopathy.

EPIDEMIOLOGY

Racquetball is a fast-paced sport, with the ball often traveling at speeds in excess of 100 miles/hour. Protecting one's eyes by wearing goggles is essential. In addition, injuries could arise from collisions on the court. Males are estimated to make up approximately 80% of injured players. The lower limb and trunk were the most commonly injured body regions for squash and racquetball players treated in emergency care settings in the United States.[4] Female players were more likely to injure their upper or lower limbs, whereas male players had a higher risk of head or neck injuries. Strains and sprains were the most common injury type for squash or racquetball players who

Medical Bag Essentials in Racquetball	
Medical Emergencies:	**Wound/Laceration/Skin Care:**
Automated External Defibrillator (AED)	Normal saline
Nitroglycerin (sublingual)	Betadine swabs
Aspirin	Neosporin, mupirocin ointment
Epi 1:1,000	Moleskin
Diphenhydramine or another	Elastic bandage
antihistamine	Tube stretch gauze
Albuterol inhaler	Sterile gauzes
Head and Spine:	Vaseline
	Steri-strips
Concussion evaluation form	Suture tray
Safe a tooth kit	Lidocaine 1%

presented to emergency rooms in the United States, making up 34% of injuries, followed by skin-level wounds which made up 17% of injuries.[4]

COMMON INJURIES

Head and Spine Injuries

Facial and ocular injuries are reported at higher rates in racquetball than in any other racquet sport. **Retinal detachment** occurs when the retina separates from the back wall of the eye.[5] Prior to the detachment of the retina from the back wall of the eye, people may see floaters and flashes. When the retina detaches, there will be an area of darkness that enters the field of vision. While some retinal detachments are treated nonoperatively, most require surgery. **Lacerations** are the most common type of injury to the head and neck, making up 49% of injuries to this region. Treatment should be focused on wound closure and preventing wound infection. **Traumatic hyphema** often occurs after blunt trauma to the eye. Traumatic hyphema is a condition in which suspected blood without any clots is present in the anterior chamber of the eye. Presenting symptoms may include pain, vision changes, and photophobia. Treatment is focused on promoting absorption of blood from the eye. **Concussions** can occur due to collisions with other players, or with the walls of the racquetball court. In the setting of a suspected concussion, a player should undergo a neurological exam, concussion specific evaluation with a validated tool like the Sport Concussion Assessment Tool 5 (SCAT 5), and be removed from play. Close follow-up is required for a guided, gradual return-to-sport protocol. **Muscle strains** and **ligamentous sprains** were the most commonly reported injuries to the trunk for players of alternative racquet sports, making up 73% of the injuries in this region. These injuries follow excessive eccentric contraction, rapid acceleration and deceleration, and overuse. They present as delayed onset soreness, which occurs 24 to 48 hours after the inciting event. Treatment is conservative management, including relative rest and core stabilization exercises.

Upper Limb Injuries

Upper limb injuries include shoulder and elbow injuries. **Rotator cuff tendinopathy** and **tears** can also occur in racquetball due to repetitive overhead maneuvers.[6] Tears occur most commonly in the supraspinatus tendon due to poor blood supply, and its anatomical location below the acromion. Individuals with curved or hooked acromions are more likely to develop tears. Rotator cuff tears commonly present as pain, clicking, or catching with overhead motion. Conservative treatment is divided into an acute phase focused on reducing symptoms, a recovery phase focused on improving scapular stabilizers and improving range of motion, and a functional phase designed to improve strength and perform activity-specific movements. Surgical intervention is warranted for full or partial thickness tears that fail conservative treatment. Patients with tendinopathy not responding to physiotherapy may benefit from a subdeltoid/subacromial bursa steroid injection or a regenerative intervention with an orthobiologics. *Lateral epicondylopathy* is an injury caused by repetitive wrist extension and forearm supination. It occurs when poor mechanics cause an overloading of the extensor and supinator tendons. In addition to poor technique, inappropriate sting tension and grip size can also lead to lateral epicondylalgia. Symptoms include tenderness just below the lateral epicondyle at the extensor tendon origin, and weakened grip strength. Treatment is most often conservative, but can also include regenerative intervention with or without an orthobiologic injection, percutaneous tenotomy, or surgical debridement of the extensor carpi radialis brevis.

Lower Limb Injuries

Lower limb injuries include acute knee and ankle injuries. *Medial meniscal tears* usually occur with cutting maneuvers which cause tibial rotation to occur when the knee is partially flexed with weight-bearing. Meniscal tears may be associated with a pop that occurs during the inciting incident. Locking of the knee may occur after the injury, and effusions may occur in the first 24 hours after the injury. Players will often complain of knee stiffness after a meniscal tear. Treatment for meniscal tears varies depending on the type of tear and symptoms, but generally physiotherapy is recommended to optimize knee function along with pain control interventions like oral NSAIDs, physical modalities, or intraarticular steroid injections. Some patients will benefit from an early surgical intervention, especially young athletes in which the meniscus can be repaired. *Ankle sprains* occur most often due to inversion of a plantar-flexed foot, which then results in ligamentous injury. Ankle sprains are categorized as either a grade I, II, or III. A grade I sprain is a partial tear of the anterior talofibular ligament (ATFL). A grade II tear is a complete tear of the ATFL and a partial tear of the calcaneofibular ligament (CFL). A grade III tear is a complete tear of the ATFL and CFL. Grades I and II sprains are treated conservatively, whereas grade III sprains can be treated either conservatively or surgically.

Other Injuries

Hematomas and *contusions* are common soft tissue injuries in racquetball due to contact with a ball moving with high velocity, contact between players, or contact with the court wall. Presenting symptoms include a focal area of tenderness and swelling. Treatment is management with nonsteroidal anti-inflammatory drugs (NSAIDs) and icing. Players can return to play when they are no longer symptomatic.

■ SUMMARY

Racquetball is a fast-paced sport that requires technical skill, can improve aerobic and anaerobic fitness, and can be played at both the recreational and elite level. In order to minimize the risk of injury, racquetball should be played with protective eyewear, a properly fitted racquet, and appropriate footwear.

■ References

1. Litsky F. Joseph Sobek, the inventor of racquetball, dies at 79. https://www.nytimes.com/1998/03/31/sports/joseph-sobek-the-inventor-of-racquetball-dies-at-79.html. Published March 31, 1998.

2. Everything about racquetball (101): in's & out. https://racquetsworld.com/what-is-racquetball.

3. Lock S. Participants in racquetball in the U.S. from 2006 to 2017 (in milions). https://www.statista.com/statistics/191922/participants-in-racquetball-in-the-us-since-2006/. Published July 2018.

4. Nah DT, Klyce W, Lee RJ. Epidemiological patterns of alternative racquet-sport injuries in the United States, 1997-2016. *Orthop J Sports Med*. 2018;6(7):2325967118786237. doi:10.1177/2325967118786237.

5. MacEwen CJ, Jones NP. Eye injuries in racquet sports. *Br Med J*. 1991;302(6790):1415-1416. doi:10.1136/bmj.302.6790.1415.

6. Ingber RS. Shoulder impingement in tennis/racquetball players treated with subscapularis myofascial treatments. *Arch Phys Med Rehabil*. 2000;81(5):679-682. doi:10.1016/s0003-9993(00)90053-4.

Erik S. Brand and Ashwin L. Rao

■ HISTORY

The sport of rowing dates to ancient Egyptian times and remains a popular competitive sport at the amateur, Olympic, masters, junior, para, and intercollegiate levels. Rowing is the second oldest intercollegiate sport in the world and the oldest in the United States, where women's rowing gained popularity with the Title IX act (1972), Olympic inclusion (1976), and National Collegiate Athletic Association (NCAA) status (1997), subsequently increasing in participants by 105% through 2018.[1] Collegiate now offers more scholarships per school than any sport other than football. This coincided with popularity of junior, para (formerly called "adaptive"), and masters rowing.[2]

■ GOVERNING ORGANIZATIONS

- International: Fédération Internationale des Sociétés d'Aviron (FISA)
- Collegiate women: National Collegiate Athletic Association (NCAA)
- National, collegiate men, junior, para, masters: United States Rowing Association USRowing)

■ PARTICIPANTS

Greater than 75,000 individuals belong to USRowing, including junior through masters levels.[2]

■ RULES AND REGULATIONS

In the United States, racing events are uniformly referred to as "regattas". Sprints are typically side by side, most commonly in multiple lanes but sometimes in 1:1 match racing format. Bumps and head races are typically rowed in succession, bow to stern. The largest standard boats have eight rowers and one coxswain, a person who steers the boat and coordinates rowing. Over time, blades have evolved with more efficient loading profiles using bigger blades, vortex edges, and other design features that re-duce slip of the blade through the water, have a stiffer feel, heavier load in the first one-third of the drive, and convert more athlete power into boat speed. This has required adjustment of rowing technique and training in order to avoid injury with heavier loads (Figure 45.1). Five kilometer head races typically take place in the fall and last approximately 17 to 23 minutes. Two kilometer Olympic distance sprint races take place in the spring and summer and last approximately 5.5 to 7.5 minutes. Adaptive, junior, and masters rowers often sprint 2,000, 1,500 and 1,000 m, respectively. Less com-mon formats include dash (which can be 500 m), bumps (multiday racing, attempting to make contact with crew ahead), marathon/ultramarathon (sometimes 160,000 to 185,000 m) and stake races (rowing to an object and back, requiring a 180° turn).

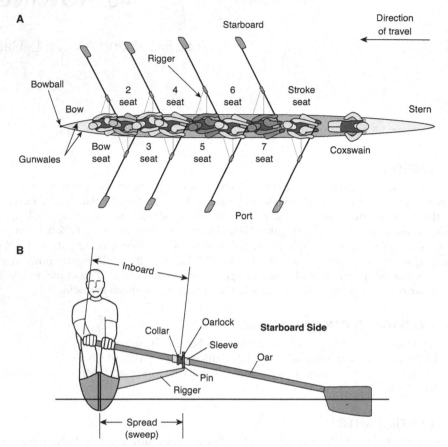

Figure 45.1 "Hatchet" style big blade oar.
Source: Reprinted with permission of (A) Niagara Rowing School and (B) Concept 2, Inc.

■ EQUIPMENT

*A **personal flotation device (PFD)*** is generally not worn by rowers. Rowing shells in the United States have a PFD exemption on waters deemed "navigable" by the U.S. Coast Guard. All other waters in the United States are under state jurisdiction including age requirements for children. Regulations for usage vary by country, state, role, and venue. Crew members should pass a physical examination by their physician, and a swim test, and may still be advised to have a PFD in some cases (e.g., unsupervised single sculling, along with cell phone in a waterproof bag). Various options include PFDs compatible with wearing versus stowing, and those activated manually versus hydrostatically. Review the USRowing safety video, safety expectations webpage, and venue rules for further details. A rubber ball or ***bow ball*** covers the sharp bow for safety. Safety rules typically require each shoe heel be attached to the stretcher (footplate) or ***heel ties***, commonly via a shoe string or something similar so rowers can pull their feet out of the shoes in case of a capsize (more common in small boats). Twelve-inch zip-ties may suffice temporarily if extra shoe laces and so forth are unavailable.

>>> Adaptive Sport Key Points: Para-Rowing Classifcation

1) PR3 (previously LTA - Legs, Trunks, Arms): Physical, visual, and intellectual impairments.
2) PR2 (previously TA - Trunk and Arms): Fixed seat. Physical impairment of legs.
3) PR1 (previously AS - Arms and Shoulders): Fixed seat. Pontoons attached to riggers.

FISA/International classification differs. Contact event Organizing Committee in advance to clarify.[2]

▪ MEDICAL COVERAGE LOGISTICS

Prior to the regatta, check the medical equipment and establish the roles of medical and support personnel in a coordinated Emergency Action Plan (EAP). Some regattas will have an ambulance with Emergency Medical Technician (EMT) personnel on-site, while others will be on-call in case of emergency. Each launch should have a map of closest ambulance access points, including docks. The medical team should practice water extraction, spine-boarding, and cardiopulmonary resuscitation (CPR) both on the water and at the dock. Time-sensitive emergency equipment such as automated external defibrillators (AEDs) should ideally be placed on every launch for ready access in the event of a sudden cardiac arrest. Team coaching and athletic personnel should take note of the nearest hospital, preferably with trauma center. Ensure that launch radios and PFDs meet venue standards. In addition to USRowing safety video and other resources, Water Emergency Training should be reviewed regularly (www.wateremergencytraining.com; www.youtube.com/playlist?list=PLHPE5cfv3zbtaAp4cjk-shFkzjRvTz2b0). On the day of regatta, providers should arrive early enough to engage with coaches, umpires, and staff, confirm access and utility of emergency medical equipment, and confirm communication lines. The equipment should be set up at a medical tent near the dock. The umpire should notify the head medical provider if an injured rower needs to be evaluated on the water.

▪ MEDICAL EMERGENCIES AND MEDICAL BAG ESSENTIALS

The collapsed or unconscious athlete is a medical emergency and proper channels (emergency medical services [EMS], CPR) should be activated. Nontraumatic deaths can be due to hypertrophic cardiomyopathy, cardiac arrhythmias, asthma, heat stroke, hypothermia, and drowning.[3] Traumatic injuries can occur during athlete ejection from the boat (called "catching a crab," when the oar gets stuck in the water, sometimes levering the rower from the seat), capsize, collisions (with boats, buoys, docks, etc.) and may include lacerations from the oar and other equipment.

▪ EPIDEMIOLOGY

Rowing is a nonimpact sport with a low incidence of injuries (1.75 and 2.01 injuries per 1,000 training sessions in senior, international, and junior rowers, respectively). Repetitive stress injuries are 2.63 times more likely than acute traumatic events in senior internationals, for whom the low back, knee, and chest/thoracic spine are the most commonly injured areas (though most injuries do not result in loss of time in training or competition). While acute traumatic injuries are less common, the highest incidence of this type of injury in senior internationals occurs on the water, whereas for juniors, the highest incidence of acute injuries arises during cross-training. Overuse injuries are mostly secondary to biomechanical alterations. Rowers sit, facing

Medical Bag Essentials in Rowing	
Medical Emergencies:	**Wound/Laceration/Skin Care:**
AED	Normal saline
Nitroglycerin (sublingual)	Betadine swabs
Aspirin	Neosporin, mupirocin ointment
Cricothyrotomy kit	Moleskin
14- and 16-G needles	Elastic bandage
Epi 1:1,000	Tube stretch gauze
Diphenhydramine or another antihistamine	Sterile gauzes
Albuterol inhaler	Vaseline
Rectal thermometer	Steri-strips
Ice baths	Suture tray
Strap to extricate an unconscious rower from a shell onto a launch and/or dock	Lidocaine 1%
	Others:
Head and Spine:	Acetaminophen
Stretcher & Spine board	Glucose tabs
Cervical orthosis	Waterproof SPF 50 sunscreen
Fractures and Dislocations:	12-in. zip ties
Immobilizers and Slings	
Crutches	

backward, on a rolling seat in tracks/slides. Sweep rowers pull one oar, whereas scullers pull two. Most work is done with the legs in a motion that resembles the power clean (weight-training maneuver) and has two basic phases. During the drive phase, from the crouched "catch" position (with oar in the water), the rower fires the legs, back, then arms, bringing the oar to the chest to propel the boat. Kicking with the feet first (as opposed to pulling with the arms) utilizes the trampoline effect (bending the oar to store and release kinetic energy, similar to a pole vault, flinging the boat forward). During the recovery phase (with oar out of the water), the rower crouches into the catch position again.[4-6]

■ COMMON INJURIES

Illnesses and Dermatologic Injuries

Rowing related illnesses include *relative energy deficiency in sport (RED-S)* which is an energy imbalance impairing metabolic, endocrine, immunological, cardiovascular, gastrointestinal, hematological, and psychological function, growth, and development. Endurance and weight-category athletes are at particular risk. A multidisciplinary approach for risk screening and addressing energy balance is required.[7] High-level rowers require 150% of sedentary caloric intake. Infection control may include influenza vaccination, nutritional consultation, and equipment cleaning. Soft tissue injuries include *calluses* on the hands (from feathering [twisting] oar), buttocks, and calves ("slide bites"). Treatment involves wound care and equipment cleaning. Prevention includes long socks, calf protectors, shorter slides, and seat cushions.

Head and Spine Injuries

Head injuries are uncommon, but *spine injuries*, especially the lower back, are the most common site of injury.[8-10] *Low back pain* can be secondary to *disk herniation* or *sponsylolysis.* A disk herniation may be predisposed by repetitive sheer, compressive, side-bending, rotational forces leading to back pain/tenderness and/or shooting pain to buttock/leg with nerve root numbness/weakness, worse with lumbar flexion. Management includes neuromuscular examination (including slump test), ruling out surgical indications and red flags, followed by relative rest, activity modification, possible medications, multidisciplinary rehabilitation including hip strengthening and mobility, symptom-limited return to rowing. X-rays and MRI are most cost effective if nonspecific low back pain is greater than 6 weeks or red flags (also useful if diagnosis is unclear and likely to change management/guide injection or surgery). Risk factors include age of less than 16 years, larger blades, free weights, erging more than 30 minutes, changing sides, weather (cross-wind, low temperature), heavy load (new line-ups, rowing with partial line-ups, ergometer damper setting greater than four, wing riggers), sitting more than 10 minutes. There is decreased incidence with stretching 10 minutes postworkout and self-care (warm-up/active stretching, foam rolling, sleep, nutrition, coach–athlete communication). Activity modification includes decreasing load (increasing rigger spread, oar inboard, stroke rate, decreasing ergometer fan setting, blade size, oar length/diameter), good technique (rowing "feet-out," on mobile head ergometer/sliders, modifying emphasis on legs/back/arms, biofeedback with tape, straws, mirrors, video, force curve analysis, etc.). **Spondylolysis** is most commonly a fatigue fracture of the fifth lumbar vertebrae pars interarticularis with overuse (including flexion and sheer) but especially the asymmetrical extension-rotation of the sweep rowing layback motion, predisposed by poor core stability/overtraining. Neuromuscular examination rules out other etiologies and most commonly finds pain with extension although unreliable in diagnosis of spondylolysis. The athlete should be removed from participation and advised to rest for 1 to 2 weeks. Nonsteroidal anti-inflammatory drugs (NSAIDs) and acetaminophen may decrease bone healing and pain biofeedback. Bracing is controversial. If persistent more than a few weeks, initial imaging is standing anteroposterior (AP)/lateral x-rays to identify gross bony abnormality/spondylolisthesis. Unusual or refractory cases should use MRI (pars protocol) in early diagnosis and CT (focused) if persistent.[10] Acute fracture requires 3 months of rest for bony union before 2 to 4 months of rehabilitation (though there is little correlation between bone healing and outcome). Alternatively, chronic fracture or stress reactions may begin rehabilitation once pain-free at rest. Return to sport once essentially normal in controlled environment (full, painless range of motion [ROM], conditioning, and sport-specific skill), is typically 5 to 7 months after diagnosis. Follow-up standing lateral radiographs are necessary if bilateral pars defects (or unilateral in a very young athlete) for symptomless slip progression. Prevention involves core stability and sufficient recovery. The *chest/thoracic* area is the third most common injury location in senior international rowers.[6] *Rib stress injury (RSI)* (commonly 5–9, possibly any rib) is due to mismatch of breakdown/repair, training load or change, RED-S, prior RSI, kinetic chain injury, poor trunk conditioning/mobility, possibly calcium/vitamin D deficiency. It is aggravated by deep breathing, pushing/pulling, sleeping on rib/compression/rolling over/initiating sit-up, coughing/sneezing. Differential diagnosis include costochondritis, costovertebral subluxation, and intercostal muscle strain. Early investigations with x-rays are often normal. Musculoskeletal ultrasound may have a role in early detection. It requires relative rest until resolution (likely 3–6 weeks), with pain-limited cross-training, possible taping, soft tissue work, ultrasound/laser, NSAID avoidance, optimizing biomechanics, risk factors, and gradual load reintroduction. Bone scan/MRI is required if diagnosis is unclear.[11]

Upper Limb Injuries

Upper limb injuries affect mostly the shoulders. Shoulder pain can be caused by positioning (anterior-placed humeral head, especially in protracted, flexed, adducted outside shoulder of sweep rowers at the catch), posture (thoracic kyphosis), tightness (neck, chest, posterior capsule, latissimus dorsi), generalized laxity, technique (over-reaching at the catch, then engaging upper trapezius instead of middle/lower trapezius and latissimus dorsi) and weakness (rotator cuff and scapular stabilizers). Symptoms include those of *impingement, instability, tendinopathy* or rarely *clavicular stress fracture*.[4] Management includes symptom-limited rowing, depending on severity, while assessing and reversing these issues. *Proximal intersection syndrome* is wrist extensor tenosynovitis/crepitus as first dorsal compartment crosses over second, about 4 cm proximal of Lister's tubercle with overuse, high stroke rate, intensity, tight grip, poor form, fatigue, and cold weather of early spring. Management includes symptom-limited rowing, depending on severity, typically participating in 2 to 3 weeks of relative rest, relaxing grip, changing handle size, erging/avoiding feathering, anti-inflammatory foods, physical modalities, splinting/bracing/taping, and possible NSAIDs/steroid injection/surgery if refractory. Prevention includes keeping warm (long sleeves, fleece pogies).

Lower Limb Injuries

Lower limb injuries include overuse of hip and knee injuries. *Femoroacetabular impingement (FAI)* is caused by cam, pincer or mixed bony overgrowth which may lead to labral/articular cartilage pathology, typically symptomatic in young, active individuals with repetitive deep squatting/twisting, resulting in diminished flexion (rowing catch position)/internal rotation, and pain commonly in the groin/lateral pelvis, possibly positive flexion, adduction, internal rotation (FADIR), scour maneuver, C-sign and other tests for internal hip pathology. Initial management may include pain-limited activity, anti-inflammatory foods (and/or medications with caution), hip strengthening and rigging adjustments to minimize repetitive uncontrolled impingement (seat cushion to diminish posterior chain pain inhibition, raising stretchers, shortening slides, orthotics to diminish foot over pronation, along with technique work). Diagnosis is commonly made by x-rays (e.g., weight-bearing AP, frog lateral and modified Dunn views), MRI (+/– arthrogram including ropivacaine, with caution due to chondrotoxicity). Refractory cases may benefit from injections and/or surgery. The knee is the second most common injury location in senior international rowers.[6] *Distal iliotibial band (ITB) friction syndrome* is pain where bowstringing lateral femoral condyle (30 degrees knee flexion), with positive Ober test, weak gluteus medius, overused tensor fascia lata, pelvic malalignment, shorter leg, foot over supination, tibial internal rotation, knee varus cause inflammation around ITB, adjacent fat. Management includes pain-limited rowing with hip strengthening, orthotics/lifts, shortening slides to allow knee extension, stretching calves/lowering shoes/balancing with oar (not knee) to avoid knee circumduction while crouching into the catch position, possible ice, heating ultrasound, and anti-inflammatory foods (and/or medications with caution). Steroid injection may risk fat atrophy. *Patellofemoral pain syndrome* can be caused by joint loading/deep flexion, patella lateral tracking, pelvic malalignment, leg length discrepancy, foot over pronation, tibial external rotation, knee valgus or hyperextension, femoral anteversion. Symptoms may include pain with stairs, theater sign, and possibly clicking while rowing. Examination may reveal edema, crepitus, tenderness of lateral patellar facet, tight quadriceps, and hip flexors. Management includes pain-limited rowing with hip/posterior chain engagement (strengthening, seat cushions to decrease pain inhibition), biofeedback (tape, straws, video/mirrors), slide/stretcher adjustment (limit knee flexion compressive forces; allow full extension engagement of vastus medialis oblique) and shoe adjustment (orthotics, in- or out-toeing).

■ SUMMARY

Rowing is a popular, inclusive, nonimpact, noncontact sport. The repetitive motions most commonly lead to overuse injuries in low back and knees but also the ribs, pelvis, wrist, and shoulder. The majority of injuries can be treated and minimized through good rowing technique and systematic activity progression.

■ References

1. Irick E. *NCAA Sports Sponsorship and Participation Rates Report.* Indianapolis, IN: National Collegiate Athletic Association; 2018:213-214.

2. http://www.usrowing.org.

3. Herring SA, Kibler W, Putukian M. Sideline preparedness for the team physician: a consensus statement-2012 update. *Med Sci Sports Exerc.* 2012;44(12):2442-2445. doi:10.1249/MSS.0b013e318275044f.

4. Thornton JS, Anders V, Wilson F, et al. Rowing injuries: an updated review. *Sports Med.* 2017;47(4):641-661. doi:10.1007/s40279-016-0613-y.

5. Hosea TM, Hannafin, JA. Rowing injuries. *Sports Health.* 2012;4(3): 236-245. doi:10.1177/1941738112442484.

6. Smoljanovic T, Bohacek I, Hannafin JA, et al. Acute and chronic injuries among senior international rowers: a cross-sectional study. *Int Orthop.* 2015;39(8):1623-1630. doi:10.1007/s00264-014-2665-7.

7. Mountjoy M, Sundgot-Borgen JK, Burke LM, et al. IOC consensus statement on relative energy deficiency in sport (RED-S): 2018 update. *Br J Sports Med.* 2018;52:687-697. doi:10.1136/bjsports-2018-099193.

8. Teitz CC, O'Kane J, Lind BK, Hannafin JA. Back pain in intercollegiate rowers. *Am J Sports Med.* 2002;30(5):674-679. doi:10.1177/03635465020300050701.

9. Tofte JN, CarlLee TL, Holte AJ, et al. Imaging pediatric spondylolysis: a systematic review. *Spine (Phila Pa 1976).* 2017;42(10):777-782. doi:10.1097/BRS.0000000000001912.

10. Standaert CJ, Herring SA. Expert opinion and controversies in sports and musculoskeletal medicine: the diagnosis and treatment of spondylolysis in adolescent athletes. *Arch Phys Med Rehabil.* 2007;88(4):537-540. doi:10.1016/j.apmr.2007.01.007.

11. Evans G, Redgrave A. Great Britain Rowing Team guideline for diagnosis and management of rib stress injury: part 1. *Br J Sports Med.* 2016;50:266-269. doi:10.1136/bjsports-2015-095126.

46. SAILING

Joanne B. "Anne" Allen

▨ HISTORY

The first sailboats date back to Phoenician times where they were used for fishing, trade, and travel. The sport of yacht racing did not begin formally until 1851, when the first America's Cup was held with schooner yachts for the oldest continuously contested trophy in the world. Over the years, the sport gained popularity not only in large yachts but also in smaller dinghies at the collegiate and Olympic level. And more recently, sailboat racing now includes high-speed foiling boats with increasing risk and technical challenges.

▨ GOVERNING ORGANIZATIONS

- International: World Sailing, formerly International Sailing Federation (ISAF) or International Yacht Racing Union (IYRU) (originally formed in 1904)
- National: US Sailing
- Major professional leagues (organizations): America's Cup, Around the World Race, Match Race, League Sailing
- University/College: Inter-Collegiate Sailing Association (ICSA)
- High School: Interscholastic Sailing Association (ISSA)

▨ PARTICIPANTS

U.S. sailing has an estimated membership of 46,000 sailors/racers aged 6 to 96, and approximately 1,700 yacht clubs and local sailing organizations participating at a variety of levels/skills in local, national, and international regattas. There are about 350 high school teams in the United States, and approximately 200 varsity and club college teams in seven conferences across the United States and Canada. In addition to the countless amateur sailors who are competing, there are professionals who race in World Match Racing Tour, compete in the prestigious America's Cup, race around the world in The Ocean Race or The Around Alone, or compete regularly on high-profile offshore teams.

▨ RULES AND REGULATIONS

The sport of sailing is governed by the World Sailing (or US Sailing) Racing Rules of Sailing and national prescriptions. Sailboat racing covers a wide spectrum of event types, from **inshore dinghy racing** and **offshore distance racing** to **global circumnavigations**, as well as including **windsurfing** and **kitesurfing**. Competition can be either "fleet" racing among many boats (Figure 46.1), or "match" racing involving a one-on-one contest, or "team" racing (several boats on each team racing against each other), and usually involves racing around "marks" (often buoys) on a designated course on the water. The races or "regatta" (a series of races) are run by a "race committee" and are often overseen by judges or umpires. However, sailing is considered a Corinthian sport, and is for the most part "self-governed," where sailors are required to absolve themselves of a rule infraction on the water by voluntarily taking a penalty.

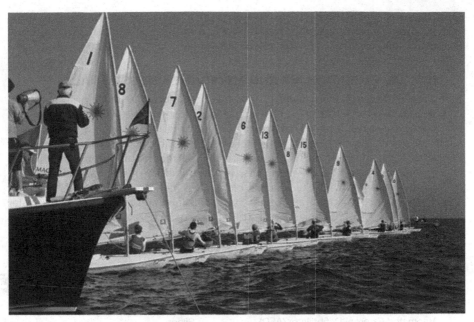

Figure 46.1 Fleet racing.

▨ EQUIPMENT

Competitions vary with specific *sailboat* types and include *Olympic classes, center-board, keelboat, multihull, yacht, boards,* and *radio-controlled sailboats.* The gear varies with weather and event conditions and may include anything from *swimsuits* to *foul-weather gear,* and often includes *water shoes, protective gloves, sun protection,* and *a cap* or *helmet. Lifejackets* are an essential part of sailboat-racing safety and are usually required to at least be in the boat, if not worn, depending on the vessel type being sailed. In the United States, they should be Coast Guard approved to be in compliance with legal requirements.

> **》》 Adaptive Sport Key Points: Paralympic Sailing**
>
> Sailing is one of the most inclusive sports in the world as boats are easily adapted for participation by sailors of all abilities. Depending on the type of boat, both able-bodied and disabled sailors can compete equally on the same playing field. Sailing became a Paralympic sport in 1996, allowing participants of all types of disabilities to race competitively on a national and international stage. Sailors are classified based on physical or visual impairments, as well as how their disability impacts their functionality while sailing. Sailboat adaptive equipment includes different types of seating systems, helm or crew adaptations, audible signaling, and stabilization devices.

▨ MEDICAL COVERAGE LOGISTICS

As the water is your "sideline," adaptations to typical medical coverage logistics often have to be made and coverage for competition should be based on each individual event, venue, and local conditions. Medical issues can occur both on the water while racing or on shore, before or after racing. Preparation for water rescue with trained rescue personnel and equipment is necessary due to the risk of falling overboard, drowning, and traumatic injury. In general, a coordinated medical and safety team, and a comprehensive emergency action plan that includes a designated access point for first responders in case of water rescue is essential.

■ MEDICAL EMERGENCIES AND MEDICAL BAG ESSENTIALS

Environmental conditions usually play a significant factor in the types of medical emergencies that can occur in the sport of sailing. Most fatalities in sailing are related to drowning as a result of falls overboard or capsizing the vessel and usually occur when the victim is not wearing a life jacket. High winds, rough seas, and operator inexperience can also be a factor in traumatic injuries that require prompt medical attention. Fractures due to sudden impacts, and amputations of fingers/limbs may occur and involve equipment like winches, blocks, and high load lines. Head, neck, and spinal cord injuries can occur and proper immobilization and removal from the water is essential. Newer foiling boats racing at high speeds may reveal a possible increase in injury rates in these classes. Other medical emergencies including cardiac arrest, hypo-/hyperthermia, seizures, and aquatic sea–life-related incidences can also occur.

Medical Bag Essentials in Sailing	
Medical Emergencies:	**Fractures and Dislocations:**
Automated External Defibrillator (AED)	Slings
Albuterol inhaler with spacer	Knee immobilizer
Epinephrine pen	**Wound Care:**
Diphenhydramine	Gauze
Pulse oximeter	Suture tray
Oxygen tank	Steri-strips
IV fluids	Lidocaine 1%
Heat blankets	Sterile saline
Ice Baths	Tegaderm
Glucometer with test strips and lancets	Betadine swabs
Thermometer	Spray disinfectant
Head and Spine:	Alcohol swabs
Concussion evaluation form	Saline eye rinse
Stretcher & Spine board	Contact lens solution
Cervical orthosis	

■ EPIDEMIOLOGY

Sailors are at risk for overuse injuries, acute injuries, and environmental illnesses from a variety of causes. The physical demands of sailing vary greatly depending on: the type of vessel and race; the crew member's position on the boat; and the wind and water conditions. Sailing-related injury rates are relatively low compared to other land-based sports. The most common injuries are contusions and lacerations due to falls or impacts from various boat parts, and repetitive overuse injuries most commonly seen in the lumbar spine, knees, and shoulders. Environmental illness also can play a factor in the sport including sun exposure, motion sickness, hypothermia and hyperthermia, and immersion injuries/drowning. Also, awareness of concussions in the sport of sailing has been increasing and more sailors are noted to be using helmets during competition.

■ COMMON INJURIES

Head and Spine Injuries

Concussions in sailing usually occur from direct trauma from the boom or contact with another boat part due to a fall. Although helmets are not required in sailing, they are suggested in youth sailing and in high-speed racing and are being used more often in high school and college teams. The Sports Medicine Committee of US Sailing states that helmets should be considered and encouraged but not mandated for aggressive competitive sailing, crew positions at increased risk for strikes to the head, and sailors who are learning the sport and thus unfamiliar with the position and movement of rigging and equipment. Although traumatic spine injuries can occur in sailing, overuse cervical and lumbar spine issues are more common. *"Trimmers neck"* is a common cause of cervicalgia due to constantly looking up at an angle to trim the sails, and low back pain is often noted with lifting and hiking out to keep the boat flat. Lumbar hyperextension may predispose dinghy sailors to **low back pain**. Addressing ergonomics and treating these injuries conservatively is recommended.

Upper Limb Injuries

Shoulder pain is a very common musculoskeletal ailment in sailors, as is elbow pain, usually from an overuse injury. Whether from hoisting sails at the mast, grinding the sail on a winch, or trimming the sail from an angled position, **subacromial impingement** and **rotator cuff issues**, along with **elbow tendinopathies** can occur. Treatment must be aimed at strengthening the shoulder and scapula thoracic stabilizers, stretching, and addressing the biomechanics of the specific motion. Hand injuries that include **lacerations, finger dislocations, contusions** have been noted usually due to handling lines under tension and operating winches under heavy forces. Proper technique and equipment use along with wearing gloves may help prevent injuries. **Carpal tunnel syndrome** has also been noted with gripping of the helm for long periods of time.

Lower Limb Injuries

Knee pain is common in sailors, particularly in dinghy classes, where hiking is needed to maintain boat performance. Straight leg hiking places high loads on the knee extensor mechanism, and droop seat hiking places forces on the knee joint in a flexed position. Both static and dynamic loads can then contribute to knee pain in a sailor. Hip injuries can occur but are less commonly noted in studies. Treatment depends on the specifics of the injury, but often will include physical therapy (PT) and strengthening muscles around the knee and hip. *Lower limb contusions* and **lacerations** are also commonly seen, particularly on larger yachts that require mobility on a wet and angled boat deck. **Fractures** and **sprains/strains** can also occur, particularly as stronger winds and hazardous seas place higher forces on the boat and rigging.

■ SUMMARY

Sailing is a dynamic and physically demanding sport which is on an ever-changing playing field and requires a knowledge of both the sport and the environment. Understanding inherent risks and water safety, in addition to common injuries and treatment, is important for the Sports Medicine team.

▓ Further Reading

Nathanson A. Sailing injuries: a review of the literature. *R I Med J.* 2019;102(1):23-27. http://www.rimed.org/rimedicaljournal/2019/02/2019-02-23-wilderness-nathanson.pdf.

Neville V, Folland JP. The epidemiology and aetiology of injuries in sailing. *Sports Med.* 2009;39(2):129-145. doi:10.2165/00007256-200939020-00003.

Tan B, Leong D, Vaz Pardal C, et al. Injury and illness surveillance at the International Sailing Federation Sailing World Championships 2014. *Br J Sports Med.* 2016;50:673-681. doi:10.1136/bjsports-2015-095748.

Iris X. Tian

HISTORY

Shooting originated in European countries and dates back to more than 500 years within German shooting clubs. It has been a mainstay of the Summer Olympic Games since the inaugural year of 1896 in Athens as one of nine events through the efforts of the French pistol champion, Pierre de Coubertin. It began with five shooting events to fifteen to date. The sport itself has grown significantly due to the advancement of firearms technology.[1]

GOVERNING ORGANIZATIONS

- International: International Shooting Sports Federation (ISSF)
- National: USA Shooting
- Major professional leagues: National Rifle Association (NRA)
- College: Nation Junior Team, College Rifle Clubs but no official associations
- High School: Youth Olympic Games (ages 15–18) but no official association

PARTICIPANTS

Two-hundred and ninety athletes competed in 15 shooting disciplines in the 2004, 2008, 2012, and 2016 Olympic Summer Games.[1]

RULES AND REGULATIONS

There is a total of 15 events in Olympic Shooting that are divided into three groups: Rifle, Pistol, and Shotgun with five events in each category. There are six men events, six women events, and three mixed team events. Each event consists of a qualification phase followed by a final phase. The rifle and pistol competitions are held on shooting ranges with targets at different distances whereas shotgun competitions involve clay targets propelled at a series of different directions and angles.[1]

EQUIPMENT

Firearms include rifle, pistol, or shotgun with variable calibers. *Shooting glasses* are made of plastic or polycarbonate with high standards to protect against high-impact/ballistic resistance. They come in a variety of colors for different indoor versus outdoor environments (yellow/amber for low light conditions, red for clay shooting, etc.) *Shooting earplugs/earmuffs*, passive or electronic, protect against hearing loss or tinnitus; the typical range for hearing protection is 15 to 35 decibels of sound attenuation or noise reduction rating (NRR). The higher the NRR, the more protection it provides. *Holsters/gun belt* are for comfort in carrying around pistols. *Gun-cleaning supplies* include cleaning rods, jag/loop, cotton patches, brushes, cleaning fluids. *Recoil shoulder pads* help decrease the impact of recoil or "kickback" onto the glenohumeral joint upon firing of firearms.

Adaptive Sport Key Points: Para Shooting

Para Sport has featured at every Paralympic Games since 1976. Athletes with physical impairments compete in rifle, pistol, and trap events. Of the 13 Paralympic shooting events, seven are open to both women and men, three are open to women only and three are open to men only. World Shooting Para Sport recently adopted the discipline of Para trap and vision-impaired (VI) shooting. The sport is governed by the International Paralympic Committee (IPC) in coordination with the World Shooting Para Sport Technical Committee and Management team. The sport follows rules of the ISSF in conjunction with its own World Shooting Para Sport Technical Rules and Regulations, which take into account considerations for Para athletes in shooting sport.[2]

 Biathlon: Cross-Country Skiing and Shooting

This is an endurance sport included as part of the Winter Olympics involving mid-distance cross-country skiing for 5 km and intermittent rifle shooting which involves shooting five targets at 50 m with five shots. Special bore rifles (5.6 mm) with open sight and manual loading are used.[3]

■ MEDICAL COVERAGE LOGISTICS

It is recommended to arrive 1 hour prior to the start of the event to introduce yourself to the organizing staff, coaches, judges, and Emergency Medical Technician (EMT) personnel, check the available equipment especially the Automated External Defibrillator (AED), and review the emergency action plan (EAP) with the medical team as well as the rules for medical intervention for the event. Review the best route to the nearest hospital with trauma center capabilities that includes neurosurgery. At least two channels of communication (radio and cell phones) among the medical team and organizing personnel should be established. Lastly, documentation of medical encounters is essential for future planning.

■ MEDICAL EMERGENCIES AND MEDICAL BAG ESSENTIALS

Although rare, medical emergencies can occur in shooting. In the case of an accidental gunshot wound, the proper channels should be activated with access to a hospital nearby, preferably one with a trauma center. Also shoulder dislocations with possible neurovascular compromise merit emergent intervention. Nontraumatic emergencies include metabolic, cardiac, and respiratory causes such as arrhythmias, asthma, heat-related illness like heat stroke, hypoglycemia, and anaphylaxis.

Medical Bag Essentials in Shooting	
Medical Emergencies:	**Wound Care:**
AED	Normal saline
Tourniquet	Betadine swabs
Epi 1:1,000	Neosporin, mupirocin ointment
Diphenhydramine or another antihistamine	Elastic bandage
Albuterol inhaler	Sterile gauzes
Glucose tabs	Steri-strips
	Suture tray
	Lidocaine 1%

▒ EPIDEMIOLOGY

Shooting was considered one of the lowest relative injury risk sports in the Summer Olympics London in 2012.[4] Most injuries occur during training secondary to overuse. Common injuries during training include shoulder dislocation, muscle strain and tears, tendinopathy, and impingement syndrome whereas ligament sprains and tears, herniated discs, and paravertebral muscle spasms are the most common injury types during competition. The shoulder and calf/thigh are the most common body parts injured during training while foot/ankle, hand/wrist, and low back are most commonly injured during competition.[5] Long training periods, placing heavy loads onto the body from the weight of the firearm, frequent flexing at the trunk/hip, staying in static shooting positions for prolonged periods, and maintaining rigid posture positions all contribute to the injury. Women are more prone to wrist and shoulder injuries due to joint laxity and commonly less upper body strength and muscle mass when compared to men. These common injuries in shooting may be prevented through an emphasis on muscle strengthening, stretching, and proprioception exercises involving the most commonly injured regions of the body (shoulder → hand/wrist →foot/ankle → calf/thigh) as part of the athletic training program. Athletes must make a conscious effort to protect their eyesight and hearing by wearing the proper protective gear.

▒ COMMON INJURIES

Head and Spine Injuries

Neck strain may result when shooting in a prone position due to the static, prolonged period that the athlete has to stay with the neck in hyperextension. Once the event is over, heat/ice, gentle range of motion (ROM) exercises, stretches, manual massage, and nonsteroidal anti-inflammatory drugs (NSAIDs) may help relieve the pain and stiffness. **Myofascial pain** with trigger points and **headaches** may result from repetitive stress on the cervical paraspinals and trapezius. Symptoms include stiffness, pain, tenderness to palpation, and decreased range of motion. Management includes range of motion exercises, massage, heat/ice, TENS (transcutaneous electrical nerve stimulation) unit, physical therapy, acupuncture, and trigger point injections. **Low back strain** and **paravertebral muscle spasms** are all common as a result of excessive loading onto the spine when shooting in a standing position while holding a rifle or shotgun. The rotational shooting position makes athletes more prone to low back injuries especially in rifle shooters. Hyperextension or hyperflexion of the hips may also lead to low back pain as these are all part of the kinetic chain. **Herniated discs** may occur due to excessive trunk flexion while holding a heavy firearm for a prolonged period which increases the pressure placed on the intervertebral discs. The rotational standing shooting position significantly increases the disc pressure in rifle shooters. Lumbar spine injuries can be prevented and managed with core strengthening, and kinetic chain training.

Upper Limb Injuries

Upper limb injuries are more common in women. **Shoulder impingement syndrome** that may evolve to **rotator cuff tendinopathy** and **tears** is the most common overuse injury in shooting due to repetitive motion sequences and maintenance of posture during shooting exercises. Furthermore, improper posture when holding a rifle or shotgun lower than normal may increase the risk of shoulder injuries. **Rotator cuff tears** are due to the repetitive recoil or "kickback" forces that result from shooting a rifle or a shotgun. The backward displacement of the firearm when discharged may lead to tendinopathies, predisposing the athlete to tears and instability of the shoulder girdle over time. Symptoms include weakness, decreased active range of motion, and pain in the shoulder joint. Management is conservative initially with pain control modalities, ROM and strengthening exercises, corticosteroid injections, or regenerative medicine interventions. In severe cases such as in complete tears, surgery may be recommended. **Shoulder contusions** result from direct repetitive forces placed onto the shoulder joint. Symptoms include pain and tenderness especially upon palpation. Management includes rest, ice, compression (wrap with bandage), elevation to reduce swelling, and NSAIDs to reduce inflammation. **Shoulder dislocations** may result due to a significant force to the glenohumeral joint. Anterior dislocation occurs in 95% of cases. Symptoms include severe pain with inability to move the arm and/or a notable bump in the shoulder. Immediate reduction to the shoulder should be performed to avoid neurovascular damage. Immobilization with a sling can be recommended for comfort for 1 to 7 days and gradually tapered off to avoid should stiffness, followed by an individualized physical therapy program focused on motion, stability, and strengthening exercises. **Elbow fractures** may result due to chronic traction placed on the triceps at its attachment points. Symptoms include pain at the elbow, weakness, and decreased range of motion. X-rays are recommended to confirm this diagnosis. Management includes rest, ice, sling/brace, and surgery for a displaced or nonunion fracture. **Hand/wrist sprain** results from prolonged maintenance of shooting positions requiring hand and wrist to be stable. Due to the copious amounts of ligaments located in the hand and wrist, it is important for athletes to participate in daily stretching, range of motion, and strengthening exercises for the hand and wrist. Symptoms include pain or tenderness to palpation over a specific joint and decreased range of motion. Management includes rest, ice, NSAIDs, temporary sling/brace for comfort, and occupational therapy. **Carpal tunnel syndrome** can occur due to overuse and increased inflammation to the flexor retinaculum which surrounds the median nerve. Symptoms include numbness/tingling or pain over the median nerve distribution and atrophy of thenar eminence (chronic). Management includes carpal tunnel brace to be worn at night or throughout the day for comfort, occupational therapy, acupuncture, corticosteroid injections, and for severe cases, carpal tunnel release surgery. **Stenosing tenosynovitis,** also known as **"trigger finger,"** may result due to repetitive movements of the index finger during shooting causing inflammation of the flexor tendons in the interphalangeal (IP) and metacarpophalangeal (MCP) joints. This narrows the space within the tendon sheath of the A1 pulley leading to tenderness at the joint, pain with finger movement, stiffness, and clicking or snapping with movement. Management includes rest, ice, occupational therapy, NSAIDs, acupuncture, corticosteroid injections, and, if conservative treatment fails, surgery.

Lower Limb Injuries

Lower limb injuries are mostly acute and mild. **Thigh/calf strains** involving the quadriceps and gastroc-soleus complex are commonly seen in shooting due to prolonged periods of kneeling and standing positions. Symptoms include stiffness and pain with movement/ambulation. Management includes rest, ice, NSAIDs, and educating athletes on proper stretching exercises for quadriceps, hamstrings, and calves before and after training or competition. **Quadriceps contusion** may result from the blunt trauma induced by heavy firearms particularly rifles and shotguns. Symptoms include pain and swelling at the site. Management includes ice and NSAIDs. **Skin abrasions** on the lower limbs may result from the heavy firearms scraping against the skin. If there is notable bleeding, wash with normal saline, place gauze over area, and secure with tape. **Foot/ankle sprains** may result from accidental loss of footing or when coming out of standing positions in active shooting after a prolonged period. Symptoms include pain at site, swelling, and pain with weight-bearing. Management includes rest, ice, NSAIDs, compression with bandage, and elevation of the foot.

■ SUMMARY

Although shooting is a low-impact, noncontact sport, it is important to be aware of the most common mechanisms of injuries, particularly overuse injuries. Understanding the different events, what is required in each, and the most common injuries is essential for sideline coverage.

■ References

1. The ISSF History. https://www.issf-sports.org. Accessed July 22, 2020

2. History of shooting para sport. https://www.paralympic.org/shooting/about.

3. Disch AC. Biathlon: acute trauma and overuse injuries. In: Doral M, Karlsson J, eds. *Sports Injuries.* 2nd ed. Berlin, Germany: Springer; 2015:2809-2815. doi:10.1007/978-3-642-36569-0_280.

4. Engebretsen L, Soligard T, Steffen K, et al. Sports injuries and illnesses during the London Summer Olympic Games 2012. *Br J Sports Med.* 2013;47(7):407-414. doi:10.1136/bjsports-2013-092380.

5. Kabak B, Karanfilci M, Ersöz T, Kabak M. Analysis of sports injuries related with shooting. *J Sports Med Phys Fitness.* 2016;56(6):737-743. https://www.minervamedica.it/en/journals/sports-med-physical-fitness/article.php?cod=R40Y2016N06A0737

Tina Bijlani

HISTORY

Speed skating initially began in the Netherlands, Scandinavia, and Northern Europe as early as the 13th century as a method of transportation across bodies of water. Initially people utilized skates made of bone or wood. The advent of metal and iron skates further popularized the activity. It soon became a form of competitive sport with the first known skating competition held in the Netherlands in 1676, as well as the first official speed-skating event in Oslo, Norway in 1863. The Netherlands hosted the first World Championships in 1889, bringing together Dutch, Russian, American, and English teams. In 1924, Speed skating appeared for the first time at the Olympic Winter Games in Chamonix with men being the only allowed participants. Later in the 1932 Olympics, women were allowed to participate as well. There are two different types of speed skating, long-track speed skating, otherwise known as "speed skating," and short-track speed skating or "short track." Short track speed skating became an Olympic event in 1992.[1]

GOVERNING ORGANIZATIONS
- International: International Skating Union (ISU)
- National: U.S. Speedskating, US Olympic Committee (USOC)

PARTICIPANTS

In this mixed-gender sport, the average age of competitive long track speed skaters is 20 to 24 years, while the average age of competitive short track speed skaters is 19 to 22 years. There are approximately 9,000 speed skaters worldwide.

RULES AND REGULATIONS

Short Track Speed Skating

Four to six racers race against each other per heat on a 111-m circuit with an internationally sized 30- by 60-m Olympic-sized ice hockey rink. The first two to finish the race are able to advance to the next heat. Body contact is prohibited, and they must skate outside the blocks. There is also a relay event in short track speed skating, consisting of four teams made up of four skaters. Skaters take turns being the lead skater and are pushed forward by the exiting skater. Only one athlete on each team may use the racing track while the others rest in the middle inside the blocks.

Long Track Speed Skating

Athletes are paired and compete in separate lanes on a 400-m oval track (Figure 48.1). They begin from a staggered lap and race in a counterclockwise direction. Athletes switch lanes during each lap at the backstretch of the oval with the outer lane racer

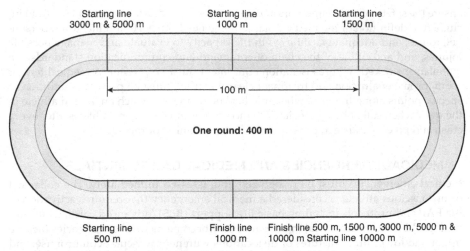

Figure 48.1 Long speed skating track with dimensions and layout.

having the right of way. Contact is not allowed in long track speed skating. In 2003, a new long track event called the "Team Pursuit" was added to the World Cup, World Championships, and the Olympic Games. Two teams consisting of three skaters each, simultaneously race against each other after beginning on opposite sides of the track. The last athlete to cross the finish line gives the team its official finish time.

▣ EQUIPMENT

Skaters should wear **skin suits** that protect them on the ice, allowing them to skate at high speeds. They are skin-tight and tailored to the individual's body shape. In short track speed skating, athletes' skin suits are required to have **kneepads, shin guards,** and **neck guards** to protect skaters from blades. In long track speed skating, **hood** is part of the skin suit with the purpose of reducing air resistance. A **hard-plastic helmet** to prevent potential head injury is required in short track speed skating. No helmet is required in long track speed skating, as a hood is a part of the body suit. **Glasses** are worn in long track speed skating to protect eyes from debris, ice chips, and to improve visibility. Skaters wear **boots with varying blades** 14 to 18 inches in length; "knap blade" in long track speed skating; fixed sharp blade skates with boots that lace high above the ankle in short track speed skating. Ceramic fingertip **gloves** in short track speed skating aid in skaters' ability to turn as well as protect hands from other blades.

> **》》》 Adaptive Sport Key Points: Speed Skating**
>
> Speed skating was first established in the Special Olympics in 1977. Skaters are required to take eight 1-hour training sessions in order to compete at state meets. Skaters with disability pair up with a partner and can take part in the Team Sprint in which both skate 500 m and 1,000 m. Times are combined into a team score. Skaters may also partake in the four-person relay. Ankle foot orthotic (AFO) ice skates and ice walkers are available.[2]

▣ MEDICAL COVERAGE LOGISTICS

The role of the race doctor is to organize and coordinate the medical staff, develop an emergency action plan (EAP), and interact with the race or event director to help ensure the safety of the competitors and spectators. Protocols and guidelines should include role definition of the medical staff, emergency transportation including personnel, routes, and adequate facilities with the capacity to evaluate and manage possible injuries, and an outline of the chain-of-command and communication standards. An ambulance stocked with resuscitation equipment must be present. A medical tent or room for fast evaluation and treatment clearly marked must be present in addition to specific points along the track where medical personnel can reach an injured athlete in the track when called by an official. The race doctor must examine athletes after every crash and give clearance to participate in further training or racing.

■ MEDICAL EMERGENCIES AND MEDICAL BAG ESSENTIALS

Medical emergencies must be recognized and assessed immediately. The collapsed or unconscious athlete is considered a medical emergency that requires activation of the EAP and protocols including basic life support (BLS)/advanced cardiac life support (ACLS). Musculoskeletal injuries that may become medical emergencies include upper and lower limb fractures or dislocations with neurovascular compromise, and traumatic brain injuries with or without spinal cord involvement. Arterial laceration from a skate blade is another potential emergency that requires immediate tourniquet proximal to the site of bleeding and pressure should be applied until Emergency Medical Services (EMS) arrives. Nontraumatic deaths can be due to hypertrophic cardiomyopathy, cardiac arrhythmias, anaphylaxis, and asthma.

Medical Bag Essentials in Speed Skating	
Medical Emergencies:	**Wound/Laceration/Skin Care:**
Automated External Defibrillator (AED)	Normal saline
Nitroglycerin (sublingual)	Betadine swabs
Aspirin	Neosporin, mupirocin ointment
Epi 1:1,000	Moleskin
Diphenhydramine or another antihistamine	Elastic bandage
Albuterol inhaler	Tube stretch gauze
Rectal thermometer	Sterile gauzes
Head and Spine:	Vaseline
	Steri-strips
Concussion evaluation form	Suture tray
Stretcher & Spine board	Lidocaine 1%
Cervical orthosis	Tourniquets
Fractures and Dislocations:	
Immobilizers and Slings	
Crutches	
Splints	

■ EPIDEMIOLOGY

Athletes race around an oval track at high velocities, making them susceptible to various injuries. Collisions are more likely to occur during short track speed skating, and thus more injuries are prevalent when compared to long track speed skating. During the 2010 Winter Olympics, 27.8% of male short track athletes sustained an injury, compared to less than 5% of long track athletes. The most common injuries sustained during on-ice competition include shoulder dislocation/separation (9%), groin strain (6.1%), concussions (6.1%), and knee contusions (6.1%). Meanwhile, the most common training injuries affect the lower limb, consisting of groin strains (22.2%), knee contusions (14.8%), and ankle sprains (12.1%).[3-5]

COMMON INJURIES

Head and Spine Injuries

Concussion is a possible injury in short track. Skaters sustain a blow to the head that results in neurologic symptoms, such as headache, confusion, dizziness, nausea, vomiting, and sometimes loss of consciousness. In speed skating, concussions may occur when athletes collide with one another or from falling on the hard ice surface. Athletes should be removed from the competition and evaluated with a full neurologic exam, in addition to the Sport Concussion Assessment Tool (SCAT). If patients become reinjured, they may suffer fatal conditions, such as cerebral hemorrhage and edema. Postconcussive syndrome is one of the more common and serious sequelae. A gradual return to sport is recommended after close follow up by a sports medicine physician in 24 to 48 hours. **Lumbar spine injuries** can be seen in speed skating, with the most common being **mechanical low back pain** of muscular etiology. Skaters may present with nonradicular low back pain, typically localized to the paraspinal region. Pain may also be caused by injury of bone, tendon, ligament, or fascia. Practitioners should inspect and palpate the spine, in addition to performing a neuromuscular exam. Conservative management is recommended, such as oral analgesics (nonsteroidal anti-inflammatory drugs [NSAIDs] or acetaminophen) or temporary activity modification. If pain is persistent, they may require to be taken out of the competition for further evaluation with imaging and treatment interventions like spine injections. When skaters make sudden movements with flexion of the spine, they may sustain acute disc herniation and nerve root compression, presenting with a **lumbosacral radiculopathy**. The spine is especially susceptible to disc herniation at the L4-L5 and L5-S1 levels. Symptoms include radiating low back pain, sensory loss, and/or weakness of the lower limbs. Examiners additionally may find a positive straight leg test. Athletes who present with acute radiculopathy and progressive neurologic deficits should be evaluated immediately with transfer to ED for neuroimaging (MRI, CT), possibly requiring surgical intervention such as discectomy or decompression. Sideline practitioners should be aware of red flag symptoms, including urinary retention, saddle anesthesia, or bilateral neurologic signs/symptoms, as these prompt emergent neurosurgical evaluation. In contrast, athletes without significant neurologic deficit may be treated conservatively. These make up the majority of cases.

Upper Limb Injuries

Glenohumeral dislocation is a common injury in speed skating. The mechanism of injury is caused by a blow to the abducted, externally rotated, and extended arm. It may also be caused by falling on an outstretched hand. Anterior dislocations are much more common than posterior. Symptoms include severe pain, swelling and bruising of the shoulder/arm, possible sensory deficits, and difficulty moving the arm. When patients present with shoulder dislocation, the primary consideration is pain control and reduction. The sideline physician should reduce the dislocation, immobilize the shoulder by placing it in a sling, and apply ice packs to the affected area. Skaters should not have anything to eat or drink in the event that they require sedation.

Lower Limb Injuries

Patellofemoral pain syndrome occurs with increased biomechanical stress of the patellofemoral joint. Weak hip abductors, external rotators, and vastus medialis can predispose an athlete to this condition. An overly rapid increase in training intensity and playing on the hard ice surface are two common risk factors for the development of patellofemoral pain syndrome in speed skaters. Symptoms include anterior knee pain, worse with knee flexion, as well as instability, clicking, swelling, and stiffness. The sideline physician should inspect for femoral anteversion, genu valgus, and foot pronation, and perform a full knee exam with special attention to the patella and patellar tendon. The step-down or single leg squat test can measure kinematic stability. Skaters should rest, apply ice, and take NSAIDs for pain control. Evaluation with an x-ray is recommended, though it is not emergent. They should be started on a physical therapy regimen and may return to speed skating once they are pain-free at rest and with activity. Patellar taping and bracing are useful adjuncts that may allow skaters to restart training regimens faster. **Patellar tendinopathy** is caused by microtears of the patellar tendon leading to a painful inflammatory condition. The mechanism of injury is due to repetitive stress on the quadriceps and patellar tendon. This is common in speed skaters due to quadriceps loading in the "crouched position." Symptoms include pain with activity and tenderness over the patellar tendon, in addition to the inferior or superior pole of the patella. Treatment is the same as for patellofemoral pain syndrome. **Peroneal tendinopathy** is specifically seen in short track speed skaters and is caused by repetitive motion. Mechanism of injury is due to chronic lateral instability and excessive subtalar rotation, as athletes must repeatedly dorsiflex and evert their feet when crossing over on tight short curves. Symptoms include pain, warmth, and swelling of the ankle along the course of the peroneal tendons. Diagnosis is aided with MRI and/or ultrasound. Management includes pain relief with anti-inflammatory medication, physical therapy, and sometimes a tendon sheath sono-guided steroid injection. **Achilles tendinopathy** is an acute or chronic condition of an impaired Achilles tendon that is commonly seen in speed skaters. The Achilles tendon originates from the gastrocnemius-soleus complex, and inserts onto the distal calcaneus. Mechanism of injury is due to repetitive eccentric overload, leading to Achilles tendon microtears and subsequent inflammation. Symptoms include difficulty plantarflexing the ankle and supinating the foot in addition to pain in the posterior ankle. Examiners should palpate the tendon for tenderness. Management includes rest, anti-inflammatory medications, bracing, and strengthening exercises. Regenerative interventions can be considered in recalcitrant cases. Careful attention should be paid to the skater suffering from Achilles tendinosis, as progression of the condition may lead to **Achilles tendon rupture**. **Medial tibial stress syndrome**, commonly known as "shin splints," is an overuse injury seen in speed skaters. Mechanism of action is repeated trauma of the connective muscle surrounding the tibia. Female speed skaters with excessive foot pronation are at risk. Symptoms include pain along the posteromedial border of the tibia. Athletes should undergo MRI to rule out a stress fracture. Skaters should rest from activity and may benefit from ice, stretching, and orthotics. They should resume skating gradually when they are pain-free for several days. Cautious training at 50% of preinjury level is recommended with a gradual increase while maintaining an adequate load/rest ratio. **Iliotibial band syndrome** is an overuse syndrome resulting in inflammation of the lateral knee. Mechanism of injury is due to repetitive flexion and extension of the knee during skating. Athletes will complain of pain over the lateral femoral condyle and/or Gerdy's tubercle, in addition to pain at the greater trochanter of the hip and along the iliotibial band. Athletes may have a positive Ober test. MRI and ultrasound can be helpful with diagnosis. Skaters should be treated with rest and physical therapy focusing on stretching of the iliotibial band (ITB), hip flexors, and the gluteus maximus while strengthening the hip abductors and pelvic stabilizers along with the foot core. Athletes can resume skating when they are pain-free for at least 2 weeks without ITB-tenderness. **Bursitis** or **bursopathy** of the foot and ankle is caused by improper skate fit or large skating volumes in properly fit skates. "Lace bite" is the phenomenon seen with skates that are laced tightly. This is otherwise known as "tibialis anterior," "extensor hallucis longus," and "extensor digitorum longus tendonitis."

Other Injuries

Other minor injuries include **bunions, calluses, hammertoes, neuritis, recurrent tinea pedis**. Skaters may sustain **lacerations** from skate blades, **contusions, fractures,** and **joint sprains** from falling.

▪ SUMMARY

Speed Skating is a high-velocity sport that has potential for several injuries. While injury is not as common compared to other sporting events, it is vital to understand the etiology and mechanism of potential injury that may arise.

▪ References

1. Vetter CS, Porter EB. Ice Skating (figure skating and speed skating). In: Madden CC, Putukian M, McCarty EC, Young CC, eds. *Netter's Sports Medicine*. 2nd ed. Philadelphia, PA: Elsevier; 2018:621-625.

2. Short track speed skating. https://www.specialolympics.org/our-work/sports/short-track-speed-skating.

3. Quinn A, Lun V, McCall J, Overend T. Injuries in short track speed skating. *Am J Sports Med*. 2003;31(4):507-510. doi:10.1177/03635465030310040501.

4. Shi S, Han J, Hu Y, et al. The validity of functional movement screening (FMS) in predicting injuries in elite short track speed skating athletes. *J Sci Med Sport*. 2018;21(suppl 1):S62. doi:10.1016/j.jsams.2018.09.141.

5. Palmer-Green D, Brownlow M, Hopkins J, et al. Epidemiological study of injury and illness in Great Britain short-track speed skating. *Br J Sports Med*. 2014;48:649-650. doi:10.1136/bjsports-2014-093494.238.

49. SWIMMING

Eliana Cardozo and Jasmine H. Harris

HISTORY

During the mid-19th century, modern day competitive swimming was established in England when the first swim clubs were formed. Formalized indoor activities within and between swim clubs would give rise to modern swimming competitions. Ultimately the link between swimming and sports was well-defined when it was included in the modern Olympic Games held in Athens, Greece in 1896. In 1908 the Fédération Internationale de Natation Amateur (FINA), which is the world's first swimming association, was formed.[1,2]

GOVERNING ORGANIZATIONS

- International: Federation Internationale de Natation (FINA; International Swimming Federation)
- National: USA Swimming
- Major professional leagues: None (International Swimming League, projected for 2019)
- College: National Collegiate Athletic Association (NCAA)
- High School: National Federation of State High School Associations

PARTICIPANTS

In the United States, an estimated total of 42,000 swimmers competed at the elite college level from 1990 to 2015.[3] A total of 314,529 high school students participated in swimming and diving events.[4]

RULES AND REGULATIONS

In a swimming competition, there are four swimming styles or strokes: butterfly, backstroke, breaststroke, and freestyle. The individual medley is an event where the swimmer swims a combination of all four strokes in equal distances. A relay is where a group of four swimmers each swim freestyle or one of the competitive strokes. All swimmers are assigned a lane number. A horn is typically sounded by a starter to signal the start of a race. Swimmers race for the fastest time using the competitive strokes at varying distances ranging from 25 to 1,500 m. Each individual stroke has specific regulations for acceptable swimming form and how swimmers may turn toward each end of the pool. There are judges of strokes and inspectors of turns who report rule violations to the referee.

EQUIPMENT

Competition swimwear consists of the *swimsuit, cap,* and *goggles*. *Swimsuits* must be made of a textile fabric with a total material thickness of 0.8 mm. The buoyancy effect may not exceed above 0.5 Newton. Men are permitted to wear a one-piece swimsuit;

women may wear a swimsuit in one or two pieces. Zippers or fasteners are not allowed. A *swimming cap* must follow the natural form of the head and cannot be made of hard material. The maximum thickness must be less than or equal to 2 mm. The cap must not be attached to the swimsuit or goggles. *Eye goggles* serve the purpose of eye protection and provide visibility. The shape or design must not provide any aquadynamic advantages.[5]

>>> **Adaptive Sport Key Points: Paralympic Swimming**

Swimming is a Paralympic sport consisting of athletes with various physical disabilities such as spinal cord injury, amputation, and visual impairment, to name a few. Swimmers are classified based on physical, visual, or intellectual impairments, as well as the extent of activity limitation due to their disability. Competition takes place in an Olympic-size swimming pool. Athletes are not allowed to use prostheses or assistive devices during competition. For the visually impaired, a "tapper" is allowed to stand at the end of the pool and use a pole to tap when the swimmer is approaching the wall.[6]

■ MEDICAL COVERAGE LOGISTICS

The FINA medical rules specify that the extent of medical support depends on the nature of the sports' activities and the level of competition. In general, medical coverage for competition should be collaborated between the physician, Emergency Medical Technician (EMT) personnel, and lifeguard. Ensure the competition venue has an equipped treatment area. Distribute a coordinated emergency action plan (EAP) including emergency procedures in case of events such as water rescue. Discuss with first response medical services the nearest designated hospital to initiate treatment for referred injured athletes. Medical personnel should be familiar and trained in water rescue and spine boarding. The medical provider with other support staff should establish an open line of communication with coaches, referees, and other staff. For elite level athletes, FINA recommends that a trained physician perform a preparticipation exam that consists of cardiovascular screening.[7]

■ MEDICAL EMERGENCIES AND MEDICAL BAG ESSENTIALS

Aquatic emergencies can occur both in or around the water due to sudden illness or injury. Medical personnel should be alert and act quickly in responding to an emergency. Drowning can be fatal and will require immediate action. Head, neck, and spinal cord injuries can occur with trauma or high-impact activity during competition. If you suspect a head, neck, or spinal cord injury and the athlete remains in water, care must be taken to immobilize the head, neck, and body while maintaining the head above water. The medical staff should work together to pull the person out of the water safely and with caution. Other serious or life-threatening emergencies of which medical personnel should be aware include seizures, hypoglycemia, cardiac arrest, and pulmonary edema.

Medical Bag Essentials in Swimming	
Medical Emergencies:	**Head and Spine:**
Automated External Defibrillator (AED)	Stretcher & Spine board
Epi 1:1,000	Cervical orthosis
Diphenhydramine or another antihistamine	
Albuterol inhaler	
Floatation devices	

■ EPIDEMIOLOGY

The highly repetitive nature of normal swimming strokes can predispose swimmers to overuse injuries, most commonly involving the shoulder. Nonfreestyle swimmers have more injuries than freestylers. Female swimmers have a higher rate of overuse injuries compared with male swimmers. The next most common injuries involve the knee and low back.[8,9] Breaststrokers experienced a higher prevalence of knee-related problems, lower back, and hip adductor injuries than nonbreaststrokers.[10]

■ COMMON INJURIES

Illnesses

Medical illnesses in swimmers include **exercise-induced bronchoconstriction, respiratory problems,** and **ear problems like otitis externa**.

Spine Injury

Cervicalgia due to neck strain or **low back pain** due to lumbar hyperextension from certain swim strokes may occur in swimmers. Treatment includes oral medications for pain control, evaluating stroke biomechanics, and physiotherapy focused on core strengthening.

Upper Limb Injuries

Shoulder pain is the most musculoskeletal ailment in swimmers. It usually stems from an overuse injury which is multifactorial. Pain can be due to a number of different injuries. In general, since it is a gradual overuse injury, the decision to compete is made depending on the level of pain and stage of recovery. **Impingement syndrome** is a biomechanical issue where the supraspinatus is being impinged under the acromion during shoulder flexion and abduction leading to supraspinatus tendinopathy and pain. In addition to this there may also be subacromial-subdeltoid bursitis contributing to the pain. Since most swim strokes include repetitive overhead motion, rotator cuff (RTC) weakness, scapular dyskinesia, and increased shoulder laxity can contribute to poor biomechanics which then lead to subacromial impingement.[11] Symptoms include lateral shoulder pain, exacerbated by overhead movements. Treatment is aimed at strengthening the RTC and scapulothoracic muscles to correct poor shoulder biomechanics and swim stroke. **Suprascapular neuropathy** occurs from repetitive traction during some swim strokes. There can also be entrapment by a cyst in the suprascapular or spinoglenoid notch. Symptoms include shoulder pain and weakness in shoulder abduction (supraspinatus) and external rotation (infraspinatus). Treatment includes physical therapy but, in some instances, may also require surgery.[12] **Labral tears** are another cause of pain in a swimmer's shoulder; they may occur posteriorly or anteriorly and are due to repetitive overhead motion during strokes. Treatment consists of conservative measures including physical therapy and in some cases surgery.[11,13]

Multidirectional instability (MDI) can predispose the athlete to injury of different shoulder structures including the rotator cuff and labrum. Some level of shoulder laxity is common in competitive swimmers, by nature of the sport, and having increased range of motion (ROM) in the shoulder has been shown to benefit swimmers.[14] As mentioned previously, treatment entails shoulder stabilization.

Lower Limb Injuries

Lower limb injuries are overuse in nature. **Adductor** and **hip flexor strains** are common, especially with breaststroke. Treatment usually includes rest, activity modification, physical therapy, and return to sport once the athlete is asymptomatic. **Knee pain** in swimmers is usually an overuse injury, most commonly seen in breaststroke.[15] It is the second most common injury in swimming after shoulder pain. In breaststroke there is a high valgus load in the knees during the extension phase; this combined with the repetitive nature of swimming, predisposes the athlete to medial knee pain from *medial collateral ligament sprain*.[15] Treatment includes rest, swim stroke optimization, and physical therapy. Anterior knee pain due to *patellofemoral syndrome* can also be seen in swimmers. It is usually treated with physical therapy aimed at strengthening the hip abductors.[10,15]

SUMMARY

Swimming is a dynamic sport which involves a great deal of repetitive motion at the shoulders and knees placing the athlete at risk for overuse injuries. Understanding common injuries and treatment is important for the sports medicine team.

References

1. Mountjoy M, Junge A, Alonso JM, et al. Sports injuries and illnesses in the 2009 FINA World Championships (Aquatics). *Br J Sports Med*. 2010;44:522-527. doi:10.1136/bjsm.2010.071720.

2. Love C. An overview of the development of swimming in England, c.1750–1918. *Int J Hist Sport*. 2007;24(5): 568-585. doi:10.1080/09523360601183095.

3. de Almeida MO, Hespanhol LC, Lopes AD. Prevalence of musculoskeletal pain among swimmers in an elite national tournament. *Int J Sports Phys Ther*. 2015;10(7):1026-1034. https://www.ncbi.nlm.nih.gov/pmc/arti cles/PMC4675188.

4. 2017–18 High School Athletics Participation Survey. National Federation of State High School Associations. https://www.nfhs.org/media/1020205/2017-18_hs_participation_survey.pdf. Published August 28, 2018.

5. Fédération Internationale de Natatio. FINA requirements for swimwear approval (FRSA). http://www.fina .org/sites/default/files/frsa.pdf. Published 2017.

6. Matsuwaka ST, Latzka EW. Summer adaptive sports technology, equipment, and injuries. *Sports Med Arthrosc Rev*. 2019;27(2):48-55. doi:10.1097/JSA.0000000000000231.

7. FINA medical rules. https://www.fina.org/sites/default/files/finamedicalrules_20132017.pdf. Published May 7, 2015.

8. Kerr ZY, Baugh CM, Hibberd EE, et al. Epidemiology of National Collegiate Athletic Association men's and women's swimming and diving injuries from 2009/2010 to 2013/2014. *Br J Sports Med*. 2015;49:465-471. doi:10.1136/bjsports-2014-094423.

9. Stavrianeas S. Aquatics. In: Caine D, Harmer P, Schiff M, eds. *Epidemiology of Injury in Olympic Sports*. vol XVI. Oxford, UK: Wiley-Blackwell; 2010:1-17.

10. Nichols A. Medical care of the aquatics athlete. *Curr Sports Med Rep*. 2015;14(5):389-396. doi:10.1249/ JSR.0000000000000194.

11. Matzkin E, Suslavich K, Wes D. Swimmer's shoulder: painful shoulder in the competitive swimmer. *J Am Acad Orthop Surg*. 2016;24(8):527-536. doi:10.5435/JAAOS-D-15-00313.

12. Kostretzis L, Theodoroudis I, Boutsiadis A, et al. Suprascapular nerve pathology: a review of the literature. *Open Orthop J*. 2017;11(suppl 1):140-153. doi:10.2174/1874325001711010140.

13. Heinlein SA, Cosgarea AJ. Biomechanical considerations in the competitive swimmer's shoulder. *Sports Health*. 2010;2(6):519-525. doi:10.1177/1941738110377611.

14. Weldon EJ III, Richardson AB. Upper extremity overuse injuries in swimming: a discussion of swimmer's shoulder. *Clin Sports Med*. 2001;20(3):423-438. doi:10.1016/S0278-5919(05)70260-X.

15. Rodeo SA. Knee pain in competitive swimming. *Clin Sports Med*. 1999;18(2):379-387. doi:10.1016/S0278-5919(05)70152-6.

Walter Alomar-Jiménez

HISTORY

Table tennis was developed during the Victorian Era in England around the 1860s as an indoor version of lawn tennis, to be played during the winter or bad weather.[1] The first patented table tennis set was developed in 1890 by David Foster. In the early 1900s, John Jacques was credited for commercializing the sport and named it "ping pong." The International Table Tennis Federation was founded in 1926 and featured in the 1988 Olympics in Seoul, Korea.[2]

GOVERNING ORGANIZATIONS

- International: International Table Tennis Federation (ITTF), founded 1926
- National: United States Table Tennis (USATT), founded 1933
- Major professional leagues: China Super League and German Bundesliga
- College: National Collegiate Table Tennis Association (NCTTA), founded 1991

PARTICIPANTS

Table tennis participants include a wide range in the age and level of participants. The ITTF have affiliated 226 national associations.[1] Table tennis is the national sport of China, having dominated most of the worldwide competitions. The sport has made enormous growth in the Americas with athletes competing at the most elite level. Although there is not an exact number of players, it is estimated that approximately 300 million people play table tennis worldwide, including 40 million competitive players.[1]

RULES AND REGULATIONS

A game shall be won by the player first scoring 11 points, unless both players score 10 points, when the game shall be won by the first player gaining a lead of 2 points. The order of service alternates every 2 points, except when both players score 10 points, or above which alternates on every point.[3] A match shall consist of the best of five or seven games, depending on the competition. Each player stands at an opposite side of the table with a racket. The play starts with a service from one of the players. The rally, which is the period that the ball is in play, continues while each player strikes the ball to the opponent's side after only one bounce. A point is scored if an opponent fails to make a correct service, return, or if the ball passes over a court without touching. Table tennis can be played with single or double players. For doubles, there are two players on each side; the service must bounce on the right half of the table for the server and receiver and players on each team must alternate hits.

EQUIPMENT

The playing surface of the *table* is rectangular, 2.74 m long and 1.525 m wide and lies in a horizontal plane 76 cm above the floor. The playing surface is divided into two equal courts. The *net assembly* consists of the net, its suspension, and the supporting posts. The top of the net shall be 15.25 cm above the playing surface. The *racket* may be of any size, shape, or weight but the blade shall be flat and rigid. The sides of the blades used for striking the ball shall be covered with pimpled rubber, with pimples outward or sandwich rubber. All equipment and rubbers must be approved by the ITTF and thus have its logo. One side of the racket must be black and the other side red. The *ball* is spherical, diameter of 40 mm, made of celluloid or similar materials, and can be white or orange. The main color of a player's *clothing*, including a shirt, skirt, or shorts has to be different from that of the ball in use. Therefore, white or orange clothing are typically not used.[4]

>>> **Adaptive Sport Key Points: Table Tennis**

Paralympic table tennis is the third largest Paralympic sport in terms of athlete numbers and been present in all Paralympic Games since 1960. These athletes compete in different classifications of categories such as: wheelchair (TT1–5), standing (TT6–10), and intellectual impairment (TT11). Paralympic table tennis has the same rules as the ITTF with minor modifications for wheelchair players such as reducing the area of the table. Some athletes with tetraplegia tape their rackets to their hands and athletes with bilateral above-elbow amputation hold the racket with their mouths.[5]

■ MEDICAL COVERAGE LOGISTICS

The role of the on-site physician leader is to organize and coordinate the medical staff, develop an emergency action plan (EAP), and interact with the coaches and officials to help ensure the safety of the players and spectators. Prior to the game, it is important to identify available medical staff, support personnel, field map, and the available medical equipment. Sports medicine physicians and Emergency Medical Services (EMS) personnel, along with sports medicine fellows, residents, medical students, athletic trainers, or physical therapists can attend expected medical needs. Establishing an EAP is the most important task. Protocols and guidelines should include role definition of the medical staff, emergency transportation including personnel, routes, and adequate facilities with the capacity to evaluate and manage head and spine injuries, and an outline of the chain-of-command and communication standards. The referee will call for medical evaluation if a player is injured. Documentation of injured player encounters is important.

■ MEDICAL EMERGENCIES AND MEDICAL BAG ESSENTIALS

The collapsed or unconscious athlete is considered a medical emergency that requires activation of the proper channels of communication and protocols including basic life support (BLS)/advanced cardiac life support (ACLS). Although rarely reported, nontraumatic emergencies can include cardiac conditions like arrhythmias and hypertrophic cardiomyopathy (HCM), anaphylaxis, asthma, and heat-related illness, specifically heat stroke.

■ EPIDEMIOLOGY

Table tennis is one of the fastest pace sports in the world, requiring fine motor skills, coordination, mental and physical fitness.[6] As a noncontact sport, most injuries are nontraumatic. The incidence of injury is low (0–3 injuries per 100 athletes).[7] Although upper limb injuries (shoulder/clavicle 29% and elbow/wrist/hand 25%) are more prevalent than lower limb injuries (knee 21% and hip/groin 11%), most severe injuries are seen on foot/ankle.[8] Additionally, 10% of injuries affect the lumbosacral spine.[9]

Medical Bag Essentials in Table Tennis

Wound/Laceration/Skin Care:

Normal saline
Betadine swabs
Neosporin, mupirocin ointment
Moleskin
Elastic bandage
Tube stretch gauze
Sterile gauzes
Vaseline
Steri-strips

Medical Emergencies:

Automated External Defibrillator (AED)
Epi 1:1,000
Diphenhydramine or another antihistamine
Albuterol inhaler

■ COMMON INJURIES

Spine Injuries

Low back strain or **sprain** is a term used to describe an episode of acute low back pain. The pain develops spontaneously or during play due to repetitive bending and lifting. It is important to evaluate all patients with low back pain for red flags such as bowel or bladder changes, weakness, fever, and history of cancer because any of those symptoms will require quick medical work-up and management. Treatment of low back pain without red flags includes remaining as active as possible, while avoiding bed rest. Most patients with acute low back pain improve over time regardless of treatment; therefore, nonpharmacologic treatment such as superficial heat is recommended. Oral medications such as nonsteroidal anti-inflammatory drugs (NSAIDs) and muscle relaxants can be used for relief of symptoms.[10]

Upper Limb Injuries

Rotator cuff injuries are among the most common in table tennis as in any racquet sport. The most common injured muscle/tendon is the supraspinatus. Symptoms include pain with overhead activity, usually above 90 degrees. Initial management includes pain control, avoiding aggravating activities, and relative rest followed by therapy to improve shoulder girdle and scapular stabilizers strength and proprioception. **Glenohumeral instability** includes a range of shoulder disorders from subluxation to dislocation and is usually due to atraumatic shoulder instability and repetitive shoulder activity. Players will report that the shoulder is being slipped out of the joint or a "dead" arm. Management could include shoulder reduction if the injury were observed, use of a sling, and therapy to restore function and prevent subsequent dislocations. Evaluation for anatomic alterations such as glenohumeral internal rotation deficit, scapular dyskinesia, is needed to establish an individualized rehabilitation plan. Recurrent dislocations are common and those that fail conservative treatment may need surgery. **Lateral epicondylopathy,** commonly known as "tennis elbow," is a condition affecting the origin of the common extensor tendons of the wrist, primarily the extensor carpi radialis brevis due to repetitive stress. Wrist motion is enormously involved during table tennis strokes, particularly forehand and backhand topspin. Symptoms include pain at the lateral epicondyle of the humerus, which is aggravated by wrist extension.

Treatment includes activity modification, anti-inflammatory medications, and ice for acute pain. In this condition, wearing a forearm band distal to the extensor muscle group origin can reduce symptoms and can be used during play. Rehabilitation should be reinforced with eccentric lengthening exercises. Other treatment options for refractory cases include regenerative medicine interventions. **Wrist ganglion cysts** are benign mucin-filled cysts. Their most common location is the dorsal wrist. The patient often presents with painless swelling, but painful wrist and grip weakness due to pain may occur. Primary treatment is reassurance. Aspiration of the cyst can be performed in symptomatic patients; however, patients should be advised that the ganglion cyst has a high recurrence rate after aspiration. **De Quervain's tenosynovitis** is an inflammation of the tendon sheath involving the first dorsal wrist compartment (abductor pollicis longus [APL] and extensor pollicis brevis [EPB]). It occurs in activities requiring forceful grip with ulnar deviation, such as table tennis. Symptoms are located over the lateral wrist and aggravated during grasp and thumb extension. Treatment of choice for this condition is bracing and corticosteroid injections. **Ulnar collateral ligament (UCL) injury**, commonly known as "skier's thumb," refers to a sprain or tear of the UCL of the thumb. Injury occurs when valgus force is applied to an abducted first metacarpophalangeal (MCP) joint. Symptoms include pain and instability in the thumb. Initial management includes ice, rest, and NSAIDs. Treatment for a grade 1 UCL sprain is taping for activity, while a grade 2 will require a thumb spica cast for 3 to 6 weeks. Surgical repair may be needed for an avulsion fracture, followed by hand therapy. **Trigger finger** or **stenosing tenosynovitis** is the locking of any finger as it flexes and extends. It is common in racquet sports, due to overuse or direct pressure at the flexor tendon sheath resulting in mechanical locking under the A1 pulley at the MCP. Symptoms include painful clicking when opening and closing the hand. Treatment includes splinting of the MCP joint at 10 to 15 degrees of flexion and corticosteroid injection targeting the flexor tendon sheath.

Lower Limb Injuries

Lower limb injuries more commonly affect the knee and ankle. **Patellar tendinopathy** is a chronic overuse injury of the patellar tendon. Table tennis players are required to adopt a flex-knee position up to 90 degrees or more for sustained periods, along with torsional torque movement of the upper limb during strokes, places the knee at severe loading situation, predisposing to patellar tendinopathy.[8] Symptoms include pain over the inferior pole of the patellar tendon during or after competition. Management includes relative rest, ice, and NSAIDs. Bracing, such as knee straps, can be useful to alleviate pain. Rehabilitation should be encouraged to correct possible biomechanical deficits such as hamstring and quadriceps weakness. **Ankle sprain** refers to injuries of the ankle ligaments, most commonly involving the anterior talofibular ligament (ATFL). The mechanism of injury is foot supination and inversion. Symptoms include pain, swelling, tenderness over the affected ligaments, and difficulty with weight-bearing activities. It is important to evaluate the patient for a high-ankle sprain and determine if further imaging such as x-rays is indicated (review the Ottawa Ankle Rules). Management involves protection, rest, ice, elevation, and compression. The use of crutches might be needed in patients who are unable to bear weight. Physical therapy after ankle sprain is highly recommended. Proprioceptive and balance exercises are very important for recovery and to prevent recurrence. Orthotic bracing is recommended for 6 months after the injury to help prevent injury recurrence.

Dermatologic Injuries

Although table tennis is a noncontact sport, minor **contusions** or **abrasions** can occur by accidentally striking the table or in rare occurrences in pair table tennis, a player hitting another player. Management consists of applying direct pressure with gauze over the area to stop any bleeding and cleaning the area with water. Depending on the severity of the laceration, steri-strips or sutures might be used.

■ SUMMARY

Table tennis is a noncontact racquet sport with low incidence of injuries; however, the repetitive motion could lead to biomechanical imbalances and predispose these athletes to overuse injuries. The sports medicine physician should be aware of the common injuries to provide adequate medical coverage.

■ References

1. Fuchs M, Liu R, Malagoli Lanzoni I, et al. Table tennis match analysis: a review. *J Sports Sci.* 2018;36(23):2653-2662. doi:10.1080/02640414.2018.1450073.

2. Milioni F, Leite JVM, Beneke R, et al. Table tennis playing styles require specific energy systems demands. *PLoS One.* 2018;13(7):e0199985. doi:10.1371/journal.pone.0199985.

3. The International Table Tennis Federation. *Handbook.* 48th ed. Lausanne, Switzerland: The International Table Tennis Federation; 2020:34-41. https://www.ittf.com/wp-content/uploads/2020/04/2020ITTFHandbook_v1.pdf.

4. The International Table Tennis Federation. *Handbook.* 48th ed. Lausanne, Switzerland: The International Table Tennis Federation; 2020:42-65. https://www.ittf.com/wp-content/uploads/2020/04/2020ITTFHandbook_v1.pdf.

5. History of para table tennis. https://www.paralympic.org/table-tennis/about.

6. Kondrič M, Zagatto AM, Sekulić D. The physiological demands of table tennis: a review. *J Sports Sci Med.* 2013;12(3):362-370. https://www.ncbi.nlm.nih.gov/pmc/articles/PMC3772576.

7. Soligard T, Steffen K, Palmer D, et al. Sports injury and illness incidence in the Rio de Janeiro 2016 Olympic Summer Games: a prospective study of 11274 athletes from 207 countries. *Br J Sports Med.* 2017;51(17):1265-1271. doi:10.1136/bjsports-2017-097956.

8. Ebadi LA, Günay M. Analysing of the types of injuries observed in table tennis players according to the some variables. *IOSR J Sports Phys Educ.* 2018;5(4):21-26. https://www.iosrjournals.org/iosr-jspe/papers/Vol-5Issue4/Version-1/E05042126.pdf.

9. Correa Mesa JF. Prevalence of musculoskeletal injuries in table tennis players. *Revista Ciencias Biomedicas.* 2014;5:48-57.

10. Qaseem A, Wilt TJ, McLean RM, et al. Noninvasive treatments for acute, subacute, and chronic low back pain: a clinical practice guideline from the American College of Physicians. *Ann Intern Med.* 2017;166(7):514-530. doi:10.7326/M16-2367.

51. TENNIS

Liza M. Hernández-González
and Richard A. Fontánez-Nieves

HISTORY

Tennis as a sport evolved from a French handball game called *"jeu de paume"* (game of the palm) during the 12th–13th century. It was later named "lawn tennis" since it was played on grass courts by the British during Queen Victoria's reign in the late 1800s. Nowadays, it is a worldwide popular sport played over a variety of court surfaces including grass, clay, and hard courts.[1]

GOVERNING ORGANIZATIONS

- International: International Tennis Federation (ITF)
- National: United States Tennis Association (USTA)
- Professional: Women's Tennis Association (WTA), Association of Tennis Professionals (ATP)
- College: Intercollegiate Tennis Association (ITA)
- High School: National Federation of State High School Associations (NFSHSA)

PARTICIPANTS

Approximately 17.9 million athletes participated in the sport of tennis in the United States in 2014.[2]

RULES AND REGULATIONS

The game is played within a rectangular court with one (singles) or two (doubles) player(s) at each side of the net (Figure 51.1). The objective is to hit the ball with the racket back and forth over the net within the established boundaries, and only one bounce is allowed for the returning player. The winner is the player who wins more points to win games, and wins more games to win sets, and therefore the match. There is no predetermined time limit, but match format requires continuous play and is usually the best of three or five sets, depending on the match type (singles vs. doubles), tournament classification, and court location. Exceptions are matches involving youth, high school, or college athletes.[3]

EQUIPMENT

The **ball** must have specific physical properties based on established regulations. The approved balls may vary from type I (slightly harder, fast speed ball); type II (standard ball); and type III (larger, slow speed ball). Ball selection will depend on the category, court surface, and location. For young athletes learning how to play the game, balls

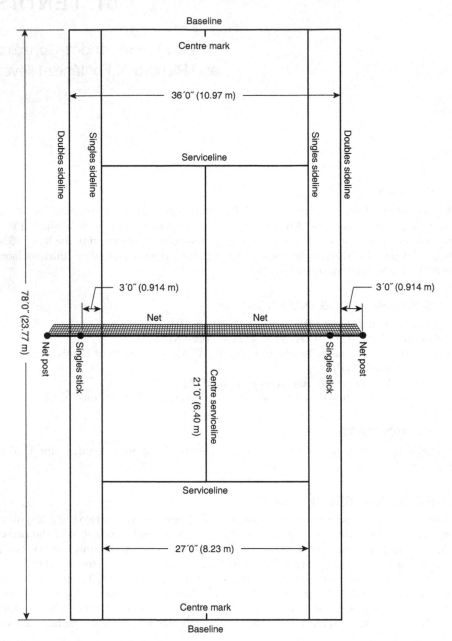

Figure 51.1 Tennis court schematics.
Source: Courtesy of the International Tennis Federation

may also vary in size and bounce to facilitate skills acquisition. The ***racquet*** is essential and is usually tailored to the athlete's style of play and preferences. It requires strings in a crossed interlaced pattern and its performance may be affected by several factors such as racquet head size, string type (natural gut or synthetic), string tension, and string gauge.

>>> Adaptive sport key points: Wheelchair tennis

In wheelchair tennis, a significant rule change is that the ball can bounce twice, if needed (in or out of the court). In addition, the wheelchair is considered a part of the body and all rules applicable to body parts apply to the wheelchair. Other adaptive equipment may vary based on individual needs and tournament requirements including court size, number of sets played, rackets, and balls.[4]

▨ MEDICAL COVERAGE LOGISTICS

The role of the medical director is to establish an Emergency Action Plan (EAP), coordinate with event personnel and referees, to ensure the safety of all players and spectators. Protocols and guidelines should include role definition of the medical staff, emergency transportation including personnel, routes, and adequate facilities, and an outline of the chain-of-command and communication standards. An accessible and centrally located area for medical evaluation, medical equipment, and personnel must be established prior to play time. Communication between medical personnel, referees, and event organizers is essential for proper medical coverage and can be facilitated by two-way radios, cell phones, or walkie-talkies. If a player suffers from a treatable medical condition, the player must communicate with the referee who will notify the medical personnel and the player may be allowed one medical time-out of 3 minutes for the treatment of each medical condition. This usually occurs during change of ends or between sets. In cases of acute injury, the player may request to be evaluated and treated immediately. Each medical encounter must be documented properly for continuity of care and planning for future events.

▨ MEDICAL EMERGENCIES AND MEDICAL BAG ESSENTIALS

Life-threatening events are quite rare in tennis. The collapsed or unconscious athlete is considered a medical emergency that requires activation of the proper channels of communication and protocols including basic life support (BLS)/advanced cardiac life support (ACLS). Attention must be paid to conditions such as hyperthermia and heat-related illness spectrum which may occur with exposure to high temperatures and humidity, especially in young and elderly athletes. Its presentation may vary from heat cramps, heat exhaustion, and eventually heat stroke, which can lead to death. Other conditions considered to be urgent include facial, dental, or eye injuries from racquets or balls. Other nontraumatic emergencies include asthma, anaphylaxis, cardiac arrhythmias, or hypertrophic cardiomyopathy.

▨ EPIDEMIOLOGY

Tennis is a sport played by athletes of all ages and levels of competition. It involves repetitive long and short bouts of aerobic and anaerobic activity for which it is considered as a great sport to improve physical fitness as well as mental and social health. Furthermore, racket sports, including tennis, have been associated with a lower incidence in all-cause and cardiovascular disease mortality compared to other sports.[5] Despite these health benefits, its biomechanics make athletes prone to a variety of overuse and acute injuries involving the lower extremities, followed by the upper extremity and trunk.[6]

▨ COMMON INJURIES

Spine Injuries

Low back pain is among the leading causes of musculoskeletal injury in both professional and elite junior players.[6] Tennis biomechanics involve repetitive trunk multiplanar

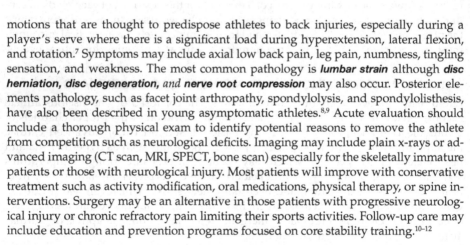

Medical Bag Essentials in Tennis

Medical Emergencies:

Automated External Defibrillator (AED)
Nitroglycerin (sublingual)
Aspirin
Epi 1:1,000
Diphenhydramine or another antihistamine
Albuterol inhaler
Rectal thermometer
Ice bucket

Head and Spine:

Concussion evaluation form
Safe a tooth kit

Fractures and Dislocations:

Immobilizers, Crutches. Slings

Wound/Laceration/Skin Care:

Normal saline
Betadine swabs
Neosporin, mupirocin ointment
Moleskin
Elastic bandage
Tube stretch gauze
Sterile gauzes
Vaseline
Steri-strips
Suture tray
Lidocaine 1%
Nasal pack
Silver nitrate

Others:

Acetaminophen
Glucose tabs

motions that are thought to predispose athletes to back injuries, especially during a player's serve where there is a significant load during hyperextension, lateral flexion, and rotation.[7] Symptoms may include axial low back pain, leg pain, numbness, tingling sensation, and weakness. The most common pathology is *lumbar strain* although *disc herniation, disc degeneration, and nerve root compression* may also occur. Posterior elements pathology, such as facet joint arthropathy, spondylolysis, and spondylolisthesis, have also been described in young asymptomatic athletes.[8,9] Acute evaluation should include a thorough physical exam to identify potential reasons to remove the athlete from competition such as neurological deficits. Imaging may include plain x-rays or advanced imaging (CT scan, MRI, SPECT, bone scan) especially for the skeletally immature patients or those with neurological injury. Most patients will improve with conservative treatment such as activity modification, oral medications, physical therapy, or spine interventions. Surgery may be an alternative in those patients with progressive neurological injury or chronic refractory pain limiting their sports activities. Follow-up care may include education and prevention programs focused on core stability training.[10–12]

Upper Limb Injuries

Upper limb injuries involve mostly the shoulder and elbow secondary to overuse. *Rotator cuff tendinopathy* and *labral pathology* are common causes of shoulder pain in tennis players. These occur secondary to repetitive overhead activities and may be related to scapular dyskinesis, muscle fatigue, joint laxity, and glenohumeral internal rotation deficits, among other factors. Symptoms include anterior or posterior shoulder pain, apprehension, weakness, or mechanical symptoms (clicking or catching). Pain usually occurs during the late cocking and early acceleration (superior labrum anterior posterior [SLAP]) or deceleration phases (rotator cuff pathology) of serve or overhead smashes. Acute evaluation includes the assessment of the strength of rotator cuff muscles, and tests for impingement, rotator cuff tears, instability and labral pathology. Diagnostic imaging is useful to confirm clinical suspicion and may include plain x-rays, ultrasound, MRI or MR arthrogram. Most patients will improve with conservative treatment including a rehabilitation program focusing on posterior capsule stretching, strengthening of rotator cuff muscles and scapular stabilizers, and proprioception exercises. Other cases may require surgical management if symptoms persist. *Lateral* and *medial epicondylalgia* are common overuse injuries seen in tennis, the latter being more common in elite players.[6] Lateral epicondylalgia, also known as "tennis elbow," usually results from repetitive activity involving the common extensor tendons during the backhand strokes. Medial epicondylalgia, or "golfer's elbow," results from repetitive overuse of the common flexor tendons during the acceleration phases of the forehand strokes and the serve. Both conditions may present with symptoms such as localized pain that may radiate to the forearm while holding objects, stiffness, and subjective weakness. Depending on the severity of injury, most will improve with activity modification, bracing, oral medications, and physical therapy. Local corticosteroid injections may be used for short-term pain relief. Also, platelet-rich plasma injections have been used for longer term benefits of pain and function.[13,14] However, refractory cases may require surgical management. Follow-up care should include education and an exercise program to increase the strength and flexibility of the wrist and forearm muscles, as well as the entire kinetic chain.

Lower Limb Injuries

Lower limb injuries are mostly acute in nature. *Thigh muscle strains* are very common in tennis including *hamstrings, adductors* and *rectus femoris muscles*.[6] These are thought to occur secondary to sudden, repetitive loading and multidirectional movements while sprinting, sliding, or lunging. Symptoms include pain, tenderness, bruising, swelling, deformity, and inability to walk, run, or play. Acute treatment includes ice packs, compression bandage, stretching, and in some cases, hematoma aspiration.[15] The ability to continue to play will depend on injury severity and in some cases, may require retiring from the match. Treatment includes oral nonsteroidal anti-inflammatory drugs (NSAIDs) and physical therapy. Return to sports must be gradual and after a rehabilitation program to avoid risk of reinjury. *Ankle sprains* are the most common lower extremity injury. The most commonly injured ligament is the anterior talofibular ligament during an ankle inversion although other lateral ankle structures may be affected with more severe injury. Symptoms include pain, swelling, ecchymosis and, sometimes, inability to walk. Acute evaluation must assess for ligament and tendon integrity, as well as neurovascular injury. Acute management includes ice packs, compression, elevation, bracing, and occasionally restricted weight-bearing. Follow-up treatment should focus on physical therapy with strengthening, stretching, balance and proprioceptive exercises to improve pain and function. Recurrent injury and chronic instability are common consequences if rehabilitation is not performed properly after acute injury.

▨ SUMMARY

Tennis is a noncontact sport that involves long-lasting and short bouts of repetitive aerobic and anaerobic activity. Sports biomechanics predispose athletes to a variety of injuries most commonly secondary to overuse syndromes. Acute evaluation and management include injury diagnosis, treatment, and the decision-making on the athlete's ability to continue play without risk of major or life-threatening injury.

▨ References

1. Lorge BS. Tennis. In: Augustyn A, Bauer P, Duignan B, et al., eds. Encyclopedia Britannica. https://www.britannica.com/sports/tennis. Published July 26, 1999. Updated April 23, 2020.

2. Tennis Industry Association. Participation category. https://cdn.ymaws.com/www.tennisindustry.org/resource/resmgr/research/4yearparticipationtrend.pdf

3. International Tennis Federation. ITF tennis. https://www.itftennis.com/en/about-us/governance/rules-and -regulations/.

4. United States Tennis Association Friend at court 2019: handbook of rules and regulations. https://www .usta.com/content/dam/usta/sections/northern-california/norcal/pdfs/leagues/resources/rules/2019 -Friend-at-Court.pdf. Published 2019.

5. Oja P, Kelly P, Pedisic Z, et al. Associations of specific types of sports and exercise with all-cause and car-diovascular-disease mortality: a cohort study of 80 306 British adults. *Br J Sports Med*. 2017;51(10):812-817. doi:10.1136/bjsports-2016-096822.

6. Fu MC, Ellenbecker TS, Renstrom PA, et al. Epidemiology of injuries in tennis players. *Curr Rev Musculoskel-et Med*. 2018;11:1-5. doi:10.1007/s12178-018-9452-9.

7. Campbell A, Straker L, O'Sullivan P, et al. Lumbar loading in the elite adolescent tennis serve: a link to low back pain. *Med Sci Sports Exerc*. 2013;45(8):1562-1568. doi:10.1249/MSS.0b013e31828bea5e.

8. Alyas F, Turner M, Connell D. MRI findings in the lumbar spines of asymptomatic, elite tennis players. *Br J Sports Med*. 2007;41:836-841. doi:10.1136/bjsm.2007.037747.

9. Rajeswaran G, Turner M, Gissane C, Healy JC. MRI findings in the lumbar spines of asymptomatic elite junior tennis players. *Skeletal Radiol*. 2014;43(7):925-932. doi:10.1007/s00256-014-1862-1.

10. Ellenbecker TS, Roetert EP. An isokinetic profile of trunk rotation strength in elite tennis players. *Med Sci Sports Exerc*. 2004;36(11):1959-1963. doi:10.1249/01.mss.0000145469.08559.0e.

11. Renkawitz T, Boluki D, Grifka J. The association of low back pain, neuromuscular imbalance, and trunk extension strength in athletes. *Spine J*. 2006;6:673-683. doi:10.1016/j.spinee.2006.03.012.

12. Correia JP, Oliveira R, Vaz JR, et al. Trunk muscle activation, fatigue and low back pain in tennis players. *J Sci Med Sport*. 2015;19(4):311-316. doi:10.1016/j.jsams.2015.04.002.

13. Chen X, Jones IA, Park C, Vangsness CT Jr. The efficacy of platelet-rich plasma on tendon and ligament healing: a systematic review and meta-analysis with bias assessment. *Am J Sports Med*. 2018;46(8):2020-2032. doi:10.1177/0363546517743746.

14. Houck D, Kraeutler J, Thornton LB, et al. Treatment of lateral epicondylitis with autologous blood, plate-let-rich plasma, or corticosteroid injections: a systematic review of overlapping meta-analyses. *Orthop J Sports Med*. 2019;7(3):2325967119831052. doi:10.1177/2325967119831052.

15. Hoftel T, Seil R, Bily W, et al. Nonoperative treatment of muscle injuries—recommendations from the GOTS Expert Meeting. *J Exp Orthop*. 2018;5:24. doi:10.1186/s40634-018-0139-3.

52. TRACK AND FIELD (RUNNING, SHOT PUT, DISCUS, JAVELIN)

Jasmine H. Harris

▉ HISTORY

Track & Field (T&F), also known as "athletics," is one of the oldest sports with its origins dating back to the ancient Greeks and Egyptians.[1] The first recorded event was a foot race for a distance of 600 ft at the first ancient Olympic Games in 776 BCE. Modern T&F resurfaced as organized competitions appearing in England and the U.S. colleges and military academies during the 1800s. With the revival of the modern Olympic Games in 1896, T&F was introduced as an international competition. Throwing events, specifically shot put and discus, also first appeared in the modern Olympic Games in 1896, followed by the javelin in 1908.[2]

▉ GOVERNING ORGANIZATIONS

- International: International Association of Athletics Federation (IAAF)
- National: USA Track & Field (USATF)
- Major professional leagues: none
- College: National Collegiate Athletic Association (NCAA)
- High School: National Federation of State High School Associations (NFHS)

▉ PARTICIPANTS

T&F has the most participants of all high school sports with nearly 1.1 million student–athletes participating each year. It has the highest number of high school participants among girls' sports and the second highest among boys' sports after American football.[3] In 2018–2019, there were nearly 60,000 men and women NCAA college athletes competing in T&F.[4]

▉ RULES AND REGULATIONS

T&F competitions are known as "meets" or "meetings." Most events are individual sports with a single victor, except for relay races which consist of four members. For **running events**, there are competition guidelines for the start, running, and finish of each event. For 400 m and shorter races, a starter block is required, and competitors must assume a different starting position on the command of "on your marks" and "set." A starter gun or electronic tone is activated as a signal to start the race. Lane rules apply depending on the race. A runner has finished the race when any part of his or her body reaches the finish line.[5] **Throwing events** involve the use of objects of various weights and shapes that are thrown for distance. The longest distance measured of three attempts is used for scoring. The shot put includes a throwing circle, a stop board, and a landing sector. The landing sector is usually located in the grass area inside the track. The shot put, typically made of metal, is thrown with one hand within a designated circle area. The discus throw includes a throwing circle, protective cage, and landing sector. They are located near the ends of the back straight and the landing sector is located in the grass area inside the track. The discus is typically made of metal or wood with a metallic rim, and it is also thrown with a flat trajectory from a circle. The javelin throw includes a runway, a throwing arc and a landing sector. Since the length of the runway exceeds the space available in the segment, it is usually extended across the track. The javelin has three parts: a metal head, a shaft, and a cord grip. The shaft is fixed to a metal head terminating in a sharp point.

■ EQUIPMENT

A competitor may compete bare feet or with *footwear*. The sole of the shoe is allowed up to 11 spikes, with varying thickness based on the events and surface of competition (synthetic vs nonsynthetic surface). *Starter blocks* are devices used at the starting position of races 400 m and shorter. They consist of two flat or sloped foot plates mounted on a frame. Athletes are allowed to use their own *throwing implements* for competition after inspected to meet required specifications. The *shot-put ball* must weigh 4 kg and 7.2 kg for female and male contestants, respectively. The *discus* measures 25 to 28.5 mm radius and weighs 1 kg and 2 kg for female and male contestants, respectively. Men's *javelin* weighs 800 g and 600 g for women.[5]

> ### ⟫ Adaptive Sport Key Points: Track and Field
>
> Track and Field is a Paralympic sport that consists of racing, throwing, and jumping events. Each athlete is classified by the type of impairment such as cerebral palsy, spinal cord injuries, amputations, short stature, visual impairments, and intellectual impairments. Athletes may compete with the aid of a visual guide, prosthesis, or a wheelchair. There are specific wheelchairs with required specifications permissible for competition. A helmet must also be worn in all wheelchair events. Throwing athletes can participate in events by standing or sitting on a throwing chair with regulated variations for position of the chair and throwing technique.[6]

■ MEDICAL COVERAGE LOGISTICS

The role of the medical director and/or on-site physician leader is to organize and co-ordinate the medical staff, develop an emergency action plan (EAP), and interact with the event ("meet") director to help ensure the safety of the competitors and spectators. Prior to a competition, it is important to identify available medical staff, support personnel, venue map, and the available medical equipment. Medical coverage for T&F competitions poses challenges as track events generally take place at the same time as field events. Onsite medical care should be located in a well-marked medical tent or room with convenient access to both track and field events. If the event is taking place outdoors, ensure there is appropriate coverage of the treatment area from the environment and ambient weather. Medical staff should be aware of injuries that may occur with throwing athletes due to the inherent heavy object used, but must also take caution with injuries to officials and spectators. Communication between individual members of the medical staff and with the meet officials, emergency medical staff, and local medical facilities is essential via two or more systems (e.g., hand-held radios and cell phones). Lastly, documentation is essential for review after the event to evaluate utilization and plan for future events.[7]

■ MEDICAL EMERGENCIES AND MEDICAL BAG ESSENTIALS

Track athletes often compete in multiple events and may be exposed to hot environments, and sometimes for long durations during competition. Serious complications such as hyperthermia and severe dehydration can occur leading to heat-related illness. Other nontraumatic emergencies include cardiac complications like arrhythmias, infarction, anaphylaxis, and asthma. Throwing events can pose serious injury and even death in both spectators and officials as a result of being struck with an object, misthrows, and distraction.

Medical Bag Essentials in Track and Field	
Medical Emergencies:	**Wound/Laceration/Skin Care:**
Automated External Defibrillator (AED)	Normal saline
Nitroglycerin (sublingual)	Betadine swabs
Aspirin	Neosporin, mupirocin ointment
Epi 1:1,000	Moleskin
Diphenhydramine or another antihistamine	Elastic bandage
Albuterol inhaler	Tube stretch gauze
Rectal thermometer	Sterile gauzes
Ice bucket	Vaseline
	Steri-strips
Head and Spine:	Suture tray
Concussion evaluation form	Lidocaine 1%
Stretcher & Spine board	
Cervical orthosis	**Others:**
Cricothyrotomy kit	Acetaminophen
	Glucose tabs
Fractures and Dislocations:	Waterproof SPF 50 sunscreen
Immobilizers, Splints, and Slings	
Crutches	

■ EPIDEMIOLOGY

The injury rate in comparison to other sports is much lower for high school T&F athletes.[8,9] There are higher injury rates in competition compared to practice regardless of gender. Sprinters have higher proportions of thigh and upper leg strains and distance runners have higher proportions of lower leg strains. Girls are twice as likely to have stress fractures than boys and tend to have a higher proportion of ligament sprains and tendinopathy.[8] For most events, the lower limbs are most frequently injured, with the ankle being the most commonly injured body part, followed by the knee, and lastly pelvis. The most common injury diagnoses were sprains and strains, followed by fractures and dislocations.[9] Hurdlers are four times more likely to injure the upper limbs due to falls. Male college throwers sustain the highest rates of upper limb overuse injuries of all college sports with the greatest proportion among shot putters.[10,11] Shoulder injuries are the most common upper limb injury, followed by the elbow, then the wrist and hand. The next most common injured body part for throwers is the ankle followed by the back.[11]

■ COMMON INJURIES

Head and Spine Injuries

Head injuries are uncommon, but **lumbar muscle strains** are commonly seen in all throwing athletes due to hyperextension and rotation of the lumbar spine often under greater than normal loads on the lumbar spine. They typically present with acute low back pain, localized to the lumbar region without neurologic signs or symptoms. Treatment is conservative with physiotherapy.

Upper Limb Injuries

Upper limb injuries are common in the throwing events. **Rotator cuff tear** and **tendinopathy** are commonly seen in all throwing athletes particularly due to repetitive stress on the shoulder. Rotator cuff tendons are under greater stress as they stabilize the shoulder throughout the explosive speed and force of throwing motions. Acute care in a track meet can consist of ice and nonsteroidal anti-inflammatory medications. Injection to continue in an event is not recommended. **Pectoralis major strain** is seen especially in shot putters due to their explosive muscle activation before release. Treatment is also conservative. **Ulnar collateral ligament (UCL) sprain** or **tears** are commonly seen in javelin throwers. Repetitive stress on the ligament during javelin throw can lead to microtrauma within the UCL. When injury occurs, athletes may describe a popping sensation with sudden pain. Physical exam findings will reveal tenderness over the UCL complex about 2 cm distal to the medial epicondyle and pain with valgus stress. Emergent radiographic imaging is warranted to evaluate for bony avulsion. Ice may be applied to the medial elbow. Caution must be taken not to place ice over the ulnar nerve. Surgical management is recommended for full tears in high level throwers. **Ulnar neuropathy at the elbow** can develop due to the valgus stress at the elbow during throwing motion. Any additional instability can potentiate the forces on the ulnar nerve and lead to a traction ulnar neuropathy at the elbow. **Medial epicondylopathy** is an overuse injury commonly seen due to repetitive forearm pronation and wrist flexion during the javelin throw. The close proximity of the ulnar nerve to the medial epicondyle can cause concomitant ulnar symptoms. In this condition, patients report a dull aching pain in the medial elbow that worsens with activity. Tenderness is present at the medial epicondyle. Pain is reproduced with resisted wrist flexion and forearm pronation. Important in the evaluation is checking the integrity of the UCL. Athletes may continue in competition if forearm taping or a fulcrum strap reduces their pain and allows correct throwing technique. **Intersection syndrome** is due to repetitive wrist extension where friction occurs between the intersection of the first and second extensor compartments of the wrist leading to tenosynovitis. This can be typically seen with shot putters as the release on a throw requires a forceful push or flick. **Carpal tunnel syndrome** is seen in shot-put athletes due to repetitive gripping. It is managed by modifying activity. **Finger dislocations** and **sprains** can be seen especially in discus throwers. Taping of individual fingers can be used acutely; however, there are strict rules on how tape can be applied to the hand. Taping of individual fingers is allowed, but taping of two or more fingers is not permissible as it may assist the throw. Taping should be reviewed by the main judge prior to the start of the event to ensure the athlete is not disqualified. **Fingertip lacerations** can be seen in all throwing athletes. Most injuries are superficial, but care must be taken to make sure no flexor tendon, digital artery, or nerve is injured. Tape is allowed to cover an open wound, but should be carefully inspected to prevent risk of disqualification from competition.

Lower Limb Injuries

Lower limb injuries are seen in running/racing events. **Hamstring strains** and **tears** are the most common lower limb injuries seen in sprinters and hurdlers usually occurring with maximal or near maximal speed and eccentric loading.[12] Athletes will typically present with sudden pain in the posterior or anterior thigh or pelvic area with tenderness to palpation on exam. Avulsion fractures should also be considered during examination, especially in younger athletes with a growing skeleton.[11] Further evaluation with radiographs of the pelvis is warranted to rule out the presence of a fracture. Acute treatment includes rest, ice for pain relief, compression, and elevation. *Patellofemoral pain syndrome (PFPS)*, also known as "runner's knee," is typically a chronic issue due to patellar maltracking. Distance runners may have an acute aggravation of their chronic PFPS and present with pain around the medial or lateral aspect of the patella. Ice massage and taping may be used for acute treatment. Athletes should be aware of potential risk of developing stress fractures should they choose to continue to compete. *Meniscal tears* are seen in shot put and discus. Rotational movements of the trunk must be perfectly coordinated with the rotation of the lower limbs. Landing after a flight phase in discus and shot put is also an injury-prone position; if the foot is not planted properly, twisting of the knee and ankle can occur. *Meniscus* and *anterior cruciate ligament (ACL) tears* can occur with this mechanism. Treatment is conservative at first, but may require surgical intervention. *Leg contusion* and *abrasions* can be seen in hurdlers, particularly in the trailing leg, due to its collision with the hurdle. Padding can be applied to the injury-prone site for protection. *Achilles tendon rupture* is a more serious acute injury in the setting of the quick and explosive nature of sprinting. Athletes will report a sudden sharp pain in the heel or calf typically at the start of a sprint. Palpation of the posterior leg may reveal a gap in the Achilles tendon accompanied by weakness in plantar flexion. Acute treatment includes placing a posterior leg splint and applying ice. Surgical repair is the main treatment in the running athlete. *Posterior tibial tendinopathy* is a common foot/ankle injury present in sprinters. Athletes will present with pain to palpation on the postero-medial ankle along the path of the posterior tibial tendon. A medial taping or wrap up on the arch may be applied for pain reduction. *Ankle sprains* are seen in shot put and discus throwers due to the physical boundary of the throwing circle as the toe board can be used as a break for the lead leg, imposing inversion and rotational forces on the ankle. Acute management involves pain modalities, and ankle support with tape or brace.

Other Injury

Another injury to consider is *urethral disruption* in a male hurdler who collides with the hurdle while each leg is on either side. Emergent evaluation is prompted if hematuria develops after contact injury.

■ SUMMARY

The challenge of medical coverage for track and field athletes is that multiple events often occur at the same time. Medical personnel should be aware of injuries that are specific to each of the athletic events. Personnel should also be especially aware of potential severe injury to athletes and spectators by contact with objects used in throwing events.

■ References

1. Galligan F. Historical dictionary of track and field. *Int J Hist Sport*. 2014;31(9):1207-1208. doi:10.1080/09523367.2012.761005.

2. Athletics. https://www.olympic.org/athletics.

3. National Federation of State High School Associations. Participation statistics. https://members.nfhs.org/participation_statistics.

4. Irick E. Student-athlete participation 1981-82–2018-19: NCAA sports sponsorship and participation rates report. https://ncaaorg.s3.amazonaws.com/research/sportpart/2018-19RES_SportsSponsorshipParticipa tionRatesReport.pdf. Published November 2019.

5. USA Track & Field. USATF 2020 competition rules. http://www.ncaa.org/playing-rules/cross-country -and-track-and-field-rules-competition. Published 2019.

6. Adaptive Track & Field USA. https://www.atfusa.org/RULES/RULES.htm. Accessed July 21, 2020.

7. Pendergraph B, Ko B, Zamora J, Bass E. Medical coverage for track and field events. *Curr Sports Med Rep*. 2005;4(3):150-153. doi:10.1097/01.CSMR.0000306198.59617.3d.

8. Pierpoint L, Williams C, Fields S, Comstock RD. Epidemiology of injuries in United States high school track and field: 2008–2009 through 2013–2014. *Am J Sports Med*. 2016;44(6):1463-1468. doi:10.1177/0363546516629950.

9. Reid JP, Nelson NG, Roberts KJ, McKenzie LB. Track-related injuries in children and adolescents treated in US emergency departments from 1991 through 2008. *Phys Sportsmed*. 2012;40(2):56-63. doi:10.3810/psm.2012.05.1965.

10. Setayesh K, Mayekar E, Schwartz B, et al. Upper extremity injuries in field athletes: targeting injury prevention. *Ann Sports Med Res*. 2017;4(1):1098. https://www.jscimedcentral.com/SportsMedicine/sportsmedi cine-4-1098.pdf

11. Meron A, Saint-Phard D. Track and field throwing sports. *Curr Sports Med Rep*. 2017;16(6):391-396. doi:10.1249/JSR.0000000000000416.

12. Comfort P, Abrahamson E, eds. *Sports Rehabilitation and Injury Prevention*. Somerset, UK: Wiley; 2010.

Francisco E. Bentz Brugal

■ HISTORY

A triathlon is an individual multisport endurance event consisting of swimming, cycling, and running executed in direct sequence. The first modern triathlon was held in 1974 in San Diego, California.[1] In 2000, the triathlon event took place at the Sydney Olympics Games for the first time.

■ GOVERNING ORGANIZATIONS

- International: International Triathlon Union (ITU)
- National: USA Triathlon (USAT)

■ PARTICIPATION

Membership in USA Triathlon grew from 21,341 in 2001 to 174,787 in 2013 with approximately an additional 342,189 1-day members for participation in sanctioned events.[2]

■ RULES AND REGULATIONS

Triathlons vary in distance from *sprint* (750 m swim, 20 km bike, 5 km run), *Olympic* distance (1.5 km swim, 40 km bike, 10 km run), *half iron* distance (2 km swim, 90 km bike, 21 km run), *iron* distance (4 km swim, 180 km bike, 42 km run), and ultradistance triathlons, which are longer than the traditional iron distance.

■ EQUIPMENT

The *tri-suit* is a multipurpose item of clothing that is worn throughout the full triathlon. The athlete will also require a *wetsuit, googles, a bicycle, helmet, race belt, sunglasses,* and *running shoes and socks*.

⟫ Adaptive Sport Key Points: Para-Triathlon

ITU has committed to support the development of paratriathlon for over 15 years. There are currently five sport classes for athletes with an impairment to compete in the sprint paratriathlon distance of 750 m swim, 20 km bike (hand bike/tandem), 5 km run (racing wheelchair). This event is part of the Paralympic games.

■ MEDICAL COVERAGE LOGISTICS

As part of the medical plan, it is important to know the number of competitors expected, and how many members of the core medical staff should be present and their specific skill sets. Medical directors should plan for the medical team to have at least two physicians in any given event or one physician per 200 participants in order to have a physician along the course if needed. There should be one medical team member (in addition to physicians) for every 100 competitors, and one medical spotter for every 200 to 400 participants.[3] The medical staff will be placed in different stations over the course. It is important to develop an emergency action plan (EAP) prior to the event and identify the safe exits without disrupting the event. There should be a command center that has map and race logistics available for the medical staff to determine strategies in case the competitor is unable to reach the medical tent and a physician should get to the area to provide assistance. Roles of the medical personnel should be defined prior to the event and different scenarios should be plotted in a way that everyone would know their role. Communication between the event personnel and medical team members is essential and should be established via at least two ways of communication (radio and cell phones). Proper documentation is imperative for postrace assessment and future event planning.

During the *swimming phase* multiple factors should be considered such as water temperature, waves, inland lakes or ocean waters, number of competitors in the water, contamination, strategies to reach the competitors in case of an emergency, and time spent in the water.[3] Water safety should be addressed prior to the event, assessing water temperature, waves and estimated time spent by competitors in water. The optimal water temperature should range between 25 to 28°C (77–82.4°F); In case of lower temperatures, wet suits should be considered, but for temperatures lower than 13°C (55.4°F) the event should be cancelled.[3] Additionally, there should be one medical person for every 25 to 50 swimmers with access to an Automated External Defibrillator (AED) at the swim venue at the exit and on the swim course.[3]

■ MEDICAL EMERGENCIES AND MEDICAL BAG ESSENTIALS

Aquatic emergencies can occur both in or around the water due to sudden illness or injury. Medical personnel should be alert and act quickly in responding to an emergency. Drowning can be fatal and will require immediate action. Head, neck, and spinal cord injuries can occur with trauma or high-impact activity during competition. If you suspect a head, neck, or spinal cord injury and the athlete remains in water, care must be taken to immobilize the head, neck, and body while maintaining the head above water. The medical staff should work together to pull the person out of the water safely and with caution. Other serious or life-threatening emergencies of which the medical personnel should be aware include head or spinal cord injury, seizures, hypoglycemia, hypothermia (swim)/hyperthermia (bike/run), limb dislocations and fractures, cardiac arrest, and pulmonary edema.

■ EPIDEMIOLOGY

Most of the triathletes have a background of running, 20% swimming, and 10% cycling.[4] During the swimming portion, contusions and lacerations, hypothermia, and envenomation/stings were the most common illnesses/injuries. During the bike portion, abrasions (road rash), contusions, and fractures due to trauma, dehydration, and gastrointestinal issues were most common. Lastly, during the run portion, heat-related illness, dehydration, muscle strains and cramps, skin blisters, and gastrointestinal issues were most common.[3] Most studies report that the lower limbs were more commonly involved, specifically the knee, foot and ankle. The lower back and the shoulder were also common. Hamstring, calf, and knee injuries were most commonly attributed to running. Achilles injuries and low-back injuries were most commonly attributed to cycling.[5]

Medical Bag Essentials in Triathlon	
Medical Emergencies:	**Wound Care/Dermal Injuries:**
AED	Normal saline
Sublingual nitroglycerin	Betadine/Alcohol swabs
Epi 1:1,000	Neosporin, mupirocin ointment
Albuterol inhaler	Gauzes
Pulse oximeter	Mole skin
Supplemental oxygen	Vaseline
Rectal thermometer	Tongue depressors/applicators
Bear huggers	Wound irrigation skit
Blankets	Sterile needle
Ice baths	Steri-strips
Sunscreen	Suture tray
Water	Topical Lidocaine
Sports drink	**Musculoskeletal:**
Pretzels	Crutches
Salt packets	Topical analgesics
I-STAT	Oral Acetaminophen tabs/caps
Syringes	
Glucometer	**Head and Spine:**
Glucose testing strips	Stretcher & Spine board
Finger lancet	Cervical orthosis
Glucose tabs	
Oral ondansetron	
IV lines	
IV bags	

In a triathlon event, between 15% to 25% of the athletes seek medical attention, especially the nonelites.[6] The most common primary diagnosis found at the ironman distance was dehydration (50.8%) followed by muscle cramps (36.1%). Similar studies categorizing triathlon injuries have corroborated that dehydration is the single most common primary diagnosis encountered in ultraendurance settings at 52%,[7] while muscle cramps (38.9%) followed by dehydration (37.7%) were more common in the half iron distance. Between 1985 and 2016, 135 deaths occurred during triathlons due to cardiac arrests, mostly in middle-aged and older men.[8] Most sudden deaths in triathletes happened during the swim segment, often secondary to a clinically silent cardiovascular disease.

For specific details about common illnesses and injuries see Chapters 41, Cycling; 43, Long Distance Running; and 49, Swimming.

■ SUMMARY

A triathlon is an endurance event consisting of swimming, cycling, and running and therefore requires the sports medicine specialist to not only understand each individual sport and associated injuries, but also as a whole event.

■ References

1. Strock GA, Cottrell ER, Lohman JM. Triathlon. *Phys Med Rehabil Clin N Am.* 2006;17(3):553-564. doi:10.1016/j.pmr.2006.05.010.

2. O'Mara K. The truth about triathlon participation in the United States. https://www.triathlete.com/culture/news/the-truth-about-triathlon-participation-in-the-united-states/. Published August 6, 2019. Accessed July 21, 2020.

3. Asplund C, Miller T, Creswell L, et al. Triathlon medical coverage: a guide for medical directors. *Curr Sports Med Rep*. 2017;16(4):280-288. doi:10.1249/JSR.0000000000000382.

4. Townsend M. Performance in component sports of triathlon events as a function of ability, age, and gender. *Percept Mot Skills*. 1995;80:274. doi:10.2466/pms.1995.80.1.274.

5. Vleck VE, Bentley DJ, Millet GP, Cochrane T. Triathlon event distance specialization: training and injury effects. *J Strength Cond Res*. 2010;24:30-36. doi:10.1519/JSC.0b013e3181bd4cc8.

6. Rimmer T, Coniglione T. A temporal model for nonelite triathlon race injuries. *Clin J Sport Med*. 2012;22(3): 249-253. doi:10.1097/JSM.0b013e318249945b.

7. Holtzhausen LM, Noakes TD. Collapsed ultraendurance athlete: proposed mechanisms and an approach to management. *Clin J Sport Med*. 1997;7:292-301. https://journals.lww.com/cjsportsmed/Abstract/1997/10000/Collapsed_Ultraendurance_Athlete__Proposed.6.aspx.

8. Harris K, Creswell L, Maron B. Death and cardiac arrest in U.S. triathlon participants. *Ann Int Med*. 2018;168(10):753. doi:10.7326/L18-0023.

54. VOLLEYBALL

Jonathan Ramin

HISTORY

Volleyball emerged as a sport in 1895 when the physical education director at the Holy-oke, Massachusetts YMCA, William Morgan, decided to create a sport with similar "athletic impulse," but less contact than the recently invented game of basketball. Morgan first referred to the sport as "Mintonette," and incorporated different aspects of basketball, tennis, handball, and baseball to form what would soon become the second most popular team sport in the world.[1]

GOVERNING ORGANIZATIONS[2]

- International: International Federation of Volleyball (FIVB)
- National: The North, Central America and Caribbean Volleyball Confederation (NORCECA)
- Major professional leagues: Association of Volleyball Professionals (AVP)
- College: National Collegiate Athletic Association (NCAA)
- High School: National Federation of State High School Associations (NFHS)[2]

PARTICIPATION

Approximately 6.3 million athletes participate in indoor volleyball and 5 million participate in beach volleyball in the United States.[3,4] These include athletes ranging from youth, high school, college, and the professional level. In the United States, volleyball continues to be more popular among female athletes, making up approximately 88% to 90% of high school and college participants.[5,6]

RULES AND REGULATIONS

A net raised to 7 ft 4 infor women and 8 ft for men separates two six-person or two-person teams in an indoor or beach volleyball match, respectively. A point is initiated by a serve, which involves an overhead strike of the ball by one player either standing or jumping from behind the service line. The serve is received by the opposing team which will have a maximum of three contacts with the ball to try to return the ball back to the other side of the net within the court boundaries. The three contacts go back and forth until one team is unable to return the ball to the opposing side and thus loses the point. An indoor volleyball match is a best-of-five game series with each game played to 25 points. The first team to reach 25 points with a minimum two-point margin of victory, wins that individual game. Should the match go to the decisive fifth set, that game is played to 15 points with a minimum two-point margin of victory. A beach volleyball match is similar to indoor except it is a best-of-three game series, with each game played to 21 points and a minimum two-point margin of victory per game. Similar to indoor volleyball, should the match go to the decisive third set, that game is played to 15 points with a minimum two-point margin of victory.

■ EQUIPMENT

Players may use **lower limb knee pads** to protect the knees from injury when diving for a ball on defense.

> ⟩⟩⟩ **Adaptive Sport Key Points: ("Sitting") Volleyball**
>
> A net raised to 1.05 m for women and 1.15 m for men separates two six-person teams on a 10 m by 6 m indoor court. The rules are similar to that of indoor volleyball, except the players' "bottoms" must be on the floor when making any attack or serve and are not allowed to stand up, take steps, or raise the body when making a play on the ball.[7]

■ MEDICAL COVERAGE LOGISTICS

Prior to a competition, it is important to identify available medical staff, support personnel, race course or venue map, and the available medical equipment. Establishing an Emergency Action Plan (EAP) is the most important concern. Protocols and guidelines should include role definition of the medical staff, emergency transportation including personnel, routes, and adequate facilities with the capacity to evaluate and manage possible injuries, and an outline of the chain-of-command and communication standards. Arrive early, at least 30 minutes prior to the game, to assess the medical equipment and support staff. The roles among the personnel need to be established before the game as well, and the EAP should be reviewed. Keep note of the nearest hospital, preferably with a trauma center.

■ MEDICAL EMERGENCIES AND MEDICAL BAG ESSENTIALS

The collapsed or unconscious athlete is considered a medical emergency that requires activation of the proper channels of communication and protocols including basic life support (BLS)/advanced cardiac life support (ACLS). Although rarely reported, nontraumatic emergencies can include anaphylaxis, asthma, and heat-related illness, specifically heat stroke. Musculoskeletal injuries that may become medical emergencies include upper and lower limb fractures or dislocations with neurovascular compromise.

Medical Bag Essentials in Volleyball	
Medical Emergencies:	Fractures and Dislocations:
Automated External Defibrillator (AED)	Immobilizers and Slings
Nitroglycerin (sublingual)	Crutches Others:
Aspirin	Acetaminophen
Epi 1:1,000	Glucose tabs
Diphenhydramine or another antihistamine	Waterproof SPF 50 sunscreen
Albuterol inhaler	
Rectal thermometer	
Ice bucket	
Head and Spine	
Concussion evaluation form	

■ EPIDEMIOLOGY

Despite being considered a "noncontact" sport, volleyball is played at high velocities with large, forceful movements of the body in all planes of motion. As a result of these forceful movements, there is a high incidence of traumatic and overuse injuries related to participation in volleyball. The overall rate of injuries in competitive- and elite-level volleyball players ranges from 2.3 to 3.8 per 1,000 playing hours.[8] The NCAA reported a study that found the rate of injuries in women's division I college players to be 8.4 per 1,000 athlete exposures over a 4-year period.[9] The rates of injuries differ greatly based on the surface on which the game is played, hard court versus sand. Some studies suggest injuries are five times more likely to occur in indoor volleyball when compared to beach volleyball.[10] The lower limbs are the most commonly injured body area, specifically the ankle followed by the knee. Injuries to the shoulder, hand, and back are also common.[10]

■ COMMON INJURIES

Head and Spine Injuries

Concussion is commonly seen in volleyball at all levels. Mechanisms of injury include ball-to-head contact during a hit/spike (most common), player–player collision, or head-floor contact.[11] Symptoms include confusion, dizziness, headaches, nausea, and in severe cases, loss of consciousness. The athlete must be removed from play and a concussion assessment must be performed. If no red flags are observed, then the player may remain on the sideline. Periodic assessment should follow until cleared to leave with a parent if under age. The player will need to follow up with a sports medicine provider in 24 to 48 hours for further assessment. **Lumbar strain** and other forms of mechanical low back pain are common injuries seen in volleyball. Mechanism of injury is repetitive jumping and landing, placing heavy loads on the muscles and ligaments of the lumbar spine. Symptoms include sharp, nonradiating pain in the low back that worsens with movement, particularly lumbar flexion, extension, or rotation. Management includes rest, ice/heat, nonsteroidal anti-inflammatory drugs (NSAIDs), and activity modification.

Upper Limb Injuries

Upper limb injuries are more often overuse injuries in the shoulder and acute in the hand. **Rotator cuff tendinopathy** is the most common shoulder injury that occurs in volleyball players. Mechanism of injury is from repetitive overhead motions involving frequent cycles of abduction and external rotation, followed by forceful internal rotation and shoulder extension as contact is made with the ball during a spike or a serve.[9] Symptoms include pain with range of motion and overhead activities. Management includes rest, ice, NSAIDs, kinesio taping, and rehabilitation exercises focusing on the scapular stabilizing muscles as well as strengthening of the rotator cuff muscles.[10] **Labral tears** in volleyball commonly include a tear in the superior portion of the labrum and extend anterior to posterior, also known as "SLAP" tears. Mechanism of injury is due to repetitive rapid, forceful overhead motions during spiking, serving, and blocking. Symptoms include pain and weakness in the shoulder joint. Management includes removal from play and, depending on severity of injury, physical therapy and bracing as well as surgery in some cases. **Suprascapular neuropathy** is commonly seen in elite-level volleyball players. Mechanism of injury is thought to be the result of repetitive "float" serves, which involves a forceful deceleration of the overhead serve upon contact with the ball. This repetitive motion can lead to compression of the suprascapular nerve at the spinoglenoid notch. Compression of the suprascapular nerve may also occur as a result of a paralabral cyst, often secondary to a torn labrum. When symptomatic, athletes will experience shoulder pain and weakness of the external rotators compared to the internal rotators. Management includes a rehabilitation and strengthening program focused on the rotator cuff, particularly strengthening the external rotators and surgery in refractory cases. ***Finger sprains*** are the most common hand injuries in volleyball. Mechanism of injury is generally from hyperextension of the metacarpal-phalangeal (MCP) or proximal-interphalangeal (PIP) joints while playing defense. The blockers and back row defenders are most vulnerable. When the ball is hit by the opposing side, the blocker has fingers spread wide at the net leaving them susceptible to a high impact strike by a ball traveling at up to 90 mph. Similarly, the back row defender who attempts to dig a ball overhead is also at high risk for finger sprains. The ***radial collateral ligament of the first MCP*** joint is the most commonly sprained finger, followed by the fifth digit. Symptoms include pain and difficulty fully flexing the injured finger. Management includes obtaining x-rays to rule out fracture, followed by either splinting or buddy taping the injured finger to an adjacent finger for more support.[12] Other hand injuries in volleyball include ***fractures, contusions,*** and ***dislocations*** which occur less commonly, but by similar mechanism when playing defense.

Lower Limb Injuries

Lower limb injuries are common in the ankle and knee. ***Ankle sprain*** is by far the most common injury in volleyball. Mechanism of injury is usually from landing during blocking or hitting at the net. Indoor volleyball rules allow for both teams to land on the center line during a block or a hit, and thus blockers/hitters are more susceptible to landing on the foot of another player. Players often experience an inversion injury to the anterior talofibular ligament. Symptoms include pain and swelling at the ankle. Management includes rest, ice, compression, elevation, NSAIDs, and possibly splinting/crutches. X-rays may also be necessary and should be considered based on the Ottawa Ankle Rules. A foot x-ray is indicated only when there is a combination of pain in the midfoot and one of the following: (a) bony tenderness at the base of the fifth metatarsal, (b) bony tenderness at the navicular, or (c) inability to bear weight for four steps both immediately after the injury and in the emergency department.[13] In order to reduce the frequency of ankle sprains, ankle taping, semi-rigid ankle supports and/or ankle coordination training exercises should be considered.[10] ***Patellar tendinopathy***, also known as "jumper's knee," is commonly seen in volleyball. Mechanism of injury is from repetitive forceful jumping during training and competition. Symptoms include pain around the patella (usually the lower pole) during jumping, running, or with flexing/extending the knee. Management includes rest, ice, NSAIDs, activity modifications (particularly jumping technique), and eccentric exercises. ***Anterior collateral ligament (ACL)*** injury is another common knee injury that occurs in volleyball. Mechanism of injury is a forceful landing from a jump that causes hyperextension or excessive internal tibial rotation of the knee.[10,14] Symptoms vary by grades of injury (Grades I–III), with Grade II as a partial ligament tear and Grade III as a full ligament tear. Athletes may feel a "pop," followed by immediate swelling of the knee when a full ACL tear occurs. Management of Grade I–II ACL injuries includes conservative treatment (rest, ice, NSAIDs). Grade III injuries require surgical intervention.

◾ SUMMARY

Volleyball is a popular high-velocity noncontact sport that can be played at all levels. Understanding the game, positions and most common injuries is essential for sideline coverage.

■ References

1. History of volleyball. https://www.volleyhall.org/page/show/3821594-history-of-volleyball.

2. The FIVB. https://www.fivb.org/EN/FIVB.

3. Lock S. Number of participants in beach volleyball in the United States from 2006 to 2018. https://www.statista.com/statistics/191708/participants-in-beach-volleyball-in-the-us-since-2006. Published January 2020.

4. Lock S. Number of participants in court volleyball. in the United States from 2006 to 2018 https://www.statista.com/statistics/191714/participants-in-court-volleyball-in-the-us-since-2006. Published January 2020.

5. Gough C. Number of participants in U.S. high school volleyball from 2009/10 to 2018/19. https://www.statista.com/statistics/268009/participation-in-us-high-school-volleyball/. Published August 2019.

6. Irick E. Student-athlete participation 1981-1982–2013-14: NCAA sports sponsorship and participation rates report. Indianapolis, IN: National Collegiate Athletic Association. http://www.ncaapublications.com/productdownloads/PR1314.pdf. Published October 2014.

7. Volleyball. https://www.disabledsportsusa.org/sport/volleyball.

8. Verhagen E, Van der Beek A, Bouter LM, et al. A one season prospective cohort study of volleyball injuries. *Br J Sports Med*. 2004;38:477-481. doi:10.1136/bjsm.2003.005785.

9. Sole C, Kavanaugh A, Stone MH. Injuries in collegiate women's volleyball: a four-year retrospective analysis. *Sports*. 2017;5(2):26. doi:10.3390/sports5020026.

10. Briner WW Jr, Kacmar L. Common injuries in volleyball. Mechanisms of injury, prevention and rehabilitation. *Sports Med*. 1997;24(1):65-71. doi:10.2165/00007256-199724010-00006.

11. Meeuwisse DW, MacDonald K, Meeuwisse WH, Schneider K. Concussion incidence and mechanism among youth volleyball players. *Br J Sports Med*. 2017;51:A62-A63. doi:10.1136/bjsports-2016-097270.162.

12. Bhairo N, Nijsten M, van Dalen KC, ten Duis HJ. Hand injuries in volleyball. *Int J Sports Med*. 1992;13(4):351-354. doi:10.1055/s-2007-1021280.

13. Stiell I, McKnight R, Greenberg GH, et al. Implementation of the Ottawa ankle rules. *JAMA*. 1994;271(11):827-832. doi:10.1001/jama.1994.03510350037034.

14. Loudon J, Jenkins W, Loudon KL. The relationship between static posture and ACL injury in female athletes. *J Orthop Sports Phys Ther*. 1996;24(2):91-97. doi:10.2519/jospt.1996.24.2.91.

55. WEIGHTLIFTING

Michelle Leong

▦ HISTORY

Comparisons of strength have occurred since prehistoric times with tribal members competing to lift the heaviest rock. The first unofficial international weightlifting competition was held in 1891. The first Olympic Games, Athens 1896 included weightlifting since it was a popular way to measure strength and power in Greek society. Modern weightlifting started off with the theatrical shows of international strongmen in the 1800s and 1900s.[1,2] In 1905, the predecessor for the International Weightlifting Federation was founded.[3] By 1928, the Summer Olympics weightlifting events had evolved to include only two-handed lifts: the clean and jerk, the snatch, and the clean and press. The clean and press was discontinued in 1972. Men were the only participants until the Sydney Olympic Games in 2000.[1] Powerlifting branched out from weightlifting as athletes wanted to participate in events other than the specified Olympic lifts. Powerlifting became progressively more popular and unofficial competitions were held across the world starting in the 1950s. In 1972, the International Powerlifting Federation was founded. The first official World Championship was held in 1973. The first women's World Championship was held in 1980.[4]

▦ GOVERNING ORGANIZATIONS
- International: International Weightlifting Federation (IWF), International Olympic Committee (IOC), International Powerlifting Federation (IPF); International Paralympic Committee (IPC); Special Olympics, Inc. (SOI)
- National: USA Weightlifting; USA Powerlifting

▦ PARTICIPANTS

Men and women participate in both weightlifting and powerlifting. The SOI recognizes athletes starting from the age of 8. The IWF/IPC recognizes athletes starting from the age of 14. IPF recognizes athletes starting from the age of 15. IOC recognize athletes starting from the age of 16.

▦ RULES AND REGULATIONS

Weightlifting: All lifts start with the barbell on the floor. Athletes stand on a wooden platform during the lift. If the athlete steps off the platform, the lift is not allowed in the score. Each athlete has three attempts per lift. The highest total combined score wins. Men compete in eight different weight categories. Women compete in seven different weight categories. *Clean and jerk:* This is a two-part lift. First, the athlete lifts the barbell from the floor to shoulders. The second movement is an explosive jerk to bring the bar overhead to arm's length. Feet movement and/or a squat is allowed during the overhead lift, but the final position must be with the body straightened and arms extended with bar in full control overhead. There is no time limit to complete the lift, but the bar must be held overhead until the appropriate signal is given before the bar can be lowered. **Snatch:** The barbell is lifted from floor to overhead in a single continuous movement. Feet movement and/or squat is allowed during the single overhead movement. The athlete must come to a fully standing position with body straightened for the lift to be complete. **Powerlifting**[5]: Similar to weightlifting, lifts are carried out on a platform. There are three attempts at each lift. The best lift score in each discipline is added to the total score. The highest total score is the winner. If two or more lifters achieve the same total score, the person with the lowest body weight is the winner. Athletes are divided by sex, age, and body weight. **Squat:** The barbell rests on a squat rack. The athlete may have aid from spotters only in removing the bar from the racks. The bar is held horizontally across the shoulders behind the neck. Hands and fingers are wrapped around the bar and a thumbless grip is allowed if preferred. The athlete moves backward into the starting position with body erect and knees locked. After receiving a signal, the athlete bends knees and lowers body until the hip joint is lower than the top of knees. The athlete must return to a body erect position. Bouncing or further downward movement is not allowed once upward movement has begun. The athlete must then rack the bar. **Bench press:** The athlete starts by lying on the bench supine. The head, shoulders, and buttocks must stay in contact with the bench surface and feet flat on the floor. Chest may be arched as long as the aforementioned parts are appropriately in contact with the bench. Hands and fingers must wrap around the bar, including the thumb. The positioning of the hands must be within 81 cm. Reverse grip is not allowed. The athlete may have aid from spotters only in removing the bar from the rack. Once the bar is removed from the rack, the athlete must stay motionless with arms straight and elbows locked until given a signal. The athlete then lowers the bar to touch the chest. When a signal is given, the athlete can bring the bar upward ending with arms erect and elbows locked. Another signal is given when the athlete can rack the bar. **Deadlift:** The barbell is horizontally laid across the athlete's feet on the floor. The bar is gripped in both hands with no specific requirements for grip. No other foot position is required except they must be between the weight plates. The athlete must lift the bar up from the floor into a body-erect position with shoulders back and knees locked. Once the lift has begun, no downward movement is allowed. After a signal, the bar can be brought back to the floor.

▪ EQUIPMENT

Olympic Weightlifting

Necessary equipment includes a bar(bell), which is a steel bar or rod, and circular disc weights with a collar to keep the weights in place. Support suit or support undergarments are not allowed. A belt, typically made of leather or vinyl, may be allowed. Tape may be worn on wrists or fingers.[1,2,6]

Powerlifting

Equipment needs are the same as Olympic Weightlifting in addition to approved squat racks and benches. Support suits and support undergarments are not allowed. A belt as just described may be allowed. In addition, neoprene knee sleeves, one-ply elastic wrist wraps or knee wraps, medical tape around thumbs (two layers only) are allowed. Baby powder, resin, talc, magnesium carbonate are also allowed.

>>> **Adaptive Sport Key Points: Paralympic Powerlifting and Special Olympics Powerlifting**

Paralympic Powerlifting: For individuals with any qualifying disability (amputee, cerebral palsty, intellectual disability, visually impaired, and *"les autres"* or others) and are elite athletes. Participants must have eligible physical impairments such as impaired muscle power, impaired passive range of motion, limb deficiency, leg length difference, short stature, hypertonia, ataxia, and athetosis. The bench press is the only event and participants are grouped into gender and weight class.

Special Olympics Powerlifting: Participants are individuals with intellectual disabilities such as cognitive delay and developmental disability. Lifting with prosthesis and orthosis with shoes is allowed. The competitive events include squat, bench press, deadlift, combination bench press and deadlift, combination of all three events, and unified sports where participant competes with a partner. Participants are divided by age, gender, and weight class.[7,8]

▓ MEDICAL COVERAGE LOGISTICS

Medical services must be provided at all official sites of the competition including competition site, warm-up area if separate, and training venue. The role of the on-site physician leader is to organize and coordinate the medical staff, develop an emergency action plan (EAP), and interact with the event director, coaches, and referees to help ensure the safety of the competitors and spectators. Medical staff must be available at least 1 hour prior to the start of competition and remain until 30 minutes after the competition has ended. The main area of care should be located close to both the competition site and warm-up area if feasible. An advanced cardiac life support (ACLS) and advanced trauma life support (ATLS)-standard ambulance should be located close to the main medical area. The local on-call physician must be available for emergencies at all times. Information on physician, local emergency services, and nearest pharmacy and hospital numbers should be available. Appropriate communications devices should be made available for all medical staff.[9]

▓ MEDICAL EMERGENCIES AND MEDICAL BAG ESSENTIALS

It is essential to understand potential medical emergencies that may arise. The collapsed or unconscious athlete is considered a medical emergency that requires activation of the proper channels of communication and protocols including basic life support (BLS)/ACLS. Although rarely reported, nontraumatic emergencies can include anaphylaxis, asthma, cardiac arrhythmia, myocardial infraction, and hypertrophic cardiomyopathy. Musculoskeletal injuries that may become medical emergencies include upper and lower limb fractures or dislocations with neurovascular compromise.

▓ EPIDEMIOLOGY

Overall, lifting athletes are at risk for acute muscle strain and chronic overuse injuries and degeneration in the back, shoulder, wrist, and knees, less commonly hips, from the repetitive movements and forces.[10-17] Research studies have gathered that on average there are one to two injuries per lifter per year or two to four injuries per 1,000 hours.[10] Injuries tend to happen more often during training sessions and during the later sessions of an actual competition.[10,11] The emergency department sees around 900,000 visits a year for general weight-training injuries.[12] Around 60% to 75% of injuries are acute and the remaining 30% are chronic.[12]

Medical Bag Essentials in Weightlifting	
Medical Emergencies:	**Wound/Laceration/Skin Care:**
Automated External Defibrillator (AED)	Normal saline
Nitroglycerin (sublingual)	Betadine swabs
Aspirin	Neosporin, mupirocin ointment
Epi 1:1,000	Moleskin
Diphenhydramine or another antihistamine	Elastic bandage
Albuterol inhaler	Tube stretch gauze
Head and Spine:	Sterile gauzes
	Vaseline
Concussion evaluation form	Steri-strips
Stretcher & Spine board	Suture tray
Cervical orthosis	Lidocaine 1%
Fractures and Dislocations:	**Others:**
Immobilizers/Splints and Slings	Acetaminophen
Crutches	Glucose tabs

■ COMMON INJURIES

Spine Injuries

Low back injuries are common among lifters. There are high compressive loads placed on the lumbosacral region with large amounts of torque. The posture of the spine during the lifts can also increase lumbar shear forces. **Herniated discs** are often reported. Symptoms include low back pain radiating down the leg, weakness, and paresthesia of the lower limb. It can be diagnosed clinically with lower limb weakness, altered dermatomal sensation, increased pain with lumbar flexion, positive straight leg raise. MRI imaging would confirm diagnosis. Conservative treatment includes physical therapy for stretching and strengthening core and back musculature. Procedures include epidural steroid injections and microdiscectomy may be needed if noninvasive treatment failed.

Upper Limb Injuries

Upper limb injuries include acute tendon/muscle tears and overuse tendinopathies. **Pectoralis tendon rupture** can occur since the pectoralis muscles provide a significant amount of power to upper limb exercises. The highest risk happens at the time of maximal eccentric contraction, such as lowering the barbell to the chest in bench press and decelerating the bar overhead in clean and jerk and snatch. Symptoms and signs include pain, ecchymosis, palpable defect in anterior axillary region, weakness and pain with arm adduction, increased fullness in the pectoral region since the muscle is not properly taut. The rupture can be confirmed with ultrasound or MRI. Complete tears at the myotendinous junction and tendon avulsions are treated surgically, while partial tears and muscle belly tears are treated conservatively. The arm is kept in a sling for immobilization in an internally rotated position for at least 3 weeks, along with symptom management. At 6 weeks, active and passive range of motion (ROM) can be started with gradual increase in strengthening exercises. An injury greater than 3 months old requires tendon reconstruction due to likely tendon retraction. **Distal biceps tendon rupture,** like a pectoralis tendon rupture, can happen during eccentric contraction, such as lowering the weight doing a bicep curl. However, it can also happen during lifts such as the deadlift when the muscle is taut with a heavy load.

Symptoms and signs are a painful pop at the elbow, ecchymosis, weakness in elbow flexion and forearm supination, palpable defect with proximal retraction of the bicep muscle. Clinically, this can be tested using the Hook test and biceps squeeze test. The diagnosis can be confirmed with ultrasound or MRI. Typically, the management is anatomical surgical repair. **Rotator cuff tear/tendinopathy** occurs due to the repetitive forces on the shoulder leading to microtrauma, outlet impingement during overhead movement (clean and jerk, snatch), and alternating eccentric and concentric contractions (bench press). There is an imbalance between the larger muscle groups, which are traditionally strengthened to complete the lifts, and the smaller muscle groups that are responsible for joint stabilization. In addition, the popular wide grip width on the barbell increases stress on the posterior shoulder stabilizers, acromioclavicular (AC) joint, and glenohumeral joint, and increases torque at the shoulder joint. Symptoms include anterior, lateral, posterior shoulder pain during overhead activity, weakness, snapping or catching sensation. The Neer-Walsh, Hawkins-Kennedy, and Jobe's provocative tests can help to clinically diagnose. Ultrasound or MRI can confirm the diagnosis. Conservative management includes rest, ice, passive range of motion exercises, physical therapy for strengthening exercises and stretching. Procedures include corticosteroid injections and surgical intervention for full thickness tears. **Wrist** or **hand sprains** occur secondary to repetitive activity and hyperextension of wrist (clean and jerk, snatch, squat, bench press). Management is conservative with rest, ice, compression, elevation, range of motion exercises, and symptom management.

Lower Limb Injuries

Lower limb injuries affect mostly the knee. It is subjected to increased compressive and shear forces with increased knee flexion, increased patellofemoral and tibiofemoral compressive forces with wide stance during a squat, and increased extensor torque at the joint. **Knee ligament tears** can happen from poor form and rapid, uncontrolled descent of knees which increases the strain and shear forces to the cruciate ligaments. Additionally, inappropriate foot placement in a squat can overload all knee ligaments. Typical signs and symptoms of a ligamentous injury include hearing or feeling a pop at the knee, knee instability, medial or posterior knee pain, effusion, tenderness to palpation. Stability is tested with drawer tests or Lachman test. The best imaging is MRI. Conservative management includes ice, elevation, and compression. Knee immobilizer or hinged knee brace can be used for initial stability. Early gentle knee flexion and extension exercises are appropriate. Eventual aggressive rehabilitation therapies have also been shown to be beneficial. Procedures include surgical ligament reconstruction. **Quadriceps tendon rupture** often occurs during the eccentric lifting phase such as descending into a squat during clean and jerk, snatch, and squat. Signs and symptoms are knee swelling, palpable defect just proximal or distal to the patella with inability to extend the knee, and inappropriate patellar elevation. This requires surgical repair.

■ SUMMARY

Weightlifting and powerlifting have a lower rate of injury during competition when compared to other sports. The majority of injuries are sprains and strains during training. However, when injuries do occur during competition, they can be severe which necessitates appropriate event coverage.

■ References

1. Weightlifting. Olympic.org. https://www.olympic.org/weightlifting. Updated 2019.

2. Augustyn A, Bauer P, Duignan B, et al. Weightlifting. In: Augustyn A, Bauer P, Duignan B, et al, eds. Encyclopedia Britannica. https://www.britannica.com/sports/weightlifting. Published July 20, 1998. Updated January 4, 2016.

3. International Weightlifting Federation. Weightlifting history. https://www.iwf.net/weightlifting_/history. Updated 2019.

4. International Powerlifting Federation. Powerlifting history. https://www.powerlifting.sport/federation/history.html. Updated 2019.

5. International Powerlifting Federation. Technical rules. https://www.powerlifting.sport/rulescodesinfo/technical-rules.html. Updated January 14, 2019.

6. International Weightlifting Federation. Technical and competition rules and regulations 2019. https://www.iwf.net/downloads/. Updated 2019.

7. World Para Powerlifting. History of para powerlifting. https://www.paralympic.org/powerlifting/about. Updated 2019.

8. Powerlifting. Special Olympics. https://www.specialolympics.org/our-work/sports/powerlifting. Updated 2019.

9. International Weightlifting Federation Guidelines Medical. https://www.iwf.net/downloads/. Updated 2019.

10. Keogh JW, Winwood PW. The epidemiology of injuries across the weight-training sports. *Sports Med*. 2017;47(3):479-501. doi:10.1007/s40279-016-0575-0.

11. Strömbäck E, Aasa U, Gilenstam K, Berglund L. Prevalence and consequences of injuries in powerlifting: a cross-sectional study. *Orthop J Sports Med*. 2018;6(5):2325967118771016. doi:10.1177/2325967118771016.

12. Golshani K, Cinque ME, O'Halloran P, et al. Upper extremity weightlifting injuries: diagnosis and management. *J Orthop*. 2017;15(1):24-27. doi:10.1016/j.jor.2017.11.005.

13. Willick SE, Cushman DM, Blauwet CA, et al. The epidemiology of injuries in powerlifting at the London 2012 Paralympic Games: an analysis of 1411 athlete-days. *Scand J Med Sci Sports*. 2016;26(10):1233-1238. doi:10.1111/sms.12554.

14. Aasa U, Svartholm I, Andersson F, Berglund L. Injuries among weightlifters and powerlifters: a systematic review. *Br J Sports Med*. 2017;51(4):211-219. doi:10.1136/bjsports-2016-096037.

15. Bangtsson V, Berglund L, Aasa U. Narrative review of injuries in powerlifting with special reference to their association to the squat, bench press and deadlift. *BMJ Open Sport Exerc Med*. 2018;4(1):e000382. doi:10.1136/bmjsem-2018-000382.

16. Keogh J, Hume PA, Pearson S. Retrospective injury epidemiology of one hundred one competitive Oceania power lifters: the effects of age, body mass, competitive standard, and gender. *J Strength Cond Res*. 2006;20(3):672-681. doi:10.1519/R-18325.1.

17. Lavallee ME, Balam T. An overview of strength training injuries: acute and chronic. *Curr Sports Med Rep*. 2010;9(5):307-313. doi:10.1249/JSR.0b013e3181f3ed6d.

INDEX

Printed in the United States
by Baker & Taylor Publisher Services